Occupational Medicine

STATE OF THE ART REVIEWS

The Workplace and Cardiovascular Disease

Guest Editors:

Peter L. Schnall, MD, MPH
Associate Professor of Medicine
University of California
Irvine, California

Karen Belkić, MD, PhD, Msci
Clinical Associate
Institute for Health Promotion and Disease Prevention Research
University of Southern California
Los Angeles, California

Paul Landsbergis, PhD, MPH
Assistant Professor of Epidemiology, Weill Medical College
Cornell University
New York, New York

Dean Baker, MD, MPH
Chief, Division of Occupational and Environmental Medicine
University of California
Irvine, California

Volume 15/Number 1
HANLEY & BELFUS, INC.

January–March 2000
Philadelphia

Publisher: HANLEY & BELFUS, INC.
210 South 13th Street
Philadelphia, PA 19107
(215) 546-4995
Fax (215) 790-9330
Web site: http://www.hanleyandbelfus.com

OCCUPATIONAL MEDICINE: State of the Art Reviews is included in *Index Medicus, MEDLINE, BioSciences Information Service, Current Contents* and *ISI/BIOMED, CINAHL database, and Cumulative Index to Nursing & Allied Health Literature.* Printed on acid-free paper.

OCCUPATIONAL MEDICINE: State of the Art Reviews   **ISSN 0885-114X**
January–March 2000   Volume 15, Number 1   **ISBN 1-56053-325-0**

OCCUPATIONAL MEDICINE: State of the Art Reviews is published quarterly by Hanley & Belfus, Inc., 210 South 13th Street, Philadelphia, Pennsylvania 19107. Periodical postage paid at Philadelphia, PA, and at additional mailing offices.

POSTMASTER: Send address changes to OCCUPATIONAL MEDICINE: State of the Art Reviews, Hanley & Belfus, Inc., 210 South 13th Street, Philadelphia, PA 19107.

The 2000 subscription price is $96.00 per year U.S., $106.00 outside U.S. (add $40.00 for air mail).

Occupational Medicine: State of the Art Reviews
Vol. 15, No. 1, January–March 2000

THE WORKPLACE AND CARDIOVASCULAR DISEASE
Peter L. Schnall, MD, MPH, Karen Belkić, MD, PhD, Msci,
Paul Landsbergis, PhD, MPH, and Dean Baker, MD, MPH, Editors

CONTENTS

   Unlike several other branches of medicine (e.g., pulmonology), primary cardiology has yet to fully develop a discipline of occupational cardiology. The authors
   outline an approach for including a focused occupational history in the CV
   work-up and present a graded, risk-stratified algorithm for occupational cardiologic assessment. This work-up can help clinicians make specific recommendations concerning working conditions, as these impact upon the patient's CV
   status. **Occup Med 15:213–222, 2000**

for enhanced prevention and clinical management, work place interventions, and social policy to reduce the impact of CVD. These strategies acquire an urgent public health dimension, given the magnitude of the CVD epidemic and the current deterioration in conditions of working life. **Occup Med 15:307–322, 2000**

Note: Authors employed by the U.S. Government have expressed their own views. Opinions and assertions contained herein are not to be construed as the offical policy of the U.S. Government.

Reprints of individual articles may be requested from: Peter L. Schnall, MD, Director, Center for Social Epidemiology, 1528 6th Street, Suite 202, Santa Monica, CA 90401

CONTRIBUTORS

Dean B. Baker, MD, MPH
Chief, Division of Occupational & Environmental Medicine; Director, Center for Occupational & Environmental Health; Professor, Departments of Medicine and Community & Environmental Medicine, University of California, Irvine, California

Mel Bartley, MSc, PhD
Principal Research Fellow, Department of Epidemiology and Public Health, University College London, London, United Kingdom

Karen L. Belkić, MD, PhD, Msci
Clinical Associate, Institute for Health Promotion and Disease Prevention Research, University of Southern California School of Medicine, Los Angeles, California

Chantal Brisson, PhD
Professor, Department of Social and Preventive Medicine, Laval University, Québec, Canada

Lawrence J. Fine, MD, DrPH
Director, Division of Surveillance, Hazard Evaluations, and Field Studies, National Institute for Occupational Safety and Health, Department of Health and Human Services, Cincinnati, Ohio

June Fisher, MD
Associate Clinical Professor, Department of Medicine, University of California, San Francisco, California

Eigil Fossum, MD
Fellow in Cardiology, Department of Internal Medicine, Ullevaal University Hospital, University of Oslo, Oslo, Norway

Paul Froom, MD, MOccH
Associate Professor, Department of Epidemiology, Tel Aviv University School of Medicine, Ramat Aviv, Israel

Regis de Gaudemaris, MD
Professor of Occupational Health, University Joseph Fourier, Grenoble, France

Birgit A. Greiner, PhD, MPH
Department of Medicine, Division of Community Medicine, University of Greifswald, Greifswald, Germany

Aud Høieggen, MD
Fellow in Nephrology, Department of Internal Medicine, Ullevaal University Hospital, University of Oslo, Oslo, Norway

Robert Karasek, PhD
Professor, Department of Work Environment, University of Massachusetts, Lowell, Massachusetts

Mark R. Kimmel, PhD
Kimmel and Associates, Oakland, California

Sverre Erik Kjeldsen, MD, PhD
Associate Professor, Division of Cardiology, Department of Internal Medicine, Ullevaal University Hospital, University of Oslo, Oslo, Norway

Niklas Krause, MD, PhD, MPH
Public Health Institute, Berkeley, California

Paul A. Landsbergis, PhD, EdD, MPH
Assistant Professor of Epidemiology, Division of Hypertension, Weill Medical College of Cornell University, New York, New York

J. Paul Leigh, PhD
Professor, Department of Epidemiology and Preventive Medicine, University of California, Davis, California

Lennart Levi, MD, PhD
Emeritus Professor of Psychosocial Medicine, Department of Public Health Sciences, Division of Stress Research, Karolinska Institute, Stockholm, Sweden

Michael Marmot, PhD, FRCP, FFPHM
Professor, Department of Epidemiology and Public Health; Director, International Centre for Health and Society, University College London, London, United Kingdom

Samuel Melamed, PhD
Head, Department of Occupational Health Psychology, National Institute of Occupational and Environmental Health, Ra'anana, Israel

Andreas Moan, MD, PhD
Consultant, Department of Internal Medicine, Ullevaal University Hospital, University of Oslo, Oslo, Norway

Kenneth Nowack, PhD
Organizational Performance Dimensions, Santa Monica, California

Yuko Odagiri, MD, PhD
Instructor, Department of Preventive Medicine and Public Health, Tokyo Medical University, Shinjuku-ku, Tokyo, Japan

Richard Peter, PhD
Department of Medical Sociology, University of Ulm, Ulm, Germany

Thomas G. Pickering, MD, DPhil
Professor, Department of Medicine, Cornell University Medical College, New York; Attending Physician, New York Presbyterian Hospital, New York, New York

Morten Rostrup, MD, PhD
Associate Professor, Department of Internal Medicine, Ullevaal University Hospital, University of Oslo, Oslo, Norway

Čedo Savić, MD, PhD
Specialist, Department of Psychophysiology and Clinical Neurophysiology, Institute of Mental Health, Belgrade, Yugoslavia

Peter L. Schnall, MD, MPH
Director, Center for Social Epidemiology; Associate Professor of Medicine, Department of Occupational and Environmental Medicine, University of California, Irvine, California

Joseph E. Schwartz, PhD
Associate Professor of Psychiatry and Sociology, Department of Psychiatry and Behavioral Sciences, State University of New York, Stony Brook, New York

Teruichi Shimomitsu, MD, PhD
Professor and Director, Department of Preventive Medicine and Public Health, Tokyo Medical University, Shinjuku-ku, Tokyo, Japan

Johannes Siegrist, PhD
Professor and Director, Department of Medical Sociology, University of Duesseldorf, Duesseldorf, Germany

Kyle Steenland, PhD
National Institute for Occupational Safety and Health, Cincinnati, Ohio

Andrew Steptoe, DPhil
Professor of Psychology, Department of Epidemiology and Public Health, University College London, London, UK

Töres P.G. Theorell, MD, PhD
Professor and Director, National Institute for Psychosocial Factors and Health, Karolinska Institute, Stockholm, Sweden

Finn Tüchsen, MSc
Senior Researcher, Department of Epidemiology, National Institute of Occupational Health, Copenhagen, Denmark

Mirjana Uglješić, MD
Belgrade City Outpatient Care Center, Center for Workers' Health Protection, Belgrade, S. R. Yugoslavia

Nicholas Warren, ScD, MAT
Assistant Professor of Medicine, Division of Occupational & Environmental Medicine, Ergonomic Technology Center, University of Connecticut Health Center, Farmington, Connecticut

Stewart G. Wolf, Jr., MD
Directors, Totts Gap Medical Research Laboratories, Bangor; Professor of Medicine, Temple University School of Medicine, Philadelphia, Pennsylvania

2000 ISSUES

**Cardiovascular Disease
in the Workplace**
Edited by Peter Schnall, MD, MPH
and Dean Baker, MD, MPH
University of California, Irvine, California;
Paul Landsbergis, PhD, EdD, MPH
Cornell University, New York, New York;
Karen Belkić, MD, PhD
University of Southern California
Los Angeles, California

Occupational Asthma
Edited by Daniel E. Banks, MD
and Mei-Lin Wang, MD
West Virginia University
Morgantown, West Virginia

**Idiopathic Environmental Intolerance
(Multiple Chemical Sensitivity)**
Edited by Patricia J. Sparks, MD, MPH
University of Washington
Seattle, Washington

**Risk and Disability Evaluation
in the Workplace**
Edited by David C. Randolph, MD, MPH
Occupational Medicine Physician
   and Consultant
Private Practice
Cincinnatti, Ohio

1999 ISSUES

Office Ergonomics
Edited by Martin Cherniack, MD, MPH
University of Connecticut
Farmington, Connecticut

Animal Handlers
Edited by Ricky L. Langley, MD, MPH
North Carolina Department of Health
   and Human Services
Raleigh, North Carolina

Special Populations
Edited by Howard Frumkin, MD
Emory University, Atlanta, Georgia
and Glenn Pransky, MD, MOccH
University of Massachusetts
Worcester, Massachusetts

**Health Issues in the Plastics
and Rubber Industries**
Edited by Richard Lewis, MD, MPH
University of Louisville,
Louisville, Kentucky

1998 ISSUES

Low Back Pain
Edited by Gerard A. Malanga, MD
University of Medicine and Dentistry
   of New Jersey
Newark, New Jersey

Workers' Compensation
Edited by T. L. Guidotti, MD, MPH
University of Alberta
Edmonton, Alberta, Canada
and John W. F. Cowell, MD, Msc
Workers' Compensation Board of Alberta
Edmonton, Alberta, Canada

Hand and Upper Extremity Injuries
Edited by Morton L. Kasdan, MD
University of Louisville
Louisville, Kentucky
and V. Jane Derebery, MD
Concentra Medical Center
Austin Texas

Managed Care
Edited by Jeffrey S. Harris, MD, MPH, MBA
J. Harris Associates, Inc.
Mill Valley, California

Ordering Information:
Subscriptions for full year and single issues are available from the publishers—
Hanley & Belfus, Inc., 210 South 13th Street, Philadelphia, PA 19107
Telephone (215) 546-7293; (800) 962-1892. Fax (215) 790-9330. Website www.hanleyandbelfus.com

ACKNOWLEDGEMENTS

We deeply appreciate the expert help, devotion, and day-to-day support of Susan Holcomb, the administrator for the Center for Social Epidemiology. Natalie Hansen was indispensable in her management of the references, for which we thank her greatly. We would also like to thank Sumita Chopra for her many diligent hours spent in the library tracking down references.

To Docent Lennart Bergfeldt and Professor Benjamin Natelson our thanks for their excellent reviews of Chapters 5 and 7 and Chapter 4, respectively.

We wish to thank the following libraries that assisted us throughout this project: Norris Medical Library at U.S.C. School of Medicine and UCLA Biomedical Library, the Karolinska Institute Medical Library (KIBIC), and the Library of the National Institute for Occupational Health in Stockholm, Sweden. Special thanks to Pam Corley, Senior Medical Information Specialist and Dr. Inga Jakobson.

Thanks are due to our publisher Hanley and Belfus and especially our editor Jacquie Mahon for their encouragement and support of this project.

We wish to express our appreciation for comments on Chapter 12 by Dom Tuminaro, Glen Shor, and Don Elisburg.

We have been inspired by our teachers, family and colleagues over the years. A special word of appreciation goes to Professors Mervyn Susser, Rochelle Kern, Jeff Johnson, Ellen Hall, Maureen Hatch, Sharon Schwartz, Bruce Link, and Ana Diez-Roux.

We wish to thank Algirdas and Joan Landsbergis, who have taught, by their example, to "do the right thing."

Professor Dževad Belkić has understood the scientific and humanitarian goals of this project from its inception and has been of crucial day-to-day support in its realization.

Partial support for Dr. Dean Baker and Dr. Peter Schnall's work was provided by the University of California, Irvine, Center for Occupational and Environmental Health.

This project was made possible by the support of the Center for Social Epidemiology. Deep thanks go to Larry Schnall whose life-long devotion to the well being of working people was the impetus for the creation of the Center for Social Epidemiology. We also wish to thank Sherry and Jane Schnall for their continued support of this ideal.

Peter Schnall, Karen Belkić,
Paul Landsbergis, and Dean Baker
EDITORS

PUBLISHED ISSUES
(available from the publisher)

WHY THE WORKPLACE AND CARDIOVASCULAR DISEASE?

by Peter Schnall, MD, Karen Belkić, MD, PhD, Paul Landsbergis, PhD, Dean Baker, MD

Cardiovascular disease (CVD) is the major cause of morbidity and mortality in the industrialized world.* While there have been trends towards lowered rates of CVD mortality in North America and Western Europe, CVD still represents a significant public health problem—indeed, a pandemic. In the former Soviet Union and other eastern European countries, CVD morbidity and mortality have increased dramatically over the last 30 years.[7] Rising prevalence rates also have been observed in many developing countries. Thus, "it has been projected that CVD worldwide will climb from the second most common cause of death . . . in 1990, to first place, with more than 36% of all deaths in 2020."[5]

In the U.S. alone, CVD is the cause of 41% of all deaths.[2] An estimated 250,000–350,000 people annually die suddenly of heart disease in the U.S.,[3,6,10,18,20,21] and at least the same number lose their lives more slowly due to manifest CVD from which they have chronically suffered.

The dominant focus of research and intervention in the medical community has been on **individual traits**, especially genetic susceptibility and risky behaviors (e.g., smoking, over-eating, sedentary lifestyle) as playing a primary role in the etiology of CVD. The underpinnings of this explanation of the CVD epidemic lie in the development of powerful engineering models. Modern advances in the physical sciences lend themselves particularly well to the study of the cardiovascular system. Namely, it has appeared that CVD could be characterized as a disturbance in hydraulic (hemodynamic) and/or electrical (electrophysiologic) function.[5] Coronary atherosclerosis (i.e., vascular obstruction) has been designated as the "prime mover" of cardiovascular disorders, such that a series of atherogenic risk factors were sought, and many were identified (e.g., hypercholesterolemia, hypertension, diabetes, obesity). According to this view, the CVD epidemic can be curtailed by: (1) better management of atherogenic risk factors, (2) use of available medical treatments and more technological advances, and (3) additional research into the molecular biology of atherogenic and other cardiodegenerative processes.

It is indisputable that this approach represents an invaluable advance in our battle against CVD. Millions of people have been protected by quitting smoking,

---

* Includes arteriosclerotic heart disease, cerebrovascular disease, and peripheral vascular disease (ICD codes 400–404, 410–414, 430–436, 440–445).

eating a "heart-healthy" diet, and exercising. And countless patients with manifest coronary heart disease (CHD) have been saved by percutaneous transluminal coronary angioplasty and coronary artery by-pass surgery, not to mention the life-saving armamentarium of pharmacologic agents we now have at our disposal. Cardiac pacemakers and automatic implantable cardioverter defibrillators provide hope for a normal life to many patients suffering from life-threatening cardiac rhythm and conduction disturbances. Only 50 years ago, nearly all of these patients would have been doomed.

Despite the optimism engendered by these achievements, we believe that a closer look at the overall public health impact of this traditional medical approach to CVD is in order. While these methods of electrical and hemodynamic systems are highly sophisticated, the etiology and pathogenesis of CVD cannot be reduced to a series of disordered pumps and electrical circuits. Furthermore, the intimate connections between the social environment and the central nervous system (CNS), and the CNS and the cardiovascular system via the autonomic nervous system, compel one to look beyond the cardiovascular system in isolation to fully appreciate how CVD develops.

In point of fact, both our understanding of the etiology of CVD and our ability to manage the epidemic are still limited. For example, the Framingham Heart Study used epidemiologic techniques to identify important risk factors (smoking, diabetes, hypertension, and cholesterol). However, these traditional risk factors explained only part of the risk for CHD.[11] In practical terms, this means that these standard risk factors fail to predict many of the new CHD cases. Note that one of these factors—essential hypertension—is of practically unknown etiology. Moreover, these traditional risk factors represent relatively "proximate" causes of CVD; each of them, in turn, has a complex set of determinants, many of which are of psychosocial origin.

New developments expand and challenge the focus on these traditional, proximate risk factors. One of these is the emergence of research into **behavioral factors** that might influence the development of CVD. A notable example has been the formulation of the concept of CVD-prone behavior—the Type A behavior pattern (TABP).[9] While initial study results from the Western Collaborate Group Study indicated that TABP was a strong independent predictor of CHD mortality,[24] subsequent research has failed to substantiate these findings.[22] More recently, hostility—a component of Type A behavior—has emerged as a possible risk factor for CVD.[30]

The importance of the TABP is not so much its contribution to the explanation of CVD, but its laying the groundwork for **social psychology** to examine the impact of the social and psychological environment on CVD. TABP was a stepping-stone to the investigation of the role of the workplace in CVD.

This formulation regarding TABP is complemented by a body of epidemiologic literature which documents the strong role of social experiences, beginning in childhood and extending through working life and beyond, in shaping human behavior. For example, recent research has demonstrated that characteristics of people's jobs, such as high or low decision-making authority, are associated with the development of specific complex behaviors and personality attributes.[4,14–16,27]

Another development that has expanded traditional cardiovascular epidemiology has been the field of **social epidemiology**, which examines factors such as social networks, social support, and social class as potential causes or modifiers of disease processes.[8,17,23,28] For example, social epidemiologists have demonstrated that lower socioeconomic status is an important risk factor for CVD.[12,19] Nonetheless, even with the inclusion of these social and behavioral factors, there is still a large amount of unexplained variance in CVD, as well as in essential hypertension.

We wish to argue that to better understand the CVD epidemic, social epidemiology needs to incorporate, in a much more prominent manner, a heretofore relatively neglected realm of social life—the workplace. We briefly present the case of essential hypertension (EH) as an illustration of our argument. EH is a major risk factor not only for CHD, but also for left ventricular hypertrophy, stroke, renal disease, and many other major pathologic processes. This disease afflicts 60 million Americans and 600 million people worldwide. The identified risk factors (i.e., obesity, salt intake, genetics, age, alcohol intake) explain only a small part of the risk.

A social epidemiologic approach suggests that EH is a disease of industrialized society.[25] There is a minimal hypertension disease burden among hunter-gatherers, nonmarket agricultural communities, and other nonindustrialized societies.[29] Within industrial society, hypertension is socially patterned by class, race, ethnicity, urbanicity, and gender. Current evidence implicates the unidentified causes of EH as most likely to include one or more ubiquitous exposures, suggesting the need to examine diet, lifestyle, work, and community. An adequate explanatory risk factor also should incorporate the social patterning of the disease.

Hypertension as an epidemic seems likely to be of relatively recent historical origins. Work organization has changed profoundly during the past 200 years. Craftwork, which predominated for many centuries, was largely replaced by the industrial revolution. Skilled workers, who had exercised substantial control over their work processes, were replaced by lower-skilled labor in new machine-based production technologies.[13] At the beginning of the 20th century, Taylorism further reshaped the workplace with its emphasis on narrow performance and efficiency using the technique of the assembly line, at the expense of employee collectivity and broader employee expertise and knowledge of the work process. Even lower-level, white-collar work, through office automation, has been shaped by the principles of the assembly line. Small businesses have been replaced by large centralized, multinational organizations. Most importantly, power to control the production process has been increasingly concentrated in the hands of management. The recent trend has been toward an acceleration of these changes in the workplace, characterized by a system of work organization known as "lean production." "These dynamics include organization restructuring, mergers, acquisitions, and downsizing, the frantic pace of work and life, the erosion of leisure time and/or the blending of work and home time. Most of these developments are driven by economic and technological changes aiming at short-term productivity and profit gain."[1]

The contemporary work environment is the locus in which adults now spend the majority of their waking hours, performing activities which are increasingly characterized, both by scientists and the workers, as demanding, constraining, and highly stressful. We know that blood pressure (BP) is elevated during working hours. We also know that performing demanding, constraining and otherwise mentally stressful activity provokes sharp rises in BP.

As will be demonstrated in this volume, an emerging body of evidence implicates specific features of work as important causes of hypertension as well as other manifestations of CVD. Chapters 2–5 explore this empirical evidence and the theoretical constructs concerning the relationship between the workplace and CVD. Psychosocial factors identified with the workplace are a particular focus. We develop the paradigm of "econeurocardiology" as a conceptual bridge which renders plausible the various theoretical constructs of work stress as they relate to CVD. The econeurocardiology concept offers a framework in which the reader can understand how these stress mechanisms give rise to various cardiovascular target organ responses. Chapter 6 explores the methodological issues in the measurement of psychosocial factors at the workplace. Recommendations are made on how to improve the reliability, validity, and feasibility of these measures. Chapters 7–10 offer the clinician a set of tools for the evaluation and management of working people at risk for heart disease. A new, more advanced approach to "occupational cardiology" is presented. Chapters 11–13 provide a public health overview, addressing economics and the legislative, legal, and preventive interventions necessary to deal with this workplace-induced CVD epidemic.

Finally, Chapter 14 summarizes the evidence, makes the case for a causal relationship between the workplace and CVD, and discusses the implications of the trends toward deteriorating working conditions (e.g., lean production, downsizing, and longer work hours). These trends may result in greater exposure to psychosocial risk factors at the workplace, which may, in turn, increase the CVD epidemic. Since this CVD epidemic is engendered, at least in part, by the social organization of work and other noxious workplace exposures, primary prevention may be possible via interventions aimed at improving the work environment. Legislative changes and public health interventions can help create a climate in which healthy work becomes the priority.

REFERENCES

1. The Tokyo Declaration. J Tokyo Med Univ 56:760–767, 1998.
2. American Heart Association: 1999 Heart and Stroke Statistical Update. Dallas, AHA, 1998.
3. Blake LM, Goldschlager N: Risk stratification of potential sudden death victims after myocardial infarction. Prim Cardiol 21:8–15, 1995.
4. Bosma H, Stansfeld SA, Marmot MG: Job control, personal characteristics, and heart disease. J Occup Health Psychol 3:402–409, 1998.
5. Braunwald E: Cardiovascular medicine at the turn of the millennium: Triumphs, concerns, and opportunities. New Engl J Med 327:1360–1369, 1997.
6. Cupples LA, Gagnon DR, Kannel WB: Long- and short-term risk of sudden coronary death. Circulation 85 Suppl I:I11–I18, 1992.
7. De Faire U: Will the decline in mortality from coronary heart disease in Sweden continue? J Int Med 242:189–190, 1997.
8. Diez-Roux AV: Bringing context back into epidemiology: Variables and fallacies in multilevel analysis. Am J Public Health 88:216–222, 1998.
9. Freidman M, Rosenman RH: Association of specific overt behavior pattern with blood and cardiovascular findings. JAMA 169:1286–1296, 1959.
10. Huikuri HV: Heart rate dynamics and vulnerability to ventricular tachyarrhythmias. Ann Med 29:321–325, 1997.
11. Kannel W, McGee D, Gordon T: A general cardiovascular risk profile: The Framingham Study. Am J Cardiol 38:46–51, 1976.
12. Kaplan GA, Keil JE: Socioeconomic factors and cardiovascular disease: A review of the literature. Circulation 88:1973–1998, 1993.
13. Karasek R, Theorell T: Healthy Work: Stress, Productivity, and the Reconstruction of Working Life. New York, Basic Books, 1990.
14. Kohn ML: Unresolved issues in the relationship between work and personality. In Erikson K, Vallas SP (eds): The Nature of Work: Sociological Perspectives. New Haven, Yale University Press, 1990, pp 36–68.
15. Kohn ML, Schooler C: Job conditions and personality: A longitudinal assessment of their reciprocal effects. Am J Sociol 87:1257–1286, 1982.
16. Landsbergis PA, Schnall PL, Deitz D, et al: The patterning of psychological attributes and distress by "job strain" and social support in a sample of working men. J Behav Med 15:379–405, 1992.
17. Link BG, Phelan J: Social conditions as fundamental causes of disease. J Health Soc Behav (Extra Issue):80–94, 1995.
18. Lown B: Role of higher nervous activity in sudden cardiac death. Jpn Circ J 54:581–602, 1990.
19. Marmot MG, Smith DG, Stansfeld S, et al: Health inequalities among British civil servants: The Whitehall II study. Lancet 337:1387–1393, 1991.
20. Mehta D, Curwin J, Gomes A, Fuster V: Sudden death in coronary artery disease. Circulation 96:3215–3223, 1997.
21. Natelson BH, Chang Q: Sudden death. A neurocardiologic phenomenon. Neurol Clin 11:293–308, 1993.
22. Ragland D, Brand R: Coronary heart disease mortality in the Western Collaborative Group Study: Followup experience of 22 years. Am J Epidemiol 127:462–475, 1988.
23. Rose G: Sick individuals and sick populations. Int J Epidemiol 14:32–38, 1985.

24. Rosenman RH, Brand RJ, Sholtz RI, Friedman M: Multivariate prediction of coronary heart disease during 8.5 year followup in the Western Collaborative Group Study. Am J Cardiol 37:903–910, 1976.
25. Schnall PL, Kern R: Hypertension in American society: An introduction to historical materialist epidemiology. In Conrad P, Kern R (eds): The Sociology of Health and Illness: Critical Perspectives. New York, St. Martin's Press, 1981, pp 97–122.
26. Reference deleted.
27. Stansfeld SA, North FM, White I, Marmot MG: Work characteristics and psychiatric disorder in civil servants in London. J Epidemiol Comm Health 49:48–53, 1995.
28. Susser M, Susser E: Choosing a future for epidemiology. I. Eras and paradigms. Am J Public Health 86:668–673, 1996.
29. Waldron I, Nowotarski M, Freimer M, et al: Cross-cultural variation in blood pressure: A qualitative analysis of the relationships of blood pressure to cultural characteristics, salt consumption, and body weight. Soc Sci Med 16:419–430, 1982.
30. Williams R: The Trusting Heart. New York, Times Books, 1989.

RESEARCH FINDINGS LINKING WORKPLACE FACTORS TO CARDIOVASCULAR DISEASE OUTCOMES

SHIFT WORK, LONG HOURS, AND CARDIOVASCULAR DISEASE: A REVIEW *by Kyle Steenland, PhD*

Data from industrialized countries suggests that irregular patterns of work, such as shift work and extensive overtime work, have become increasingly common. In conjunction with this trend, there are more epidemiologic studies of the health effects of such irregular patterns of work, a number of which focus on heart disease. The following is a review of the literature, with comments on possible mechanisms linking irregular hours and heart disease as well as on the methodologic difficulties of studying this topic. Shift work and heart disease are the primary focus here, because most of the epidemiologic efforts have been directed at this area, but the epidemiology of overtime work and heart disease also is reviewed.

Shift Work and Heart Disease

DEFINITION AND PREVALENCE OF SHIFT WORK

Shift work refers to work patterns other than the standard day shift. It therefore includes both rotating shifts in which the worker works a rotating pattern of days, evenings, and nights, and permanent shift work in which a worker works steadily during evenings or nights (second or third shift). Most of the epidemiology regarding the health effects of shift work has focused on rotating shifts. There are many forms of rotating shifts. A worker may work a week of days, a week of evenings, and a week of nights, with weekends off. He or she may work three shift rotations changing more frequently, including sometimes double shifts (16 hours), or perhaps alternative day and night work.

The prevalence of shift work varies from country to country, but most data suggest that in Western industrial countries approximately 10–20% of workers now work rotating shifts. Taylor and Pocock cite a figure of 25% for England in 1968; Tenkanen, et al. cite an estimate of 15–20% for Europe currently; and Knutsson, et al. report an estimated 10–12% in Sweden in the early 1990s.[134,254,256] Gordon, et al. cite a figure of 26% for men and 18% for women in the United States in 1980.[80] It appears that in both Europe and the U.S. the proportion of workers on rotating shifts has been increasing since WW II.[80] For some particular occupations such as nursing, the proportion of workers on rotating shifts is very high. In Boston, for example,

OCCUPATIONAL MEDICINE: State of the Art Reviews—
Vol. 15, No. 1, January–March 2000. Philadelphia, Hanley & Belfus, Inc.

7

60% of nurses reported in 1988 that they had a history of shift work.[127] Permanent shift work appears to be more rare than rotating shift work; for example, Akerstedt, et al. report Swedish data showing a prevalence of only 7% for permanent shift work.[2]

MECHANISMS FOR SHIFT WORK AND HEART DISEASE

Shift work might reasonably be considered a risk factor for heart disease because: (1) shift work, especially rotating shift work, disrupts **circadian rhythms**, which are are linked to a number of CV risk factors such as blood pressure, heart rate, and catecholamine levels, (2) shift work is either correlated with or leads to poorer **lifestyle factors** which in turn are related to increased CV disease, e.g., reduced physical activity, poorer diet, increased cigarette consumption, and less social contact, and (3) shift work involves more **occupational stress** because such jobs are more demanding and often involve less control on the part of the worker, and increased stress may increase heart disease. These possible mechanisms clearly are not exhaustive. For example, Harma mentions the known decrease in fibrinolysis in early morning hours which might preferentially affect night workers, or some unknown aspect directly related to sleep deprivation itself.[92] Bøggild and Knutsson provide a more thorough review of potential mechanisms.[25] Note that for the second pathway described above, shift work could be either causal or simply a marker for confounders (standard heart disease risk factors), which when controlled would eliminate any association between shift work and heart disease.

The (continual) disruption of circadian rhythm for rotating shift workers is probably the strongest proposed mechanism, with important and documented effects on the CV system (see Chapter 5 for a review). However, key questions remain about exactly how this disruption might lead to increased disease in shift workers, and whether they can adapt to such disruption.

Shift work could cause either acute or chronic effects on the heart, i.e., acute effects while performing shift work, or chronic effects years later. Disruption of circadian rhythms might be suspected of having acute effects, although chronic alterations of blood pressure, for example, might lead to heart disease at a later date. A worse pattern of lifestyle characteristics and increased stress could reasonably be associated with either acute or chronic effects on the heart. Whether the presumed effects are acute or chronic, they may be more easily observed in younger men, during working ages, simply because single risk factors for heart disease are more easily detected at younger ages before a large number of risk factors begin to cause much higher heart disease rates.[108] On the other hand, if the effects were chronic, they might not become apparent until older ages and perhaps not until after workers had left the workplace.

METHODOLOGIC ISSUES IN STUDYING SHIFT WORK AND HEART DISEASE

As a general recommendation, in light of the potential for a long lag period between shift work and overt CV disease, studies should include followup of workers after leaving work. Analyses should pay careful attention to different possible lag times between the beginning of shift work and observable heart disease. Assuming some appreciable lag, studies restricted to workers currently employed might more profitably focus on the development of intermediate CV risk factors (e.g., blood pressure, cholesterol) rather than manifest CV disease (which in many cases will cause the worker to leave the workforce). However, cross-sectional studies of intermediate risk factors among the currently employed are limited due to the usual problem of determining temporal sequence, so longitudinal studies with baseline measures before shift work would be far preferable.

There are several additional aspects of shift work that potentially complicate any epidemiologic study of its relation to heart disease. Shift workers may be a select population, and it may be difficult to find a comparable reference population of day workers. Shift workers may be selected into shift work because they are healthier to begin with and the employer believes they are better adapted to shift work. However, the opposite scenario is also possible—shift workers may already have an unhealthy lifestyle and, therefore, may be willing to work irregular hours because they won't suffer any lifestyle change. There are few data on this issue. McNamee, et al. found a significantly reduced risk of ischemic heart disease in the first 10 years after starting shift work, which then was no longer apparent, suggesting an initial selection of shift workers for good health.[172] Knuttson and Akerstedt studied 53 men who applied for day work or shift work and found that the applicants for shift work were more accustomed to irregular sleep patterns, but there were no differences in traditional CV risk factors.[135]

In addition to selection into shift work for health-related reasons, shift workers may have unhealthier lifestyles and lower educational backgrounds than day workers, biasing upwards studies of heart disease. Such biases are minimized if one compares workers to workers, making the same general social class likely, especially if they are in the same workplace. This potential bias is more of a concern in broad-based studies such as population-based case-control studies including many social classes, or in cohort studies including subjects from many different workplaces.

There is reasonable evidence that some percentage of new shift workers switch back to day work because they cannot tolerate shift work. Harma, et al. provide evidence that 20% of shift workers switch back to day work within a year due to intolerance of shift work.[93] Koller reports cross-sectional data indicating 22% of workers with a history of shift work had abandoned shift work due to health or family problems.[140] Akerstedt, et al. cite evidence from Sweden in the 1940s that approximately 10% of workers with a history of shift work had transferred back to day work for health reasons within 10 years.[2] Angersbach, et al. report in a study of 600 workers that 11% had switched from shift work to day work, two-thirds of whom did so for health reasons.[11] These same authors found a higher prevalence of health problems in these workers who had dropped out of shift work, compared with day workers or workers who had stayed in shiftwork. McNamee, et al. found an increased risk of heart disease death in the first 5 years after a shift worker switched back to day work (odds ratio 2.69 [1.04–6.96]).[172] On the other hand, Bøggild, et al. found no increased risk for shift workers who switched back to day work.[26] Nachreiner has provided an overview of the recent literature on workers' tolerance of shift work.[182]

The phenomenon of workers, particularly unhealthier workers, switching back from shift work to day work is an example of a **healthy shift-worker survivor bias**, which tends to create a bias towards the null in studies of shiftwork and CV disease. This potential bias is particularly important in prevalence studies comparing shift workers to non-shift workers, and in longitudinal studies that seek a trend in risk with shift work duration rather than compare those ever employed in shift work to those never employed in shift work.

While the healthy shift-worker survivor bias concerns workers switching from shift work to day work, there is also the more general problem of the **healthy worker survivor bias**, which refers to the tendency of sick workers to leave the workforce altogether. Heart disease is a serious illness that often results in the removal of workers from the workplace. One approach, when comparing shift workers to day workers, is to compare illness or mortality rates when both groups are working or when both groups are not working.[245]

It is difficult to summarize these possible biases to say that the overall "net" likely bias is negative or positive. Judgement of the likely sum effect of such biases depends on study design and can best be done for each study individually

EPIDEMIOLOGIC STUDIES OF SHIFT WORK

Cardiovascular Risk Factors. Disruption of circadian rhythms, poor lifestyle, and increased stress presumably operate via a worse profile of CV risk factors among shift workers versus day workers. However, the healthy shift-worker survivor bias and the healthy worker survivor bias might make it more difficult to observe such a worse profile, particularly in prevalence studies. The data on CV risk factors as shown in Table 1 do not indicate a consistently worse profile of risk factors among shift workers. Almost all of these studies are cross-sectional, assessing the prevalence of risk factors at a given point in time. Shift work is defined in these studies by either current status as a shift worker or by a history of shift work. Some studies excluded day workers who had ever been shift workers, but most did not, thereby allowing a possible healthy shift-worker survivor bias.

Blood pressure usually exhibits a trough at night and peak during the day. The study by Baumgart, et al. listed in Table 1 shows that shift workers rapidly alter this pattern and exhibit a peak at night while working; other investigators have duplicated these findings.[44,250,294] However, most studies do not indicate that shift workers have a higher mean blood pressure, which would be expected to lead to more heart disease (an exception is the study by Prunier-Poulmaire, et al., but it is somewhat suspect due to a small day worker referent group that was doing a different kind of job, and the fact that 18 of 21 self-reported health conditions were significantly worse in shift workers, suggesting a possible selection bias). It is possible that a different diurnal pattern of blood pressure troughs and peaks could increase risk of heart disease, but this is currently unknown.

The lack of consistent prevalence findings of more CV risk factors does not strengthen the case that shift work increases CV risk, but neither does it fatally weaken it. First, the evidence is not totally negative; second, the healthy worker biases may play a role in negative studies. Even if a consistent profile of worse CV risk factors (either lifestyle factors such as smoking or physiologic measures such as blood pressure) was found among shift workers in prevalence studies, the question would still be open as to whether shift work was *directly responsible for* the increased prevalence of risk factors or simply *associated with* such factors. In the former case, shift work would truly be a cause of CV disease, and epidemiologic analyses would not control for risk factors because they would be intermediate variables on a causal pathway. In the latter case, shift work might or might not be a true cause of heart disease, but if it were, it would not operate via causing an increase in known risk factors. Thus, epidemiologic analyses would have to control for known risk factors because they would be considered confounding variables. This problem—whether known risk factors for an outcome should be considered intermediate or confounding variables—is a common one in epidemiologic studies.[281] Adequate studies to sort out this problem require a longitudinal design in which shift workers and day workers are studied at baseline and then followed to determine whether CV risk factors develop preferentially in shift workers.

Cardiovascular Disease. The principal epidemiologic studies comparing CV mortality or incidence among shift workers and day workers or non-shift workers are listed in Table 2. The focus is on studies of *rotating* shift workers. There is only one study of permanent shift workers in the literature; this study focused on fatal

TABLE 1. Selected Recent Studies of Cardiovascular Risk Factors in Shift Workers*

Study†	Population	Design	Findings, Shift Versus Day Work; Comments
Nakamura, et al. 1999	66 male Japanese blue-collar shift workers, 239 day workers, same plant	Prevalence data measured in annual health checkup	Workers rotating 3 shifts, but not those rotating 2 shifts, had significantly higher cholesterol and obesity than day workers
Prunier-Poulmaire, et al. (1998)	French custom officials, 262 shift workers, 40 day workers working in airplanes	Prevalence data, self-reported high blood pressure	Older workers with more rotating shifts reported significantly higher blood pressure; however, they also reported significantly increased health problems for 16 of other 19 health conditions
Knuttson and Nilsson 1998	Sample of 2548 men and 2836 women from 1990 Swedish census, 17% shiftworkers or nightworkers	Prevalence data on current smoking	More current smoking for shift or night workers, odds ratio 1.3 (1.1–1.6), controlling for age, stress, sex
Tenkanen, et al. 1997	1806 Finnish workers (564 shift workers) in several industries, age 40–55 in 1982	Prevalence data in 1982 for risk factors, shift work as of 1982	No differences in smoking, alcohol, obesity, physical activity, or cholesterol; more reported stress
Lasfargues, et al. 1996	676 male and 524 female night workers vs. pair-matched controls, both from 150,000 volunteers for health checkup in France, aged 30–50, 1991–3	Prevalence data, matching on broad socioeconomic strata (manual worker, clerical, manager), age, and sex	No difference in blood pressure, alcohol, self-reported health status. Cholesterol significantly lower in male night workers. Significantly higher triglycerides, smoking, obesity, WBC, sleep problems in night workers. Not clear whether night workers rotated shifts.
Kawachi, et al. 1995	79,109 U.S. nurses age 30–55 in 1976, 60% current or past shift workers as of 1988	Prevalence data in 1988 for risk factors, any history of shift work (both self-reported)	More smoking, high blood pressure, diabetes, obesity, physical activity, less alcohol, no difference in high cholesterol (all age-adjusted)
Skipper et al. 1990	464 U.S. nurses, 54% rotating shifts, 23% days, 12% evenings or nights	Self-reported 1988 prevalence data, age-adjusted, shift work as of 1988	No differences between rotating shift workers and others for physical or mental health, except increased stress for rotating shifters
Romon, et al. 1992	71 French shift workers with more than one year vs. 70 age-matched day workers with no past shift work	Prevalence data, measured in 1988	Higher triglycerides, less alcohol, no differences in cholesterol obesity, cigarettes, blood pressure, nutrients
Knutsson, et al. 1990	12 shift workers, 13 day workers, Swedish paper mill	Prospective over 6 months, shift work as of time of study	No difference in change in lipids or blood pressure over 6 months
Bursey 1990	57 English shift workers (> 5 yr), 57 day workers over 40 (never shift work)	Prevalence data measured at time of study, matching on age, cigarettes, blue-collar status	No difference in obesity, blood pressure, cholesterol, EKG

Table continued on next page.

TABLE 1.   Selected Recent Studies of Cardiovascular Risk Factors in Shift Workers* (*Cont*).

Study†	Population	Design	Findings, Shift Versus Day Work; Comments
Baumgart, et al. 1989	17 English shift workers serving as their own controls	Continuous blood pressure measured morning and night shifts	No difference in mean blood pressure between night and day shifts; evidence of an 8-hour lag in the diurnal variation of blood pressure as soon as night work began
Costa, et al. 1990	158 toll collectors night or shift work vs. 44 day workers, same company, aged 35 or older	Prevalence data	No difference in cholesterol, obesity, blood pressure, triglycerides unadjusted for age, no difference in summary measure of cardiovascular risk factors after age adjustment
Knutsson, et al. 1988	361 shift workers, 240 day workers, blue-collar workers at 3 Swedish plants	Prevalence data measured 1975–1976, shift work as of time of study	More smoking, higher triglycerides, no differences in age, cholesterol, obesity, blood pressure
Gordon, et al. 1986	828 men, 833 women, random sample of U.S., 22% rotating shift workers	Prevalence data self-reported 1980, shift work self-reported as of 1980	Men and women reported more drinking, job stress, emotional problems. No association with age, education, or income, or smoking. Women reported more tranquilizer use.

* For a more complete review of such studies, including non-English publications, see reference 25.
† McNamee et al. 1996 omitted because of lack of age-adjusted data.

heart disease while working (assuming an acute effect) and showed no harmful effects of evening or night work.[246]

The data in Table 2 are rather sparse, and the results are not consistent. Four studies show a significant increase in CV disease for shift workers, while four do not. The 1997 study by Tenkenen, et al. is one of the strongest because it was done within a clinical trial and had good data on heart disease risk factors and outcomes (data were analyzed with and without treated subjects, to make sure results were not confounded by drug treatment).[256] Subjects worked at a variety of workplaces and represented different social classes (restriction of the data to blue-collar workers lowered the relative risk about 25%, indicating some confounding by social class). Overall, analyses indicated that the excess risk shown by shift workers (approximately 40%, borderline significant) was not much affected by adjustment for risk factors such as blood pressure, cholesterol, smoking, or occupational stress. This finding suggests that shift work does cause heart disease, but not via an increase in prevalence of any known or suspected risk factors (e.g., occupational stress), at least as measured in this study. Indeed, Tenkanen, et al. hypothesize another mechanism possibly related to both stress and circadian rhythms—an alteration of fibrinolysis among shift workers. They provide some data showing that the heart disease risk of shift workers versus day workers was somewhat less for those who were taking gemfibrozil as part of a clinical trial. (Gemfibrozil is a lipid-lowering drug that subsequently was found to increase fibrinolysis.) In a followup paper, Tenkanen, et al. found that higher relative risks occurred for shift workers who smoked, suggesting an interaction.[255] However, they did not provide a test of significance for this interaction.

TABLE 2. Studies of Shift-Work and Cardiovascular Disease*

Study†	Population	Design	Findings, Shift Versus Day Work; Comments
Bøggild, et al. 1999	5249 men aged 40–59 in 1971, from 14 companies	Cohort study with 22-yr followup, fatal/non-fatal IHD	RR 1.0 (0.9–1.2) for shift workers, control for most risk factors
Knutsson, et al. 1999	2006 cases first myocardial infarction, 2642 controls	Population based case-control study	RR 1.3 (1.1–1.6) for men and RR 1.3 (0.9–1.8) for women for shift work in last 5 years. Control for smoking, education
Tenkanen, et al. 1997 Tenkanen, et al. 1998	1806 Finnish workers (564 shift workers) in several industries, age 40–55 in 1982, generally long-term shift workers	Cohort study with 6-yr followup, IHD, (ICD 410-414) via death or hospital discharge	RR for IHD 1.4 (1.0–1.9), adjustment for cigarettes, lipids, blood pressure, obesity, alcohol, job strain. No analysis by duration of shift work
McNamee, et al. 1996	Male manual workers at single plant, age < 50 when first employed between 1950–1992, 467 IHD deaths as per death certificate, 467 controls	Nested case-control study, shift work based on personnel records, any history > 1 mo (2/3 exposed)	OR 0.5 (0.3–0.8) in first 10 years after shift work began, OR 0.9 (0.7–1.2) thereafter. No trend with duration of shift-work, control for BP, smoking, job status, obesity measured before employment
Kawachi, et al. 1995	79109 female nurses aged 42–67 in 1988, free of IHD, 60% with history of shift work	Cohort study with 4-yr followup, 292 fatal and nonfatal CHD	RR 1.3 (1.0–1.7) for shift work, RR 1.2 (0.9–1.6) for < 6 yr shift work, RR 1.5 (1.1–20) for 6 yr. Adjustment for risk factors in 1990 (little effect of adjustment on RRs)
Knutsson, et al. 1986	504 paper mill workers in 1968, 394 shift workers, few ex-shift workers, at a single plant	Cohort study 15-yr followup, 43 cases of IHD (angina or MI)	RR 1.4 (n.s.), increasing risk of IHD with increasing duration of shift work until 20 years (RR 2.8, 16–20 yr.), when RR drops possibly due to survivor effect, control over smoking, age
Angersbach, et al. 1980	210 shift workers, 142 day workers, 41 ex-shift workers, all who stayed employed over 11 years, at a single plant	Followup morbidity study over 1966–77 based on company medical records	No differences in cardiovascular complaints registered in company clinic; study limited by restriction to active workers
Taylor and Pocock 1972	Male manual workers with 10+ years employment after 1946 and born before 1920, from 10 companies, 4188 shift workers with 10+ years shift work, 3869 day workers with 10+ years day work and < 6 mo shift work, 555 ex-shift workers with 6+ mo shift work	Cohort study with followup through 1968, 444 CHD deaths, comparison to general population via SMRs	SMR 0.9 (0.8–1.1) for day workers, 1.0 (0.9–1.2) for shift workers, 1.2 (0.9–1.7) for ex-shift workers SMR 1.2 (1.0–1.5) for shift workers under age 60, primarily in one company adjustment only for age, no analysis by duration of shift work

* Cross-sectional studies are omitted.   † Three studies potentially relevant to rotating shift workers are omitted (Alfredsson, et al. 1982, Alfredsson, et al. 1985, Tuchsen 1993) because they are not based on a well-defined population of shift workers. The exposure variable in these three studies is defined as work in an occupation presumed to involve more frequent shift work than other occupations. These studies all show some increase in mortality among workers in jobs presumed to involve more shift work. However, the imprecision of the definition of shift work and the possibility of confounders related to occupation make these studies of less value than the ones listed. (IHD = ischemic heart disease, ICD = ischemic coronary disease, CHD = coronary heart disease, MI = myocardial infarction)

The study by Kawachi, et al. of U.S. nurses is a second well-designed study with a positive result (RR = 1.31, 95% CI 1.02–1.68).[127] Adjustment for traditional risk factors generally did not change results much, again suggesting that any shift work effect is not mediated through the risk factors usually considered for heart disease, although in this study only self-reported data on risk factors was available. A significant trend of increased risk with increasing duration of rotating shift work was shown. There is no suggestion in the data that those who left shift work shortly after entering it (the "drop-outs") had a higher heart disease risk. This could be because few nurses were able to switch back to day work, even if they had health problems.

The third positive study, by Knutsson, et al., is a smaller study without extensive control over conventional CV risk factors.[136] It is consistent with the Kawachi, et al. study in that there is an overall excess risk of about 40% for shift workers, and a significant increasing trend in risk with increasing duration of shift work, at least until 20 years. Employees who have been shift workers for more than 20 years show a decreased risk, which the authors interpret as a survivor effect—shift workers who survive more than 20 years are a particularly hardy group unaffected by heart disease. However, no such survivor effect was seen in the Kawachi, et al. study.

The fourth positive study, also by Knutsson, et al. is unusual in that it is a population-based case-control study in which shift work in the last five years was determined by interview.[134] Shift work (14–15% did shift work, about the same for men and women) in this study is not rotating shifts per se, but includes those reporting night work (about 3–4% did night work). The limited time window for shift work and the lack of detailed information on the reported shift work are limitations in this study. The categorization of exposed (shift work) versus nonexposed is likely to be less precise than in cohort studies; this fact would ordinarily bias findings towards the null. Nonetheless, a modest but significant relative risk of 1.3 was found for both men and women. Adjustment for self-reported job strain did not change the findings, nor was there any interaction with the job strain variable. The principal concern in this study is possible upward bias in the odds ratio due to uncontrolled confounding. Shift workers were of lower socioeconomic class than non-shift workers, and smoked more. Education and smoking (current, former, never) were controlled in the analysis, but residual confounding by social class may have occurred, and there was no control for risk factors such as obesity, blood pressure, and cholesterol. While it could be argued that these last factors might be intermediate variables which should not be included in the model, this case has not been proved, and it is at least equally plausible that these variables act as confounders.

The four remaining studies in Table 2, in contrast, are largely negative. There are no obvious flaws in the designs of the studies by Bøggild, et al., McNamee, et al., and Taylor and Pocock to explain why they are negative.[26,172,254] The Bøggild, et al. study is one of the better analyses overall, as it is a cohort study with good baseline data on possible confounders, some validation data indicating that self-reported data on shift work were reasonably accurate, and a recontact of 75% of the cohort 15 years after baseline to again ascertain shift-work status.[26] Workers worked in 14 different companies and came from different social classes. Although workers with any night work are mixed with rotating shift workers, evidence presented suggests that most shift workers rotated. There is no suggestion of any excess risk for shift workers in this study, with or without controlling for traditional risk factors. There is some evidence in these data that inadequate control over social class, in studies with heterogenous populations of workers, might be an important confounder in shift-work studies.

The McNamee, et al. study was done in a workforce at a single plant.[172] This study showed no effect overall of shift work, nor with duration of shift work (in contrast to Kawachi, et al. 1995 and Knuttson, et al. 1986). McNamee, et al. conducted a number of time-specific analyses, including analyses by years since beginning shift work; the latter revealed a significant excess risk for ex-shift workers shortly after leaving shift work (odds ratio 2.69, 1.04–6.96, 14 cases, 6 controls) compared to day workers. However, this finding may have been a reflection of sick workers leaving employment rather than a health effect specific to shift work.

The Taylor and Pocock study is an older study that is limited by the lack of a direct comparison between shift workers and day workers (all groups are compared to the general population), but which is based on large numbers and had a good division of workers between long-term shift workers, day workers, and ex-shift workers.[254] Despite the lack of a direct comparison between worker groups, this study can be considered negative. There is an interesting finding of a modest excess for shift workers under 60 years of age, but the authors state that this is largely due to one particular company and that there may be additional reasons (not specified) why young workers at this company might have high heart disease rates.

The final study in this group, by Angersbach, et al., is a morbidity study based on company medical records and restricted to workers who remained employed during an 11-year period.[11] This is an important limitation in so much as the effects of shift work on the heart might cause workers to leave employment, or might first occur only after employment, so this study must be given less weight than the others. A similar study of illness among active workers was conducted, but it did not report CV disease separately.[253]

SUMMARY OF EPIDEMIOLOGIC EVIDENCE FOR HEART DISEASE–SHIFT WORK LINK

Taken as a whole, the epidemiologic data suggest that a modest association between shift work and heart disease may exist. There are plausible biological mechanisms (via disruption of circadian rhythms) by which shift work could result in heart disease. However, the epidemiologic studies are still relatively few in number, and they are not consistent. Therefore a causal relationship between shift work and heart disease cannot be inferred. It is a difficult subject to study epidemiologically, and we must wait for additional data before drawing more definitive conclusions.

Those studies that do show a shift work effect do not suggest that this effect is mediated by changes in conventional heart disease risk factors; however, these risk factors may not have been well measured or may not have been the true risk factors of interest. Furthermore, there may be effects of shift work on the CV system that are not well understood and are not well explained by the current proposed mechanisms. There is some evidence of selection biases operating that could bias findings towards the null, but there is other evidence that some positive findings in general populations may have been confounded positively by social class.

REGULATIONS CONCERNING SHIFT WORK

Kogi recently reviewed international regulations on the organization of work, principally the recommendations of the International Labor Organization (ILO) dating from 1990, and the directive of the European Council of 1993 which (at least in theory) must be enforced within the European Economic Community. These regulations apply more generally to all work organization, but a number of points are directly relevant to shift work. The ILO recommendations call for: (1) advice to the worker at regular intervals on how to cope with shift work, (2) transfer to a similar day job when the worker is found unfit for shift work, (3) special compensation for shift work, (4) consultation between worker and employer on the details of the shift work, and (5) at least 11 hours rest in each 24-hour period (no consecutive full-time shifts). The European directive is similar. It calls for: (1) a minimum daily rest period of 11 hours in a 24-hour period, (2) a rest period of at least 35 consecutive hours per 7-day period, (3) maximum of 48 work hours per week, and (4) transfer to day work when problems with night work are recognized.

In the U.S. there are no general regulations covering shift work, although there are some regulations for particular sets of transportation workers (pilots, truck drivers, and railroad workers). The U.S. National Institute for Occupational Safety and Health has published guidelines for shift work.

Overtime Work and Heart Disease

Overtime work is commonly thought to be stressful and fatiguing and may be correlated with sleep deprivation, thereby involving two of the same mechanisms hypothesized for heart disease and shift work. There are data indicating that, in general, being at work (versus not being at work) increases blood pressure, so that longer working hours implies more time with increased blood pressure.[210] Finally, there are more recent data indicating that long hours of overtime may increase average blood pressure as measured over 24 hours. One model for an effect of long hours on heart disease suggests that this increased blood pressure contributes to an acute myocardial infarction.

Studies of long hours and heart disease involve many of the same methodologic issues as studies of shift work and heart disease; it is important to compare populations of workers that are as similar as possible with respect to potential confounders to avoid selection biases, and longitudinal studies with careful attention to temporal sequence of exposure are preferred.

Overtime work as a risk factor for heart disease is difficult to separate from the more general literature regarding stress, since overtime work generally is considered stressful. There are a few early studies suggesting that long working hours are among the stressful factors that increase the risk of heart disease.[224,264] More recently, Falger and Shouten studied cases of male acute myocardial infarction versus hospital and neighborhood controls.[68] With hospital controls (but not neighborhood controls), they found that self-reported prolonged overtime (time period not defined) caused a significant two-fold excess risk for acute myocardial infarction after controlling for smoking, age, education, and self-reported exhaustion. The focus in these studies has been more on stress rather than on overtime work per se.

There are two other studies in which working long hours is inferred for study subjects based on occupational category, using ancillary surveys of work habits by different occupations.[37,88] These studies can provide only indirect evidence and are not reviewed here.

The most important studies to date attempt to separate the independent effects of long hours and stress, either by explicit attempts to measure both these variables and by matching, or by quantitatively measuring hours worked.[95,111,243] Two of the studies concern long hours and blood pressure, while one is a case-control study of long hours and myocardial infarction. All three come from Japan, where working long hours is common and where death from overwork, or "Karoshi," is a publicly recognized phenomenon, despite the lack of formal epidemiologic evidence.

Hayashi, et al. studied 10 normotensive men working long hours (more than 60 hours overtime a month) and 11 normotensive controls (less than 30 hours overtime a month) (Group A).[95] Blood pressure was recorded during a routine checkup. Investigators also studied 15 exposed men and 11 controls who had mild hypertension (group B), as well as a group of normotensive men whose hours varied between heavy overtime and light overtime (group C). Groups A, B, and C all worked for the same company, and group C members worked in the same department; exposed and controls were similar with respect to age, body mass, and smoking habits. Hourly blood pressure, recorded over a month and averaged, showed significantly higher blood pressure for the exposed versus controls in groups A and B. Group C, perhaps the most interesting because it was studied longitudinally and avoided potential confounding (subjects were their own controls), showed a significant increase in blood pressure (diastolic and systolic) and a significant decrease in sleep when working more overtime (average 96 hours/month, versus 43 hours/month during the control period).

Iwasaki, et al. studied systolic blood pressure among 71 salesmen in the same company divided into two groups by length of work week in the previous month.[111] Based on a single blood pressure measurement, the group with more hours (65 hours/week) had higher systolic blood pressure for one age group (age 50–59) than did the group with shorter working hours (57 hours/week), despite the fact that the difference in hours worked was not extreme. Smoking and body mass were comparable between exposed and nonexposed. This study provides only weak evidence of an exposure effect due to its cross-sectional nature, the possibility of confounding, and reliance on a single blood pressure measurement.

In the most thorough study to date, Sokejima and Kagamimori compared 195 Japanese survivors of first heart attacks to 331 controls who were free of heart disease and matched by age and occupation to the patients.[243] Controls were chosen via lists of workers who had had yearly routine medical exams. Occupational matching was by eight broad occupational categories. Data on medical history, blood pressure, cholesterol, glucose tolerance, body mass, and smoking habits were obtained for both cases and controls, as were data on psychosocial conditions at work and time spent in sedentary work. The last two factors were not associated with heart disease in the analysis, while the former, more established risk factors were. Working hours in the month before infarction or interview (for controls) did not differ between cases and controls (average 9.2 hours). However, when the data were categorized, patients had significantly increased likelihood of having worked either short or long hours in the previous month (either > 11 hours on the average, or < 7) compared to controls, suggesting a U-shaped relationship between working hours and heart disease. The authors speculated that the increase in risk for those with short working hours might have been due to these subjects suffering from early disease (and therefore working less), or from a protective effect of working a full work day. The authors also found that there was a significant trend of increasing risk of infarction with a larger increase in working hours during the year prior to infarction, so that a change towards longer working hours increased risk. This finding is consistent with a postulated increase in blood pressure contributing to a heart attack.

In summary, although the literature is sparse, there is some suggestion that long hours can increase blood pressure and lead to increased heart disease, independent of other stressful conditions at work. These findings must be viewed as preliminary, but are intriguing enough to warrant more studies on overtime work and heart disease.

CHEMICAL AND PHYSICAL FACTORS   *by Larry Fine, MD, PhD*

Recently, much of the interest in the relationship between work and cardiovascular disease (CVD) has focused on psychosocial factors. However, there are a host of occupational chemical and physical factors that have been studied to investigate their possible relationship to CVD. Some of these exposures, such as cold weather, noise, and passive smoking, are common.

Cold Weather

Several epidemiologic studies have observed a definite relationship between environmental exposure to temperature below 18°C and small increases in the acute mortality from coronary artery disease (CAD) and CVD in individuals older than 50 years.[66] These increases in risk of death from cold exposures in Europe occurred to a greater degree in regions with warmer winters, in populations with cooler homes, and among people who wore fewer clothes and were less active outdoors. In a large study of 50- to 69-year-old men in London between 1986 and 1992, it was found that cold exposures of normal life are sufficient to induce prolonged hemoconcentration and increases in both systolic and diastolic blood pressure (BP). These changes occurred on the first cold day and persisted for a few days.[55] The increases in mortality appear preventable by adequate indoor heating and adequate protection against cold while outdoors.

In a study of the population of Yakutsk, which has extremely cold winters with mean October to March temperatures of –27°C, mortality from CVD and CAD among individuals 50–59 years old did not change. In comparison to other Siberian cities, this lack of mortality associated with cold stress seemed to result from the wearing of exceptionally warm clothing and the reduction of outdoor excursions at temperatures below –20°C.[54] These studies suggest that older workers who have regular or intermittent outdoor exposure in the winter may be at slightly increased risk of mortality from CVD and CAD; however, the excess risk seems to be prevented by adequate clothing (e.g., overcoats, gloves, and hats) and opportunities to rest in warm indoor environments. The mortality of older workers with outdoor exposures is an area for future study.

The relationship between mortality and cold exposure may be of interest in climates with mild winters, since the effects observed in Europe are seen in, for example, Italy and Greece. In addition, studies of cold temperatures may be of interest even in workers with exposures below 20°C, whether indoors or outdoors. ST-segment depression with or without anginal symptoms during ambulatory electrocardiac monitoring is suggestive of transient myocardial ischemia. Results from the CORDIS study found significant increases in the rate of silent ST-segment depression among women workers working at ambient temperatures lower than 20°C after adjusting for possible confounding factors such as age, type of work, smoking, and relative weight. It seems biologically plausible that sudden exposure to cold could induce coronary artery spasm, since the cold pressor test can provoke abnormalities of myocardial perfusion not only in patients with structural coronary disease or variant angina, but also normal subjects.[124a,221a]

Heat Exposures and Warm Weather

Acute myocardial infarction (MI) may occur (although rarely) after severe heat exhaustion or heat stroke, as they are associated with widespread tissue injury.[77] The risk of acute ischemia with heat stroke or heat exhaustion in working populations is unknown. In a study of Hajj pilgrims suffering from heat stroke, 21% had localized

ST-T electrocardiographic changes consistent with acute myocardial ischemia.[3] Heat waves in the United States are clearly associated with increase in overall mortality among the elderly. One European study found excessive total daily CV mortality among males between the ages of 45 and 65 when maximum air temperature exceeded 33°C.[240a]

Heat stroke and exhaustion are certainly acute risk factors for myocardial ischemia in an individual with CAD. For exposures less intense than those that cause heat stroke or exhaustion, the risk of cardiac ischemia in an individual with CAD appears to be related to the magnitude of the heat stress.[230,251c] One epidemiologic study of open-hearth steelworkers did not find an elevated risk of death from CAD.[217] However, a second study of French Potash miners concluded that there was an increased risk of IHD from the hot underground mining environment. One possible reason for the negative study is the selection of strong, healthy workers, both at hire and during employment.[288]

Further studies of heat waves to determine if active working adults have elevated mortality patterns and more studies of occupational groups with intermittent exposures to high temperatures would be interesting. Prompt recognition and therapy for heat stroke and heat exhaustion may prevent or limit myocardial ischemia in workers with underlying coronary disease.[50]

Noise

Research on noise exposure and hypertension or elevations in blood pressure has focused on two aspects: objective measures of noise exposure, usually exceeding 80 dB, and duration of exposure. A few studies have defined noise as any exposure that is considered by the exposed worker to be an annoyance. Two recent reviews have reached somewhat different conclusions about the relationship between objectively measured noise exposure and hypertension.[65,267] Experiments in animals suggest that noise exposure in spontaneously hypertensive rats can increase the number of ischemic myocardial lesions.[99] This issue is not entirely resolved, but there may be a dose-response relationship between noise and hypertension; the importance of duration of exposure has not been clarified.[70,101,295] The proponents of a causal relationship between noise and hypertension have noted that the likely increases in BP would result in modest increases (1.1–1.2) in the relative risk for CAD.[65] Overall, there is considerable, if conflicting, evidence that prolonged exposure to high noise levels causes significant, chronic elevation of BP.

A few studies address the effect of noise on other cardiac risks, such as cholesterol. However, the results are not definitive, but raise the hypothesis that noise exposure could affect lipid levels.[174] One interesting and provocative study found a borderline significant relationship in men between transient episodes of ST-depression on ambulatory electrocardiac monitoring and industrial noise exposure.[81] Since noise exposure is still common, further research on the relationship between CVD and chronic, high-level noise exposure is important.

Passive Smoking

A review by Kristensen underlined the importance of passive smoking at work as a risk factor for premature CVD in Denmark.[65] A risk assessment based on measured levels of environmental tobacco smoke (ETS) in office air and salivary cotinine in nonsmoking U.S. workers estimated that 4000 heart disease deaths occurred annually among office workers from occupational exposures to passive smoking.

This number was based on an estimated prevalence of unrestricted smoking in U.S. office workplaces of 28%.[221]

In some workplaces with particularly high levels of exposure to passive smoking, such as casinos, CAD risk may be even greater.[268] Environmental sampling was performed to evaluate occupational exposure to ETS among casino employees. The geometric mean serum cotinine level of the 27 participants who provided serum samples was 1.34 nanograms per milliliter (ng/ml) pre-shift, and 1.85 ng/ml post-shift. Both measurements exceeded the geometric mean value of 0.65 ng/ml for participants in the third National Health and Nutrition Examination Survey (NHANES III) who reported exposure to ETS at work.[268] This evaluation demonstrates that a sample of employees working in a casino gaming area were exposed to ETS at levels greater than those observed in a representative sample of the U.S. population, and that the serum and urine cotinine of these employees increased during the working shift. The number of these high-exposure environments in the U.S. is unknown.

Physical Exercise and Vibration

Numerous studies consistently find that higher levels of physical activity, whether at work or leisure, are associated with lower risks of CAD and CVD.[158] The biological processes proposed to explain the beneficial effect of higher levels of physical activity are very plausible.[158] Because of the negative effect of a lack of physical activity, sedentary work can be viewed as an occupational risk factor for CAD.[65] The relative risk of death from CAD is about 2.0 for sedentary compared with active occupations. Unfortunately, the level of physical activity in the population may be on the decline overall because of changes on the job and in transportation.

Uncertainty exists about the level and type of physical activity on the job may be protective.[284] Three specific physical occupational factors have been suggested as possible risk factors.[246] While increasing the level of physical activity is beneficial in preventing CAD, *irregular* heavy physical exertion (such as 6 or more metabolic equivalents) is associated in most studies with substantially increased risk of an acute MI in the first hour after the exertion.[289a] However, while the relative risk is high, the absolute risk is low, and habitual physical activity greatly reduces the risk of heavy physical exertion.

Evidence that lifting may be an occupational risk factor is limited. Associations with lifting may be due to some other confounding factor.[246] However, a significant increase in SMR for MI related to heavy lifting has been found; when combined with hectic work, the risk was even higher. Resistance weight training has been used safely in the rehabilitation of patients with cardiac disease.[19]

Both segmental and whole body exposure to vibration have been postulated to have acute effects on the CV system. Since there are some data supporting this hypothesis, further investigation of this association would be of some interest.[8a,61a]

Chemical Exposures and Cardiovascular Disease

A few occupational exposures, such as carbon monoxide, carbon disulfide (CS_2), methylene chloride, and nitrate esters, have been definitely linked to selected CV conditions. The evidence for these exposures is by far the strongest when the level of occupational exposure is high. For some chemicals (e.g., lead, arsenic, and 2,3,7,8-tetrachlorodibenzo-p-dioxin) evidence is more limited or substantial occupational exposures are less common. Low-level exposures to carbon monoxide, lead, and carbon disulfide are common.

CARBON DISULFIDE

CS_2 was definitively associated with increased risk of CAD in Finnish epidemiologic studies which showed that higher exposures before 1970 were linked to high relative risks for CAD, and that following substantial reduction in exposure the risk declined to less than 1.[192] Overall, the several other epidemiologic cohort mortality studies strengthen the evidence that CS_2 can cause CAD in workers exposed for long time periods and at high levels.[166,251b] The mechanism may be primarily a direct adverse effect on the CV system, since the risk of dying from heart disease has been largely restricted to currently or recently exposed workers in some of the cohort mortality studies. The importance of this hypothesis is that the adverse effect may be reversible to some extent.

There is some debate about the level of exposure associated with increased risk of CAD.[211] The most recent cohort mortality study concluded that exposure to relatively low levels of CS_2 increases the risk of CV mortality.[251a] As with many occupational adverse effects, the precise shape of the dose-response curve between mortality from CAD and exposure to CS_2 remains an important area of research.

CS_2 has been associated with several effects that suggest direct and indirect mechanisms for the increased risk of CAD. Interestingly, in both Belgian and Japanese CS_2 workers, but not Finnish workers, an increased prevalence of microaneurysms of the retinal artery has been reported.[196a,277] The other effects that have been noted are ECG abnormalities, a negative inotropic effect, an increase in LDL-cholesterol, and increased diastolic BP.[57,62,147]

NITRATE ESTERS

Nitrate esters such as nitroglycerin (NTG) and ethylene glycol dinitrate (EGDN) caused angina and more rarely cardiac sudden death in highly exposed workers in the past.[18,105,244a] Following withdrawal from exposure, coronary artery spasm has been postulated as occurring. In the occupational setting, skin exposure to the nitrate esters is the principal route of exposure. In the studies of mortality from CAD in exposed explosives workers, it is not clear whether the effects are solely acute after withdrawal from exposure or also occur during acute overexposure. There are substantial case studies and epidemiologic evidence to confirm this hypothesis of an acute effect of nitrate esters. Only one study found evidence that there may be a chronic effect that persists several years after exposure ceases.[105] This study suggested that CV effects of NTG and EGDN might be more complex than simply the precipitation of coronary spasm after acute withdrawal from exposure. It is possible that the nitrates also lead in some manner to increased diastolic BP, since one study also found, in addition to a chronic increase in CAD mortality, a nonsignificant increase in CVD mortality.[106] Older clinical reports suggested that sudden death rarely occurs in exposed workers without pre-existing CAD. However, Stayner found that workers hired after 1970 who were screened every 6 months for hypertension as well as resting and exercise ECG abnormalities did not have an excess risk of death from NTG exposure.[244a] This absence of an effect could be due to a combination of lower exposures and effective screening to identify more high-risk workers. Prospective studies of currently exposed workers are needed to determine whether there is any remaining excess risk.

CARBON MONOXIDE

Substantial exposure to carbon monoxide (CO) is more common than substantial exposure to either nitrate esters or CS_2. CO exerts its adverse effects via its avid binding to hemoglobin, resulting in decreased delivery of oxygen to the tissues.[58] In addition, CO binds to the cytochrome oxidase system in the mitochondria of cardiac muscle, raising the possibility that CO exposure could directly decrease myocardial contractility. A limited number of occupational exposures to CO can result in carboxyhemoglobin levels greater than 25%. When the carboxyhemoglobin level exceeds 25%, the reduction in tissue oxygen delivery can cause myocardial ischemia or infarction, dysrhythmias, or even sudden death.[58] These high levels of exposure can occur from exposure to combustion sources, such as during fire fighting activities or use of gasoline engines in confined spaces (e.g., gasoline-powered washers for cleaning of flood debris in basements). For example, in one study of structural fire fighting, 10% of the samples exceed 1500 ppm of CO.[112]

The acute cardiac effects of CO even at low levels of exposure are dependent on the ability of the coronary arteries to increase blood flow to the myocardium in response to the hypoxic stress of CO. Workers with significant CAD may be affected at lower levels of exposure. In addition, CO exposure from workplace combustion sources are additive with the CO exposure that smokers receive from their cigarettes. One study showed that smokers in workplaces with low levels of CO exposure (3–12 ppm), far below the OSHA exposure limit (50 ppm or 55 mg/m^3), had carboxyhemoglobin levels of 2.1–7.6%.[285] Levels above 4% carboxyhemoglobin have been associated with reduced time to onset of angina during exercise tests.[132] Higher workplace exposures, for example at the OSHA recommended exposure limit, could raise the carboxyhemoglobin level of the nonsmoker above 4%. Workers with CAD may have an increased number of angina attacks in occupational environments with CO exposure.

Overall, mortality studies of exposed workers provide some evidence that CO exposure may be associated with an increase in mortality from CAD while the exposure continues. Some of these studies are positive and others are negative.[90,141,249a] Some of the positive studies involved workers who are exposed to more than one agent. For example, one found a significant increase in mortality from sudden death presumably due to CAD in furnace workers in ferroalloy plants.[104] The increase was not explained by smoking or alcohol consumption; however, these workers were exposed to manganese, CO, and heat. Interestingly, two studies have found evidence of an increase in hypertension morbidity or mortality; however, in both studies workers did have multiple exposures.[104,141] The latter observation raises the hypothesis that chronic CO exposure could potentiate other CV effects.

One of the few studies with a detailed exposure assessment for CO, no other potential cardiac toxic exposures, and a good internal comparison group is that comparing tunnel workers to toll booth operators.[249a] The tunnel workers had a 35% increased mortality from CAD. The excess declined after 1970 when the CO levels were reduced by improved ventilation (prior to 1970, levels averaged over 50 ppm). The excess mortality was limited to the first few years after employment ceased.

Overall, the epidemiologic studies do suggest that high-level CO exposure may cause at least moderate increases in the risk of CAD. It is not surprising that studies of the adverse effects of CO in physically active occupations with intermittent exposures, such as fire fighting and foundry work, have had mixed results. Acute exposures in fire fighting or to a combustion source in a confined space and that cause carboxyhemoglobin level above 25% may pose a cardiac hazard even for individuals with a normal CV system, while lower levels of exposure may pose a hazard for individuals with significant CAD. These lower exposures in the individual with CAD would be potentially more hazardous if other factors were present that could increase the risk of cardiac ischemia, such as cigarette smoking, high altitude, or substantial physical exercise.

METHYLENE CHLORIDE

Methylene chloride (dichloromethane) is metabolized to CO. Any worker who presents with a clinical picture consistent with CO toxicity and a history of solvent exposure should be evaluated for methylene chloride exposure. Exposures as low as 75 ppm of methylene chloride can produce similar levels of carboxyhemoglobin as exposure to CO at 35 ppm. Methylene chloride has been a common solvent in furniture-stripping solutions.[171] The risk of methylene chloride exposure is related to the duration and intensity of the exposure. Two epidemiologic studies of occupationally exposed chemical workers involved in the production of methylene chloride have not found an association with CAD.[75,198]

LEAD

Occupational exposures to lead are still common in some industries, such as construction and manufacturing of lead batteries. The identification of subtle subclinical effects of lead at low exposure levels has led to reduction in recommended occupational exposure limits from 80 to 40 micrograms/dl.[80a] At these lower levels of exposure it is possible that lead may be contributing to hypertension.[150] This concern was first raised by studies in the general population. One recent review of the animal, epidemiologic occupational, and general population studies concluded that there is a weak positive relationship between both systolic and diastolic BP and lead exposure. A two-fold increase in blood lead concentration was associated with a 1 mm increase in systolic pressure and 0.6 mm increase in diastolic pressure.[244b] The reviewers were not sure that the relationship was causal. They believed that there were several possible plausible mechanisms, including interference of lead with calcium metabolism, a possible direct effect of lead on the vascular smooth muscle, or potentiation of sympathetic stimulation by lead. The most recent cross-sectional studies of workers are also inconsistent. The issue of whether occupational exposures to lead contribute to hypertension is not totally resolved.

SOLVENTS AND DYSRHYTHMIAS

A limited number of chemicals have been associated with atrial and ventricular dysrhythmias by mechanisms unrelated to ischemia; such events may occur even in individuals with anatomically normal coronary vessels.[286] Some organic solvents, particularly fluorocarbons such as chlorofluorocarbon 113, are implicated in the occupational setting.[189] Suspected proarrhythmic agents are bromofluorocarbons, methyl chloroform, methylene chloride, and trichloroethylene.[126] The strongest evidence for this relationship is from case reports following very high, intentional exposures (e.g., glue sniffing).[51] Other evidence comes from clinical studies and experimental animal investigations.[126] The animal studies suggest that a wide range of solvents at very high levels of exposure are cardiac toxins; however, the risk in usual working situations is probably small.[220]

The pathogenesis of solvent-related dysrhythmias likely involves potentiating the effect of endogenously secreted catecholamines to cause arrhythmias. The combined effect of the solvent and catecholamines results in atrial or ventricular arrhythmias.[126] At very high levels of exposure other mechanisms are possible, such as decreased myocardial contractility or hypoxia from respiratory depression.

There are several case reports of sudden death or atrial fibrillation following exposure to chlorofluorocarbon 113 in confined spaces. The most volatile fluorocarbons are the most hazardous. Epidemiologic studies of workers exposed to fluorocarbons in nonconfined spaces and presumably at lower levels of exposures are not consistent.[61] A positive study found an association between history of episodes of palpitation among pathology residents and exposure to fluorocarbons in the preparation of frozen sections from surgical specimens.[244] A negative study involved ambulatory EKG monitoring and exposure measurements to fluorocarbon-113 in sixteen sedentary aerospace workers. The frequency of ventricular and atrial premature beats and other evidence of dysrhythmias on a low exposure day (64 ppm personal time-weighted average [TWA]) were compared to a higher exposure day (442 ppm TWA).[62] There is also an equivocal study among refrigerator repairmen.[61]

In summary, occupational exposures to fluorocarbon-113 at levels below the OSHA standard of 1000 ppm have not been associated with cardiac dysrhythmias.

Several epidemiologic mortality studies of solvent-exposed workers have been conducted, principally in aerospace, rubber, chemical, and dry cleaning industries. Each of these studies has limitations in determining if there is an association between acute solvent exposure and cardiac mortality. Most were designed to concentrate on the relationship between chronic solvent exposure and cancer rather than acute exposure and CVD. The majority of cardiac deaths occurred years after exposure ceased. Most did not have detailed exposure measurements; therefore, the potential for misclassification of exposure is substantial. A review of the epidemiologic literature shows no *consistent* association between solvents, with the exception of CS_2, and elevated risks of mortality from heart disease.[286]

A few studies do indicate one or more positive associations. A case-control study in the rubber industry found no evidence of association between the most solvent exposures and heart disease, but did find limited evidence of an association between ethanol or phenol exposure and mortality from CAD.[287] A recent cross-sectional study reported associations between occupational exposures to benzene or xylene, but not to phenol, and the prevalence of hypertension, atrial, and ventricular ectopic beats.[142] A significant but slight increase in mortality from CAD was reported among aerospace workers exposed to trichloroethylene or toluene.[22] This study had an internal reference group and careful exposure assessment. The 10–20% increases in this study generally were not dose related, and there were overlapping exposures to several solvents. In another study of trichloroethylene there was no evidence of an increased risk from CV mortality in the workers with long duration or higher levels of exposure.[13]

PSYCHOSOCIAL FACTORS: REVIEW OF THE EMPIRICAL DATA AMONG MEN   *by Karen Belkić, MD, PhD, Paul Landsbergis, PhD, Peter Schnall, MD, Dean Baker, MD, Töres Theorell, MD, PhD, Johannes Siegrist, PhD, Richard Peter, PhD, and Robert Karasek, PhD*

In 1958, a case-control study by Russek and Zohman revealed that of 97 male coronary patients under age 40, 91% were judged to have been exposed to "occupational stress and strain," based on a detailed occupational history, compared to 20% of healthy controls.[224] In the same year, Friedman, Rosenman and Carroll published their seminal paper demonstrating a significant relation between serum cholesterol and blood clotting times, and cyclic variation in occupational stress among accountants.[76] Since these early studies there has been a burgeoning body of evidence demonstrating a relationship between psychosocial factors at the workplace and cardiovascular disease (CVD).

Approximately 20 years ago, the **Job Strain Model** was introduced by Karasek.[123] Systematic investigation of psychosocial workplace factors and CVD was dramatically advanced by this model, which can be readily applied in epidemiologic studies. The first hypothesis is that strain occurs when there is excessive psychological workload demands together with low job decision latitude. This combination provokes arousal, as well as distress, activating both the sympathoadrenomedullary and adrenocortical axes, and yielding a highly deleterious combination.[71,74] A third dimension, social isolation, was later added to the Job Strain Model.[114] The second hypothesis is that high demands together with high decision latitude lead to active learning of new behaviors, and possibly improved health through long-term positive changes in coping behaviors. (See Chapter 3 for a detailed discussion of the theoretical construct.)

More recently, the **Effort-Reward Imbalance (ERI) Model** was introduced by Siegrist and colleagues.[233-235] In comparison to the Job Strain Model with its emphasis on moment-to-moment control over the work process (i.e., decision latitude), the ERI Model provides an expanded concept of control, emphasizing macro-level long-term control vis-à-vis rewards such as career opportunities, job security, esteem, and income. The ERI Model assesses the balance between these rewards and effort, positing that work stress results from an imbalance between high effort and low control over long-term rewards. Effort is seen to stem both extrinsically from the demands of the job and intrinsically from the individual's tendency to be overly committed to these work demands. (See Chapter 3 for further discussion.) In addition to research using these two models, several other psychosocial risk factors are being examined for their potential explanatory value with regard to CV outcomes. Threat-avoidant vigilant work, also termed "disaster potential," represents a plausible construct for which there is some empirical data, reviewed herein.

The following review results from *in extenso* English language publications in peer-reviewed journals as these pertain to samples of men, in whom the majority of this research has been conducted. The empirical evidence with regard to workplace psychosocial factors and CVD outcomes among women is described toward the end of this chapter.

The Job Strain Model

ISCHEMIC HEART DISEASE AND OTHER HARD CVD ENDPOINTS

Table 3 presents the data concerning exposure to job strain and/or its major dimensions, in relation to ischemic heart disease or other hard CVD endpoints. A brief description of how the job strain variable was assessed in each study, the variables for which adjustment is made, and significant positive as well as null and negative findings are shown. (For more details concerning methods for evaluating job strain and other psychosocial workplace factors, see Chapter 6.)

There were eight case-control studies of job strain and CVD. Those investigations which obviated self-report bias by imputing job strain exposure on the basis of occupational title revealed major significant findings with regard to aspects of control[6,8,87,265] and/or to exposure to high psychological demands together with low control.[6,8,88] The other five studies, relying on self-report data, also revealed primarily significant positive associations. An exception is the very small study of Emdad, et al., which, unlike the others, restricted itself to a single occupational group (professional drivers) having a limited range of variation on demands and control, and, thus, less statistical power to detect an effect of job strain.[64]

Self-report data of Hallqvist, et al. provided another important facet of causal evidence by showing a dose-response relationship between strength of exposure to job strain and relative risk of myocardial infarction.[87] The significant, positive Synergy Index reveals that exposure to the combination of high demands and low control confers greater risk than the additive effects of the dimensions.

TABLE 3. Studies of Job Strain and Ischemic Heart Disease among Men

			Case Control Studies		
First Author (Year)	Study Participants	Form(s) of Job Strain Variable	Illness Outcome	Significant Positive Associations (Adjusted Confounders)		Null or Sig. Negative Assoc. (Adjusted Confounders)
Alfredsson, et al. (1982 & 1983)	Swedish, < 65 y.o. N = 334 cases, N = 882 population controls	Imputed: Hectic/various aspects of control as quadrant terms	Hospitalized and/or fatal MI	Total study (Age): Monotony Rushed tempo + low influence over work tempo Rushed tempo + not learning new things 40–54 y.o. (Age & immigrant status or education) Hectic work + no influence on pace Hectic work + few possibilities to learn new things	RR 1.32 1.35 1.45 ≈ 1.7 ≈ 2	Rushed tempo = NS Low influence over work tempo = NS Not learning new things = NS Rushed tempo + monotony = NS (Age)
Billing, et al. (1997)	Swedish, < 70 y.o. Cases: N = 531 male, 236 female Population controls: N = 34 male, 15 female	Self-report: PSJSQ Main effects only	Chronic, stable angina pectoris, clinic patients	Skill discretion Control (Age)	p < .001 < .01	ψ demand = NS Decision authority = NS (Age)
Bobák, et al. (1998)	Czech, 25–64 y.o. N = 179 cases N = 784 controls All full-time employed	Self-report: ψ Demands (3 items) Decision-latitude (8 items) Quartile term (21% job strain)	First nonfatal MI	Highest decision latitude quartile (Age, district, education, hypertension, other coronary RF)	RR 0.43	Job strain = NS Highest ψ demands quartile RR = 0.52 (Age, district, education, hypertension, other coronary RF)
Emdad, et al. (1997)	Swedish, < 52 y.o. N = 13 cases N = 12 hypertensive controls, All professional drivers	Self-report: PSJSQ Demand/control Quotient term	Hospitalized IHD			Job strain = NS ψ demand = NS Decision latitude = NS Skill discretion = NS Control = NS (Age)

(Table continued on next page.)

TABLE 3. Studies of Job Strain and Ischemic Heart Disease among Men *(Continued)*

First Author (Year)	Study Participants	Form(s) of Job Strain Variable	Illness Outcome	Significant Positive Associations (Adjusted Confounders) (Quartile) RR / (Optimal) RR	Null or Sig. Negative Assoc. (Adjusted Confounders)
Hallqvist, et al. (1998), Theorell, et al. 1998)	Swedish, 45–64 y.o. N = 1047 cases N = 1450 population controls	Self-report: PSJSQ Quartile term and optimal term (reflects optimum balance between exposure contrast and power) Imputed: PSJEM Decision latitude Quartiles	First hospitalized and/or fatal MI	Self-report: (Quartile) RR / (Optimal) RR Job strain 2.2 → 9.2 Synergy index 4.0 → 7.5 • Manual workers Job strain 10.0 → 46.1 Synergy index 11.1 → 23.9 Decision latitude 2.3 (Hypertension, smoking, BMI) Imputed OR Decision latitude (Age, catchment area) 1.7	Self-report: • Non-manual workers Job strain = NS ψ demands = NS Decision latitude = NS • Manual workers ψ demands = NS (Hypertension, smoking, BMI) Imputed Decision latitude = NS (Age, catchment area, social class, coronary RF)
Hammar, et al. (1994)	Swedish, 30–64 y.o. N = 13,205 cases N = 22,599 population controls	Imputed: Hectic/aspects of Decision-latitude Quadrant term (relaxed quadrant as referent)	First MI	White collar Hectic work and low influence over work hours (Age, county, calendar year) RR 1.4	Blue collar Single factors = NS Hectic work and other factors = NS White collar Single factors = NS (Age, county, calendar year)
Sihm, et al. (1991)	Danish, < 55 y.o. N = 52 cases N = 72 community and hospital controls	Self-report: Workload/elements of control Quadrant term	Survivors of MI	RR Heavy workload + contradictory demands 1.96 Heavy workload + low responsibility 1.78 Low workload + good social interaction 0.58 (Age, SES)	Workload = NS Autonomy = NS Influence = NS Contradictory demands = NS Growth + development = NS (Age, SES)
Theorell, et al. (1987)	Swedish, < 45 y.o. N = 85 cases N = 116 community controls	Self-report: 3 Quotient terms: Demands (2 items) ÷ Influence (3 items) Intellectual discretion or variety (1 item each)	Hospitalized nonfatal MI Coronary artery atheromatosis	p Variety of work tasks 0.01 ψ demands/variety of work tasks 0.01 ψ demands/intellectual discretion 0.04 (Age, education, coronary risk factors)	ψ demands = NS Influence over work = NS Intellectual discretion = NS ψ demands/influence over work = NS (Age, education, coronary risk factors) Degree coronary atheromatosis and quotient terms or main effects = NS

(Table continued on next page.)

TABLE 3. Studies of Job Strain and Ischemic Heart Disease among Men (*Continued*)

Cross Sectional Studies

First Author (Year)	Study Participants	Form(s) of Job Strain Variable	Illness Outcome	Significant Positive Associations (Adjusted Confounders)		Null or Sig. Negative Assoc. (Adjusted Confounders)
Johnson, et al. (1988)	N = 7165, Swedish, 16–65 y.o. population sample	Self-report: ψ Demands (2 items) Control (11 items) Support (5 items) Quadrant term (relaxed quadrant as referent)	Self-reported CVD (N = 409)	Blue collar High ψ demands/low control High ψ demands/low control/ low support White collar High ψ demands/low support (Age, dimensions of isostrain) 3-Factor multiplicative interaction ratio = 1.09	PR 3.55 7.22 1.81	All High ψ demands = NS Control = NS White collar High ψ demands/low control = NS (Age, dimensions of isostrain)
Johnson, et al. (1989)	N = 7219, Swedish, 25–65 y.o. population sample	Self-report: ψ Demands (2 items) Control (11 items) Support (5 items) Compare high to low quintile	Self-reported CVD (N = 407)	All Isostrain Blue collar Isostrain (Age)	PR 1.77 2.04	White collar Isostrain (Age) = NS
Karasek, et al. (1987)	N = 5000, Swedish, mean age 37.1 ± 12.1, white collar, trade-union members	Self-report: Workload (3 items) Decision latitude (4 items) Main effects only	Self-reported heart disease	(Age, marital status) Workload Conflict Clarity Decision/latitude Social support	SOR 1.24 1.18 1.12 0.92 0.90	
Karasek, et al. (1988)	U.S., 18–79 y.o. N = 2409 HES, N = 2424 HANES population sample (87% white)	Imputed: QES Quadrant term (20% job strain)	MI (N = 39 HES) (N = 30 HANES)	Job strain—HES —HANES ψ Demands—HANES Decision latitude—HES —HANES (Age, race, education, SBP, other coronary RF)	SOR 1.5 1.6 2.1 -1.5 -2.0	ψ Demands—HES = NS (Age, race, education, SBP, other coronary RF)

(Table continued on next page.)

TABLE 3. Studies of Job Strain and Ischemic Heart Disease among Men (*Continued*)

First Author (Year)	Study Participants	Form(s) of Job Strain Variable	Illness Outcome	Significant Positive Associations (Adjusted Confounders)	Null or Sig. Negative Assoc. (Adjusted Confounders)
Hlatky, et al. (1995)	N = 1132 males, N = 357 females U.S. patients undergoing coronary angiography (88% white, 60% white collar)	Self-report: JCQ Predefined cutpoints: (23% job strain men, 43% in women) Job strain index = quotient	Degree of coronary atheromatosis		Job strain = Quadrant term = NS Index = NS (*Age, gender, blood pressure, coronary risk factors, history of MI, typical angina*)

Cohort Studies

First Author (Year)	Study Participants	F/u (y)	Form(s) of Job Strain Variable	Illness Outcome	Significant Positive Associations (Adjusted Confounder)		Null or Sig. Negative Assoc. (Adjusted Confounder)
Alfredsson, et al. (1985)	N = 958,096 total*, Swedish, 20–64 y.o., population-based	1	Imputed: Hectic/various aspects of control as quadrant terms	Hospitalized MI (N = 1059)	(*Age*) Punctuality Few possibilities to learn new things Hectic and monotonous work Hectic work and few possibilities to learn new things (*Age + marital status, nationality, income, smoking or heavy lifting at work*)	SMR 121 113 118 ≈ 125	(*Age*) Hectic work = NS Monotonous work = NS

* Total not by gender, gender-stratified analysis done—males in this table

| Bosma, et al. (1997 & 1998) | N = 6896, U.K., 35–55 y.o. civil servants | 5.3 | Self-report: ψ Demands (4 items) Control (15 items) Median cutpoint quadrant Term and interaction term Observer: 4 items | Self-report Angina, CHD event, Dx. IHD | (*Age & f/u time*) Low control (SR) & angina pectoris Low control (SR) & diagnosed IHD Low control (SR) & any CHD event Low control (O) & any CHD event Job strain (SR) & any CHD event | OR 1.54 1.6 1.55 1.43 1.45 | Job strain (SR) & angina pectoris = NS Job strain (SR) & diagnosed IHD = NS Job strain (O) & all outcomes = NS (*Age & f/u time*) |
| Johnson, et al. (1989) | N = 7219, Swedish, 25–65 y.o. population-based | 9 | Self-report: ψ Demands (2 items) Control (11 items) Support (5 items) Compare high to low quintile | CVD mortality (N = 193) | (*Age*) Isostrain: Total group Blue collar | RR 1.92 2.58 | Isostrain: White collar = NS (*Age*) |

(Table continued on next page.)

TABLE 3. Studies of Job Strain and Ischemic Heart Disease among Men (*Continued*)

First Author (Year)	Study Participants	Flu (y)	Form(s) of Job Strain Variable	Illness Outcome	Significant Positive Associations (Adjusted Confounders)		Null or Sign. Negative Assoc. (Adjusted confounders)
Johnson, et al. (1996)	N = 12,517, Swedish 25–74 y.o. population-based (nested case-control N = 2422 controls)	14	Imputed: ψ Demands (2 items) Control (12 items) Support (4 items) Interaction terms	CVD mortality (N = 521)	Low control Low control/low support (*Age, class, nationality, physical job demands, education, exercise, smoking, last year employed*)	RR 1.83 2.62	ψ demands = NS Job strain = NS (*Same adjustment as for positive findings*)
Karasek, et al. (1981)	N = 1461, Swedish, 15–61 y.o., population-based (Nested* case-control: N = 66 controls)	9	Self-report: ψ demands (2 items) Intellectual Discretion (2 items) Personal Schedule Freedom (3 items)	CVD & cerebro-vascular mortality (N = 22)	High ψ demands High ψ demands & low personal freedom schedule (*Age, education, smoking, CHD sx at baseline*)	OR 4.0 4.0	Low intellectual discretion = NS Low personal freedom schedule = NS (*Same adjustment as for positive findings*)
		6		Self-report CHD	High ψ demands Low Intellectual Discretion (*Age, education, smoking, overweight*)	SOR 1.29 1.44	Personal Schedule Freedom = NS (*same adjustment as for positive findings*)
Theorell, et al. (1991a)	N = 79, Swedish, <45 y.o. employed, first MI survivors	5	Self-report: 3 Quotient terms: Demands (2 items) + Influence (3 items), Intellectual discretion or variety (1 item each)	Mortality from repeat MI (N = 13)	Demands + variety (univariate) Demands + intellectual discretion (*Biomedical risk factors*)	P 0.03 0.02	Demands = NS Single aspects of decision latitude = NS
Alterman, et al. (1994)	N = 1683 U.S., 38–56 y.o. Chicago Western Electric healthy employees of European ancestry (74% blue collar)	25	Imputed: QES Tertile term (7% job strain))	CHD mortality	High decision latitude (*Age, SBP, cholesterol, smoking, alcohol, family history CVD*)	RR 0.76	Job strain (*Age*) = NS ψ Demands (*Age*) = NS Decision latitude (*Education + age, SBP, cholesterol, smoking, alcohol, family history CVD*) = NS

(Table continued on next page.)

TABLE 3. Studies of Job Strain and Ischemic Heart Disease among Men (*Continued*)

First Author (Year)	Study Participants	F/u (y)	Form(s) of Job Strain Variable	Illness Outcome	Significant Positive Associations (Adjusted Confounders)	Null or Sig. Negative Assoc. (Adjusted Confounders)
Hlatky, et al. (1995)	N = 1132 men, N =357 women U.S. patients undergoing coronary angiography (88% white, 60% white collar)	4	Self-report: JCQ (Cutpoints: ψ demands > 32, decision latitude < 28) Men: 23% job strain Women: 43% job strain Job strain index = quotient term	Incident nonfatal MI (N = 70) Cardiac deaths (N = 42)		In patients with significant CAD: Job strain index & quadrant term = NS for cardiac death & cardiac events ("*Established prognostic factors*" *including ejection fraction, CAD extent, myocardial ischemia*) In patients without significant CAD: Job strain index & quadrant term = NS for cardiac events (N = 6 total) (*Age, gender, ejection fraction, insignificant CAD*)
Reed, et al. (1989)	N = 4737, U.S. Hawaiians of Japanese descent, 45–65 y.o. population-based	18	Imputed: QES Quartile Term Multiplicative Score Vector Score	Incident definite CHD (N = 359)		All calculated forms of Job Strain = NS ψ Demands = NS Decision latitude = NS In acculturated group: Low job strain (vector score) p < 0.05 (*Age, blood pressure & other coronary risk factors*)
Steenland, et al. (1997)	N = 3575, U.S. 25–74 y.o., population-based 58% blue collar	12–16	Imputed: QES Quartile term (17% job strain)	Incident heart disease (N = 519)	Job control (highest compared to lowest quartile) (*Age, education, blood pressure, other coronary risk factors*)	OR 0.71 Stratified analysis blue and white collar: Job strain, ψ Demands, Low control = NS High control & high demand OR = 0.69 for blue collar (*As for positive findings*)

Notes: Significant positive associations require a lower limit of the 95% confidence intervals > 1.0 and/or p < 0.05. The N for women is indicated only if the analysis was *not* gender stratified.
ψ = psychological, Dx = diagnosed, HES = Health Examination Survey, HANES = Health and Nutrition Examination Survey, IHD = ischemic heart disease, JCQ = job content questionnaire, NS = nonsignificant, OR = odds ratio, PSJSQ = psychological job strain questionnaire (Swedish), PSJEM = Psychosocial Job Exposure Matrix, QES = quality of employment surveys, RF = risk factors, RH = relative hazard, RR = relative risk, SES = socioeconomic status, SMR = standard mortality ratio, SR = self-reported.
* The study by Karasek, et al. (1981) analyzes incident cases of CVD death compared to matched controls selected from the cohort. As per Hulley, et al.,[109] we term this a "nested case control study" and include it within the cohort studies.

Of the five cross-sectional investigations of job strain and CVD, four relied upon self-report of exposure to the job strain dimensions and of the disease outcome. Johnson and Hall found that the interaction among demand, control, and support was more than multiplicative (by 9%), with a three-factor multiplicative interaction ratio = 1.09.[114] Karasek, et al. used the imputational method to assess exposure to job strain, together with objective verification of the presence of myocardial infarction (MI).[124] Thus, this population-based, cross-sectional data can be considered free of self-report bias of any kind and reveals a significant positive association between exposure to job strain, as well as each of its main dimensions, and MI.

Among the ten cohort studies of job strain and CVD, six report significant positive results with regard to exposure to various types of low control,[7,9,29,30,116,247] and four show significant associations with exposure to some form of high psychological demands coupled with low control.[7,29,30,119,259a] Significant positive results were seen for exposure to high psychological demands alone[119] and for isostrain (high psychological demands, low control and low social support at work).[115]

Four cohort studies had predominantly null results.[9,103,218,247] Three of these had followup periods of 12–25 years without assessment of employment status subsequent to intake, such that the participants were likely to have been temporally far removed from these job exposures.[9,218,247] In two of these the mean age at CHD occurrence is high, and with advancing age the impact of CVD risk factors declines.[9,218] The three also used the imputation method for determining exposure to job strain (see Chapter 6). While providing a convenient means of converting coded occupational titles into exposure data and obviating self-report bias, the imputation method provides no assessment of within-occupation variability and, due to nondifferential misclassification, underestimates actual associations between job characteristics and health outcomes.[143] Thus, while significant positive associations found using the imputational method provide powerful evidence for the model, negative or nonconfirmatory studies may be due, at least in part, to loss of statistical power.[226] This is particularly problematic with respect to psychological demands, which show the largest amount of variance within rather than between occupations, and this variance is therefore not reflected in the averaged values.[261]

Particular attention in the clinical cardiologic arena has been paid to the study of Hlatky and colleagues in which exposure to job strain was reported not to be significantly associated cross-sectionally with degree of angiographically-assessed coronary atherosclerosis, nor prospectively with cardiac events.[103] In immediate response to the publication of these results, the American Heart Association issued the following statement: "Although psychological stress in the workplace is widely believed to increase the risk of coronary heart disease, scientific evidence supporting this belief 'is relatively sparse' according to scientists publishing a new study. Their research suggests that job strain is not an important coronary risk factor."[10] We believe that this conclusion is incorrect. This study does not appear to have been designed initially to test the job strain hypothesis. The original purpose of this research seems to have been to examine employment patterns among patients with coronary artery disease.[168] The sampling technique used (evaluation of all patients with chest pain undergoing coronary angiography) may have been suitable to that purpose. However, it is not appropriate for research intended to explore the role of psychosocial stress factors in CVD.

A close examination of the study reveals a number of major, interconnected flaws which inextricably undermine its internal validity. By choosing consecutive stable patients with chest pain, who were undergoing coronary angiography at a university hospital, as the study sample, with the cross-sectional endpoint being degree of coronary atherosclerosis, the chances are high that the etiologic relationship between exposure and outcome is severely distorted.[109,215] This overreporting of chest pain would lead a large number of patients without coronary artery disease (CAD), but *with* self-reported job strain, to present to the medical system, and insofar as a substantial number of these persons were sent to angiography, this would lead to a lowered odds ratio for CAD related to job strain. This form of **selection bias** is an example of *differential* misclassification, which tends to bias the results negatively. Existing effects between job strain and CAD are less likely to be detected because the frequency of reported chest pain is higher, by at least an order of magnitude,[219] in the study patients than in the population of a similar age.

Patients with chest pain and normal coronary arteries have been recognized as a group with a high prevalence of occupational and behavioral difficulties.[42,154,195,200,206,208] Major problems with confounding also exist in the Hlatky, et al. study. The patients with normal coronary arteries or insignificant CAD more often had white-collar jobs than did the patients with significant CAD ($p = 0.0001$), and yet no adjustment for socioeconomic status was made. Lack of gender stratification further obfuscates etiologic relations. By self-report data, 43% of the women fell into the job strain category compared to 23% of the men. Women comprised 48% of patients with normal coronary arteries versus 14% of those with significant CAD. No mention was made of Syndrome X, characterized by enhanced ventricular pain sensitivity,[199] and whose prevalence among women is high.[282] There is also evidence that the CAD patients reporting low decision-latitude and/or job strain had disproportionately stopped working at 1 year followup[168]; this further attenuates any association between point exposure to job strain at entry into the study and subsequent cardiac events.

One cohort study examined the important issue of cumulative exposure to psychological demands, control, and social support.[116] These authors emphasize that the etiological fraction for CV disease mortality attributable to long-term exposure to low work control is substantially larger (35%) than previously estimated for job strain assessed at a single point in time (7–16%). By assessing cumulative exposure it becomes apparent that the magnitude of the CV effects due to unhealthy work conditions has been heretofore largely *underestimated.*

These studies, taken together, predominantly demonstrate a significant, positive relation between exposure to low control and/or job strain and subsequent CVD. The evidence, while limited, suggests the existence of a dose-response relationship (both in terms of intensity of point exposure[87] and temporal duration[116]) between exposure to job strain or low control and CVD outcomes. The cohort studies provide another important piece of confirmatory evidence of causality, based upon their demonstration that the temporal nature of the association is in the expected direction.

BLOOD PRESSURE

Ambulatory Blood Pressure Studies. As elaborated in Chapter 5, there are numerous potential mediating mechanisms by which psychosocial workplace factors can increase the risk of developing ischemic heart disease. Elevation in arterial blood pressure (BP) and hypertension represent one of the most well-recognized and important risk factors, with ambulatory, as opposed to casual, clinic BPs being of greatest prognostic importance, particularly when recorded during work.

Table 4 summarizes the data relating job strain and/or its major dimensions to ambulatory BP. Of the 11 cross-sectional ambulatory BP studies, five reveal a significant positive effect of exposure to job strain upon ambulatory systolic blood pressure (SBP) recorded during work.[41,159,227,228a,276] In the four of these five studies in

TABLE 4.   Studies of Job Strain and Ambulatory Blood Pressure among Men

Cross-Sectional Studies

First Author (Year)	Study Participants	Form(s) of Job Strain Variable	Significant Positive Effects: SBP (Adjusted Confounders)	Significant Positive Effects: DBP (Adjusted Confounders)	Null or Sig. Negative Assoc. (Adjusted Confounders)
Blumenthal, et al. (1995)	N = 61, U.S., 29–59 y.o. mild, unmedicated hypertensives	Self report: JCQ Quadrant term (24% job strain) (% men not specified)			− 4 SBP (significance unspecified) DBP = NS *(Age, education, income, job status)*
Cesana, et al. (1996)	N = 527, No. Italian, 25–64 y.o. population sample	Self-report: JCQ Quadrant and tertile terms	Quadrant Tertile Normotensives: Work + 3.4 → + 4.2 24 h + 2.8 → + 4 *(Age, education, overwt index, PA)*		Borderline hypertensives Quadrant term work and 24 h: SBP and DBP = NS Tertile term: SBP work: −4.6, 24h: −3 DBP work: −1.7, 24h: −1 Normotensives Quadrant and tertile term: Work & 24 h DBP = NS *(As SBP)*
Härenstam, et al. (1988)	N = 66, Swedish, (age unspecified), prison staff	Self-report: Job demands (14 items) Decision-latitude (2 items) Skill discretion (6 items) Main effects only	Skill discretion predicts Work SBP p < 0.01 Leisure SBP p < 0.001 *(Age, status, nightwork, ETOH, BMI)*		
Knox, et al. (1985), Theorell, et al. (1985)	N = 71, Swedish, 26–32 y.o. from military recruit lists	Imputation: Hectic (1 item) Control over work pace (1 item) Quadrant term (28% job strain)			SBP: Work and home = NS DBP: Work and home = NS
Light, et al. (1992)	N = 65, U.S., 18–47 y.o. 58% white, 42% black 71% white collar	Self-report: JCQ Quadrant term (23% job strain-men)	Job strain: Work + 6.0 *(Age, BMI, status, PA, posture, race)*	Job strain: Work + 4.0 *(As SBP)*	ψ demand, decision latitude, skill discretion work SBP + DBP = NS *(As SBP)*

(Table continued on next page.)

TABLE 4. Studies of Job Strain and Ambulatory Blood Pressure among Men (*Continued*)

First Author (Year)	Study Participants	Form(s) of Job Strain Variable	Significant Positive Effects: SBP (Adjusted Confounders)	Significant Positive Effects: DBP (Adjusted Confounders)	Null or Sig. Negative Assoc. (Adjusted Confounders)
Schnall, et al. (1992), Landsbergis, et al. (1994)	N = 262, U.S., 30–60 y.o. from 8 worksites, 84% white	Self-report: JCQ, Quadrant term (21% job strain) and 9th cell term	Job strain Quadrant 9th cell Work +6.7 → +11.5 Home +6.5 → +8.6 Sleep +6.2 (no data) ψ demands Work (p = 0.015) (Age, race, education, BMI, smoking, PA, urine Na+, TAB, worksite, ETOH)	Job strain Quadrant 9th cell Work +2.7 → +4.1 (As SBP)	Job strain: DBP home & sleep = NS ψ demands = NS (except work SBP) Decision latitude = NS (As SBP)
Schnall, et al. (1998)	N = 195, U.S., 33–63 y.o. from 8 worksites, 84% white	Self-report: JCQ, Quadrant term (16% job strain)	Job strain Work +6.4 Home +6.9 Sleep +5.0 (Age, race, BMI, smoking, ETOH)	Job strain Work +5.0 Home +4.9 (As SBP)	Job strain sleep DBP = NS (As SBP)
Steptoe, et al. (1995)	N = 49, U.K., 20–29 y.o. firefighters	Self-report: ψ demands (3 items), Control (3 items), Skill utilization (4 items) (51% job strain)	Job strain & systolic reactor: Afternoon work +12.4 (Groups with and without job strain, high-low reactivity did not differ significantly in age, BMI, ETOH, smoking, baseline BP, inter alia)		Job strain: Work SBP & DBP = NS (Age, BMI)
Steptoe, et al. (1999)	N = 60 men, N = 102 women* UK, mean age = 39 teachers	Self-report: 10 items/quotient term with cutpoints (49% job strain total) (% in men unspecified)	Low job strain: Evening work +3.1 (Age, BMI, baseline SBP)	Low job strain: Evening work +2.1 (Age, BMI)	Job strain: Work SBP & DBP = NS Evening SBP & DBP = NS (Age, BMI)
Theorell, et al. (1991b)	N = 161, Swedish, 35–55 y.o. borderline HTN (DBP = 85–94) employed	Imputed: ψ demands (2 items), Control (12 items), Quotient term with 3 levels: high, medium, low		Low physical demand: Job strain Medium High Work +7.4 → +11.9 Leisure +5.9 → +9.9 Sleep +7.4 → +10.2	High physical demand: DBP work, leisure & sleep = NS High & low physical demand SBP work, leisure & sleep = NS

* Results not gender-stratified

(*Table continued on next page.*)

TABLE 4. Studies of Job Strain and Ambulatory Blood Pressure among Men (*Continued*)

First Author (Year)	Study Participants	F/u (y)	Form(s) of Job Strain Variable	Significant Positive Effects: SBP (Adjusted Confounders)	Significant Positive Effects: DBP (Adjusted Confounders)	Null or Sig. Negative Assoc. (Adjusted Confounders)
van Egeren, et al. (1992)	N = 17, U.S., 21–52 y.o. university employees, sedentary work, (88% white)		Self report: JCQ Cutpts of Schnall, 1990 (24% job strain-men N = 4)	Job strain Work +9 Home +5 (Age, baseline BP, BMI, TAB, caffeine)	Job strain Work +4 (As SBP)	Home DBP, sleep SBP & DBP = NS (As SBP)

Cohort Ambulatory BP Studies

First Author (Year)	Study Participants	F/u (y)	Form(s) of Job Strain Variable	Significant Positive Effects: SBP (Adjusted Confounders)	Significant Positive Effects: DBP (Adjusted Confounders)	Null or Sig. Negative Assoc. (Adjusted Confounders)
Schnall, et al. (1998)	N = 195, U.S., 30–60 y.o. from 8 worksites, 84% white	3	Self report: JCQ Quadrant term (21% job strain)	Job strain at T1 & T2 vs. at neither Work +11.1 Home +11.1 Sleep +10.8 Job strain at T1, not at T2 Work −5.3 Home −4.7 (Age, BMI, race, smoking, ETOH)	Job strain at T1 & T2 vs. at neither Work +9.1 Home +7.3 Job strain at T1, not at T2 Work −3.2 Home −3.3 (As SBP)	Job strain at T1 & Tw vs. at neither DBP sleep = NS Job strain at T1, not at T2 SBP & DBP sleep = NS (As SBP)
Theorell, et al. (1988)	N = 40, Swedish, 26–60 y.o., 6 different occupations	1	Self report: PSJSQ Quotient term—4 levels	Highest repeated job strain Work +4		Highest repeated job strain: Work DBP = NS Leisure SBP & DBP = NS

Case-Control Ambulatory BP Study

First Author (Year)	Study Participants		Form(s) of Job Strain Variable	Significant Positive Effects (Adjusted Confounders)		Null or Sig. Negative Assoc. (Adjusted Confounders)
Schnall, et al. (1990)	N = 215, U.S., 30–60 y.o. from 8 worksites, 84% white		Self report: JCQ Quadrant term (21% job strain)	Job strain OR Case defined at work ambulatory BP > 85 — 3.1 Case defined at work ambulatory BP > 90 — 3.6 Case defined at work ambulatory BP > 95 — 24.4 (Age, BMI, type A behavior, 24 h urine Na$^+$ excretion, physical activity on the job, education, smoking, ETOH, work site)		

BMI = body mass index, ETOH = alcohol, JCQ = job content questionnaire, NS = nonsignificant, OR = odds ratio, PA = physical activity, PSJSQ = psychosocial job strain questionnaire (Swedish), TAB = Type A behavior.

which recordings were continued outside work, ambulatory SBP was found to be significantly elevated during leisure, nonwork time among those exposed to job strain. One additional study, in which only main effects were assessed, shows that low skill discretion is a significant, independent predictor of ambulatory SBP during work, as well as during leisure time.[91] High psychological demands also were found to be associated with a significant elevation in ambulatory SBP during work.[228a] Ambulatory diastolic blood pressure (DBP) was significantly higher during work among those exposed to job strain, with a "carry-over effect" to leisure time in two studies.[159,227,228a,259,276]

Significant dose-response relationships were reported in three studies: when job strain was defined at a more extreme level (e.g., the top tertile of demands or the bottom tertile of latitude, or their combination—the 9th cell term; see Chapter 6), the blood pressure effect also was greater. Thus, analyzing the Schnall, et al. 1992 study and the Landsbergis, et al. study together, when job strain was defined by the usual quadrant term work ambulatory SBP showed a +6.7 mmHg effect, but when the 9th cell was used the effect rose to +11.5.[152,228a] In the study of borderline hypertensives by Theorell and colleagues, exposure to "medium" levels of job strain (and low levels of physical demand) was associated with a +7.4 mmHg effect on ambulatory DBP during work, compared to +11.9 among those exposed to "high" job strain.[259] Self-report bias was obviated in this study by use of the imputation method.

In contrast, both Blumenthal, et al. and Cesana, et al. obtained null or negative results when job strain was assessed by self-report among borderline, unmedicated hypertensives.[23,41] The latter group of authors have suggested that this may reflect a denial phenomenon. This formulation is concordant with Theorell's observations that an underreporting of a stressor may be associated with overreaction physiologically, among those with a positive family history of hypertension.[257]

In the Knox, et al. study and the Theorell, et al. 1985 study, use of the imputation method based upon single items to define the major job strain dimensions may have contributed to nondifferential misclassification.[133,262] Two single-occupation studies by Steptoe and colleagues also reveal a number of null cross-sectional ambulatory BP findings. In a group of firefighters, 51% were deemed to have been exposed to job strain, based upon a small number of items for each dimension.[249] Using similar methodology, 49% of teachers (not gender stratified) were said to have been exposed to job strain.[248] Nondifferential misclassification due to limited range of variation of actual job characteristics may explain these results. Nevertheless, when job strain exposure status was combined with systolic reactivity, a significant positive effect upon afternoon work SBP was found (+12.4) among the firefighters. Among the teachers, the difference in BP between evening and day work was significantly less among those with high (−0.64/−2.45) versus low (−3.72/−4.5) job strain (not gender stratified).

The case-control study of Schnall, et al. reveals a significant positive relation between exposure to job strain and hypertensive status, as defined by work ambulatory BP.[228] Furthermore, as the definition of hypertension was made progressively more rigorous (work ambulatory BP > 85, 90, and 95 mmHg), the odds ratio for exposure to quartile-term job strain increased correspondingly (3.1, 3.6, and 24.4, respectively).

Both cohort ambulatory BP studies report significant positive findings. In the Schnall, et al. 1998 study, exposure to job strain at baseline and 3 years later showed a +11.1 mmHg effect on workplace and home ambulatory SBP compared to those unexposed at both times.[227] The DBP effect also was marked. Furthermore, those men who reported being exposed to job strain at baseline but not 3 years later showed a significant drop in work and home ambulatory BP at 3-year followup, after controlling for major confounders.

Casual Blood Pressure Studies. Studies of job strain in relation to casual BP (usually measured in the clinic or other unspecific setting outside the workplace) are generally less consistent than those using ambulatory recordings at the workplace. Significant positive effects of exposure to job strain among men were found with respect to casual SBP in the cross-sectional studies of Cesana, et al., among normotensives but not borderline hypertensives, and of Melamed, et al., in which exposure to hectic, short-cycle, repetitive work was compared to jobs with substantial variety or longer cycle.[41,173] Kawakami and colleagues reported a significantly elevated SBP and DBP among day workers exposed to job strain, but not among those working rotating shifts.[130] In only one of the five large databases assessed by Pieper, et al. was exposure to job strain using the imputation method significantly associated with casual SBP and DBP.[209] However, a summary estimate of all five working population samples revealed a significant relation between a low decision-latitude and SBP. In a similar vein, Curtis, et al. found a significant inverse relation between hypertensive status based on casual BP readings and self-reported decision latitude at work.[52]

In contrast, in other studies neither exposure to job strain nor its major dimensions (when analyzed) were associated with hypertensive status or BP levels, based on casual BP readings.[4,9,40,64,110,252] (In the Carrère, et al. study, BP was measured immediately pre- and post-work.) In the investigations of Greenlund, et al. and Netterstrøm, et al., nonsignificant relations (gender-adjusted but not stratified) between job strain or its major dimensions and casual BP measures were found, with a few unexpected inverse relations in the latter study.[82,186] A cohort study by Chapman, et al. revealed that exposure to deadlines at work was associated with a significant increase in SBP, while other single or interaction terms reflecting job strain and/or its major dimensions showed no significant relations to SBP nor DBP among men.[43]

The papers of Albright, et al., Carrère, et al., and Emdad, et al. are on single occupations, and therefore are of limited range of variance.[4,40,64] The major issue, however, for most of these studies, is that casual BPs are highly variable and, in the clinic setting, may be influenced by psychosocial factors related to the clinic visit itself, the so-called "white coat effect."[207] Worksite point measurements of BP appear to be more reliable than casual clinic BP (see Chapter 7). Schnall and colleagues found that workers exposed to job strain showed an increased likelihood of having hypertension, classified on the basis of worksite point measurements of BP.[228] Furthermore, as the definition of hypertension was made more stringent, the odds ratio increased, providing additional evidence of the reliability of workplace point estimates, as well as the criterion validity of the relation between job strain and BP elevation.

Thus, with respect to casual BP, we find limited evidence that job strain or its dimension(s) has a major impact. This is in contradistinction to studies that measure ambulatory BP and examine averaged BPs during work, as well as other periods, as the outcome. These studies show strong, consistent effects of job strain or its major dimension(s) on BP. Furthermore, there is some evidence, albeit not totally consistent, of a dose-response relationship with respect to ambulatory BP and exposure to increasingly severe job strain. In addition, there is cohort data demonstrating not only the expected temporal relationship between exposure and outcome,[227] but also the effect of cumulative exposure. Finally, the data, albeit observational rather than a controlled intervention, indicate that "*a change in exposure* is associated with a *change in morbidity*."[227] Hernberg has categorized the latter as "the most conclusive evidence of causality."[100]

OTHER CARDIAC RISK FACTORS

Some studies indicate that exposure to job strain and/or its major dimensions is associated with other standard cardiac risk factors among men. There are theoretical background discussions on how work organizations can influence health-related behaviors that impact upon the CV system.[113,151]

With regard to **cigarette smoking**, it has been proposed that workplace stressors have less impact on smoking prevalence than on smoking intensity, since people often begin smoking before entering the labor market.[283] Accordingly, the focus here is on results concerning smoking intensity among current smokers. Green and Johnson found, after controlling for sociodemographic factors, that male chemical plant employees in higher-strain work smoked significantly more cigarettes, and more of them had increased the number of cigarettes smoked, compared to those with lower-strain jobs.[81] Hellerstedt and Jeffery also reported a significantly greater number of cigarettes smoked per day among men in high-strain jobs compared to passive jobs, after sociodemographic adjustment.[98] Kawakami, et al. found that high-strain jobs *and* passive jobs with low social support were associated with increased smoking intensity.[130] Other studies also reveal a significant positive association between job strain and/or its major dimensions and smoking intensity among men.[176,209]

However, in a study of young adults, after adjusting for age, education, and type A behavior, Greenlund and colleagues found no significant relation between self-reported job demands, decision latitude, job strain, and smoking intensity.[82] Among male professional drivers, no significant relation was found between self-reported job strain, psychological demands, decision latitude, and smoking intensity.[63] Two imputational studies, in which sociodemographic adjustment was not made, also reveal no association between exposure to job strain and/or its major dimensions, and how much workers smoke.[9,218] In the one prospective study in which changes in smoking prevalence were examined, men whose job decision latitude increased over 3 years had a substantial reduction in cigarette smoking. The greatest increase in decision latitude was found among those 13 men who quit smoking.[151]

Sedentary behavior during nonwork time was found to be significantly associated with less social interaction at work, as well as with fewer opportunities to learn new things on the job (an integral part of the decision-latitude), in a population-based sample of Swedish men, after adjusting for age and education.[113] Similarly, another study found a significant inverse relation between low decision-latitude and number of exercise sessions per week, after sociodemographic adjustment.[98] However, no significant association was found between sedentary leisure time and job strain or its major dimensions in the study of Landsbergis, et al.[151]

Obesity, as assessed by detailed anthropometric measurements, has been found among Hispanic men in the U.S. (HHANES study) to be significantly associated with exposure to job strain, decision authority, and psychological demands (imputation method), after adjusting for age, education, and smoking status.[78] Netterstrøm and colleagues reported that both self-reported and imputed exposure to job strain were associated with a significantly elevated body mass index (BMI) in a sample of men and women; these results were adjusted for, but not stratified by, gender.[186] In contrast, a number of other studies relying upon BMI show no relation between job strain or its major dimensions and BMI among men.[98,110,151,218] In a study of male professional drivers, an inverse relation was found between self-reported job strain and self-reported BMI.[63] This finding was attributed to denial, which has been shown to deleteriously impact upon cardiac risk among professional drivers.[187,292]

Hellerstedt and Jeffery found a significant relation between **high-fat diet** and exposure to high psychological demands, as well as job strain.[98]

Psychosocial stressors may promote atherogenic processes (see Chapter 5). Here, we briefly summarize the epidemiologic data concerning these metabolic parameters and job strain and/or its major dimensions. Ishizaki, et al. found that low psychological demands significantly predicted tissue plasminogen activator levels, independently of traditional cardiac risk factors.[110] Elevated fibrinogen was reported by Brunner and colleagues in the Whitehall II study to be associated with low workplace control, as assessed both by self-report and external observer.[36] In the former case, this effect remained after adjustment for socioeconomic status. However, Ishizaki, et al. found neither job strain nor its major dimensions significantly associated with plasma fibrinogen levels. Moller and Kristensen also failed to find that job strain was a significant, independent predictor of plasma fibrinogen levels, using a multivariate model that included social class.[178]

Of the studies that have examined the relations between serum cholesterol and/or its constituent fractions, and job strain or its major dimensions, no significant results among men have been reported.[9,67,82,110,130,173,180,186,218] Netterstrøm, et al. reported that HbA1C was significantly associated with imputed exposure to job strain in a sample of men and women; these results were adjusted for, but not stratified by, gender.[186] Other studies assessing glucose intolerance showed no significant relation to job strain or its major dimensions among men.[67,82,110,173]

Thus, there is preliminary evidence that job strain or its major dimension(s) may impact on cardiac risk factors besides BP. Some noteworthy results are seen regarding smoking intensity. There are some suggestive data regarding links to the coagulation mechanisms and other metabolic indices contributing to the atherogenic process; however, there are also substantial null findings. Much additional research is needed before definitive conclusions can be reached in this area.

The Effort-Reward Model

ISCHEMIC HEART DISEASE AND OTHER HARD CVD ENDPOINTS

Measures of effort-reward imbalance (ERI) at work have been found to predict new manifestations of coronary heart disease in Germany, Finland, and England (Table 5). In a prospective study of 416 German factory workers aged 25–55, a number of measures of high effort and low reward independently and strongly predicted CHD incidence over 6.5 years after adjusting for other behavioral and somatic risk factors.[239] These measures included status inconsistency (OR 4.4), job insecurity (OR 3.4), work pressure (OR 3.5), and overcommitment (OR 4.5). A combined "low reward/high effort" variable was also a significant predictor (OR 3.4) in a separate analysis. If advanced, subclinical CHD (OR 6.2) or stroke (OR 8.2) is added to the case definition, the association with ERI becomes even more substantial.[233]

Among men in the British Whitehall study, exposure to a combination of high effort and low reward more than doubled the risk of newly reported CHD over 5.3 years.[30] Finally, in a prospective study of Finnish men, those facing high work demands, low work resources, and low income had a more than doubled risk of myocardial infarction or dying from heart disease after 8.1 years, compared to men with low demands,

TABLE 5. Studies of the Effort-Reward Imbalance Model and Cardiovascular Outcomes for Men

Cohort Studies

First Author (Year)	Study Participants	Form(s) of Exposure Variable	F/u (y)	Illness Outcome	Significant Positive Associations (Adjusted Confounders)		Null or Sig. Negative Assoc. (Adjusted Confounders)
Siegrist, et al. (1990)	416 male German blue-collar workers from 3 factories	Low security, career opportunities: job insecurity or status inconsistency. High effort: work pressure or overcommitment	6.5	Acute MI or SCD (n = 263 in analysis)	Status inconsistency Overcommitment Low security, career opportunities *or* high effort Low security, career opportunities *and* high effort (Age, BMI, SBP, lipids)	OR 4.4 4.5 4.5 30.6	Job instability, piecework, shiftwork, noise, increase in workload = NS; low promotion prospects Not significant controlling for other measures of low security, career opportunities and high effort Job insecurity Work pressure
Siegrist & Peter (1994); Siegrist (1996)				Acute MI, SCD, or advanced (subclinical) CAD (n = 329 in analysis)	Work pressure Low security, career opportunities, *or* high effort Low security, career opportunities, *and* high effort	2.5 2.4 6.2	Overcommitment
Siegrist, et al (1992); Siegrist (1996)				Acute MI, SCD, or stroke	Overcommitment Status inconsistency Low security, career opportunities, *and* high effort (Age, BMI, BP, lipids, smoking, exercise)	3.6 2.9 8.2	
Lynch (1997a)	N = 940, Eastern Finnish men, 42–60 y.o., population-based	• Stress from work demands scale (11 items split at high 20%) • Economic rewards scale (income, split at low 20%)	4.2	Progression of carotid atherosclerosis (plaque height, max. & mean IMT)	High demands, low income For change in max. IMT For change in plaque height (Age, baseline IMT) For change in plaque height (Age, HDL, LDL, triglycerides, smoking, alcohol, BMI, SBP, treated hypertension or hyperlipidemia)	p 0.03 0.008 0.04	Groups with other combinations of demands and income = NS (Age, baseline IMT)

(Table continued on next page.)

TABLE 5. Studies of the Effort-Reward Imbalance Model and Cardiovascular Outcomes for Men *(Continued)*

First Author (Year)	Study Participants	Form(s) of Exposure Variable	F/u (y)	Illness Outcome	Significant Positive Associations (Adjusted Confounders)	Null or Sig. Negative Assoc. (Adjusted Confounders)
Lynch, et al. (1997b)	N = 2297, Eastern Finnish men, 42–60 y.o., population-based	• Stress from work demands scale (11 items) • Resources scale (5 items) (skill discretion/emotional rewards of work; interesting, enjoyable, meaningful work) • Economic rewards scale (income, split at low 40%) Referent = low, high, high	8.1	Acute MI CVD mortality	High demands, low resources, low rewards — RH 2.3 *(Age, alcohol, smoking, physical activity)*; 2.2 *(Age, depression, marital status, hopelessness)*; 1.9 *(Age, fibrinogen, SBP, BMI, CV fitness, lipids, other bioRF)* High demands, low resources, low rewards — 2.6 *(Age, alcohol, smoking, physical activity)*; 2.3 *(Age, fibrinogen, SBP, BMI, CV fitness, lipids, other bioRF)*	Groups with other combinations of demands, resources, rewards = NS *(Age)*
Bosma, et al (1998)	10,308 British civil servants (33% women), 35–55 y.o.	High effort: competitiveness, overcommit, hostility. Low reward: poor promotion prospects, blocked career	5.3	Newly reported CHD (results for men)	High effort and low reward — OR 2.2 *(Age, BMI, smoking, BP, lipids, employment grade, negative affectivity, length of followup, job control)*	High effort *or* low reward

Cross-Sectional Study

First Author (Year)	Study Participants	Form(s) of Exposure Variable	Illness Outcome	Significant Positive Associations (Adjusted Confounders)	Null or Sig. Negative Assoc. (Adjusted Confounders)
Peter, et al (1999b)	2098 Swedish men and women, 45–64 y.o., population-based case-control SHEEP study	Effort-reward imbalance: ratio > 1 Job strain: latitude bottom 25% or demands top 25%	Acute nonfatal MI (results for men)	Effort-reward imbalance (no job strain) — OR 1.4; Effort-reward imbalance *and* job strain — 2.3 *(Age, BMI, smoking, HPT, lipids, exercise, diabetes, family history, SES)*	

bioRF = biological risk factors, CAD = coronary artery disease, CVD = cardiovascular disease, HPT = hypertension, IMT = intima-media thickness, MI = myocardial infarction, SCD = sudden cardiac death.

high resources, and high income.[165] In addition, in this sample a combination of high work demands and low income was significantly associated with progression of carotid atherosclerosis.[164] (In the German and Finnish studies, some measures of high effort or low reward were not associated with heart disease, as shown in Table 5.)

BLOOD PRESSURE

As seen in Table 6, in the cross-sectional study of 179 male German middle managers aged 40–55, forced job change (low reward) (OR 3.3) and a variable combining frequent interruptions (effort) and forced job change (OR 5.8) were strongly associated with hypertension.[205] Similarly, in a cross-sectional study of Stockholm area residents, an effort-reward ratio greater than one was associated with hypertension (OR 1.6) among men.[202] The combination of ERI and shiftwork among Stockholm men led to an even stronger association (OR 2.2) with hypertension.[203]

In the prospective study of 416 German blue-collar workers from three factories, low promotion prospects at work (OR 2.7), competitiveness at work (OR 2.8), and feelings of sustained anger (OR 5.4) predicted coronary high risk status.[238] (High risk was defined as the 13.6% of the sample with both hypertension and high lipid levels.) In addition, a variable combining overtime work (effort) and fear of job loss, job instability, and layoffs (low reward) was similarly associated (OR 3.3) with a comanifestation of hypertension and atherogenic lipids.[233] (In all of these studies of hypertension, some of the measures of high effort or low reward were not associated with hypertension; see Table 6.)

OTHER CARDIAC RISK FACTORS

Cardiac risk factors other than hypertension may represent additional pathways by which ERI may contribute to CVD. Among German blue-collar workers, LDL/HDL ratio was associated with high work demand, increased workload, and job insecurity, combined with occupational instability.[235] In German managers, LDL cholesterol was predicted by a combination of workload and lack of support.[237] In Swedish men, cholesterol/HDL ratio, but not plasma fibrinogen, was associated with ERI.[202,203] Among the German managers, fibrinogen was associated with a combination of overcommitment and lack of social ("reciprocal") support, but not with combinations of other measures of effort or reward.[237]

COMMENTS ON THE NULL FINDINGS AND GENERAL INTERPRETATION

Despite the positive findings, some questions remain about which specific work factors are responsible for increasing CHD risk, and whether these variables are additive or interactive.

Specific Predictors of Risk. In the earlier studies, the set of variables used to measure effort and reward was not always identical, as some studies used "proxy" measures.[30,164,165] In addition, Siegrist, et al. applied a less restrictive measurement approach where subjects were considered "exposed" to ERI when at least one of the effort and one of the reward variables were positive.[238,239] Thus, we cannot be sure which work characteristic contributed to this combined risk factor. More recently, a standardized summary measure of ERI has been constructed based on a predefined algorithm.[202–204] To illustrate this issue, in the three studies of hypertension (Table 6), only the German middle-manager study found associations between outcome and measures of extrinsic effort.[205] Extrinsic effort was not associated with hypertension in the Swedish WOLF study.[202] In the German blue-collar study, work pressure was not associated with outcome, and forced piecework was not in the analysis (due to

TABLE 6. Studies of the Effort-Reward Imbalance Model and Hypertension for Men

Cohort Studies

First Author (Year)	Study Participants	Form(s) of Exposure Variable	F/u (y)	Illness Outcome	Significant Positive Associations (Adjusted Confounders)		Null or Sig. Negative Assoc. (Adjusted Confounders)
Siegrist, et al. (1991); Siegrist (1996)	416 male German blue-collar workers from 3 factories	Low security, career opportunities: job instability, low promotion prospects. Overcommitment: competitiveness, sustained anger. High effort-low reward: overtime *and* job instability *or* fear of job loss	6.5	Comanifestation of hypertension and high LDL-cholesterol (n = 314 in analysis)	Low promotion prospects Competitiveness Sustained anger High effort-low reward *(Age, BMI, smoking, exercise)*	**OR** 2.7 2.8 5.4 3.3	Work pressure, job instability; forced piecework and status inconsistency were not in the analysis, due to attempts to find the most parsimonious model

Cross-Sectional Studies

First Author (Year)	Study Participants	Form(s) of Exposure Variable	Illness Outcome	Significant Positive Associations (Adjusted Confounders)		Null or Sig. Negative Assoc. (Adjusted Confounders)
Peter & Siegrist (1997); Siegrist (1996)	179 healthy German male middle managers, 40–55 y.o.	High extrinsic effort: time pressure, frequent interruptions. High intrinsic effort: overcommitment (upper tertile), sustained anger. Low reward: lack of support, status incongruence, status discrepancy, forced job change	Hypertension (≥ 160/95 mmHg) (n = 170 in analysis)	**Bivariate analysis:** Time pressure Frequent interruptions Forced job change Freq. interruptions + forced job change **All exposure variables in model:** Forced job change **Effort-reward imbalance measures:** Freq. interruptions *or* forced job change Freq. interruptions + forced job change *(Age, BMI, smoking, exercise)*	**OR** 3.3 2.3 5.8	Overcommitment Sustained anger Lack of support Status incongruence Status discrepancy Time pressure Frequent interruptions
Peter, et al (1998)	N = 2228, Swedish men, 30–55 y.o., population-based WOLF study	Effort-reward imbalance: (ratio > 1): overcommitment (upper tertile), extrinsic effort (above median), low reward (above median)	Hypertension (≥ 160.95 mmHG) (results for men)	**Bivariate analysis:** Effort-reward imbalance Low reward *(Age, smoking, BMI, exercise)* Effort-reward imbalance *(Age, smoking, BMI, exercise, lipids, SES)*	**OR** 1.7 1.6	Overcommitment Extrinsic effort
Peter, et al (1999a)		Rotating shift workers (vs day shift)		Effort-reward imbalance + rotating shift *(Age, smoking, BMI, exercise)*	2.2	

BMI = body mass index, SES = socioeconomic status.

colinearity).[238] Only in one later analysis of the sample was overtime (plus low reward measures) associated with high CHD risk.[233] Similarly, "forced job change" in the middle manager study and "low promotion prospects" in the blue-collar study were the only low reward measures associated with hypertension. ("Status inconsistency" was not in the analysis of the blue-collar sample due to colinearity with other reward measures.)

In the CHD studies (Table 5), no extrinsic measure was included in the Whitehall study analysis,[30] and a very broad measure of work demands was used in the Finnish studies.[164,165] Low status control (low job security) was essentially the measure of low reward in the German blue-collar sample and the Whitehall study, while economic reward and social support were added as measures of reward in the Finnish and the Swedish SHEEP studies.

Interaction Versus Additive Burden.   As with the Job Strain Model, the question arises as to whether measures of high effort and low reward combine with each other additively to increase CHD risk, or whether they interact with each other ("synergism," see Chapter 3). In some analyses, as seen in Tables 5 and 6, synergism appears to exist. In the blue-collar study and the middle manager study, for example, the relative risk of CHD due to measures of high effort combined with low reward is substantially greater than the sum of the risks due to these two components separately.[205,233] However, no statistical tests of interaction were conducted. A number of more recent analyses used a combined high effort-low reward ratio variable, which prevents observation of possible interaction.

In summary, several studies, both cross-sectional and prospective, have shown significant positive associations between measures of high effort/low reward and elevated lipid levels, hypertension, and CVD. The magnitude of the relationship is similar to that typically found for job strain with respect to these outcomes. Furthermore, preliminary evidence indicates that the effects of job control and ERI are statistically independent of each other in prediction of CHD[30] and that the combined effects of exposure to job strain and ERI upon CVD are much stronger than the separate effects of each.[204]

Threat-Avoidant Vigilant Work

A particularly heavy psychological burden occurs when one must continuously maintain a high level of vigilance to avoid disastrous consequences, which could occur with a momentary lapse of attention or a wrong decision. Among several of the occupations shown to be at high risk for CVD (e.g., bus, taxi, and truck drivers; air traffic controllers; sea pilots), threat-avoidant vigilant activity is a prominent aspect of work. Experimental animal studies have shown an association between performance of threat (shock) avoidance tasks and cardiac electrical instability.[46,162]

A few epidemiologic studies have specifically examined aspects of threat-avoidant vigilant activity with regard to CVD outcomes. In a cohort study by Menotti and Seccareccia of 99,029 Italian men employed by the railroad system, occupational psychologists rated jobs with respect to level of "responsibility at work."[175] Levels were based on the "economic and financial implications of decisions taken at work, as well as the relevance of possible damage and hazards both economic and for human life as a consequence of possible mistakes made at work." The age-adjusted mortality rates due to MI were significantly greater ($p < 0.001$) for each of three ascending levels of responsibility at work compared to the lower levels. Job dimension data from expert ratings were imputed to a CV disability data base (N = 9855).[181] For the dimension of having to be "alert to changing conditions," age-adjusted ORs of

1.85, 2.17 and 2.8 were found for the second, third, and highest quartiles, respectively. The "hazardous job situation" dimension showed age-adjusted ORs 2.07, 3.32, and 4.09, for the second, third, and highest quartiles, respectively. (Confidence intervals were not provided; the author identified job dimension scores having an OR of at least 2 as meriting additional research attention.) In the imputational study by Alfredsson, et al., an SMR of 132 (116–149) was calculated for hospitalization for MI, among Swedish men whose jobs entailed risk of explosion.[7] Occupational titles were used to impute job characteristics based upon observational analysis and interviews in a study of 6213 Finnish municipal employees.[251] These authors identified requisites for "alertness of the senses" and dangerous work as quantitatively important stressors among male transport workers, with high prevalence of self-reported hypertension and CHD.

These epidemiologic studies provide suggestive evidence for an association between aspects of threat-avoidant work and CVD outcomes. Further investigation is needed, with more precise, well-controlled risk estimates, and accounting of biomedical and psychosocial risk factors.

SOCIAL CLASS, OCCUPATIONAL STATUS, AND CVD *by Michael Marmot, FFPHM—Supported by an MRC research professorship and by the John D. and Catherine T. MacArthur Research Foundation Research Network on Socioeconomic Status and Health*

A dominant feature of the occurrence of cardiovascular disease (CVD) in most industrialized societies is the higher rate in people of lower socioeconomic position. The Whitehall studies of British civil servants showed that the link between socioeconomic position and CVD was not confined to higher rates among the poor.[169,170] The poor do have high rates, but there is a social gradient: the lower the social status, the higher the CV risk. A review by Kaplan and Keil covers a wealth of studies showing a similar social gradient in the U.S.[118]

What implications does the social gradient have for questions of etiology and in particular for the role of work? In the U.K., we traditionally used Registrar General's social classes, which are based on occupation. It has never been clear whether the differences in CVD observed using these classes are due to occupation or to other features correlated with occupational status.

Elsewhere in this volume we show how ideas on the effects and meaning of social stratification have been shaped by Marx, Durkheim, and Weber. It is useful to think of three "meanings" of socioeconomic position, in terms of the ways they may affect health. First, low social position may be related to **material deprivation**, and absolute material deprivation (poverty) may be related to risk of illness. Second, socioeconomic position may be related to **standing in society** which may, in turn, relate to shared values, culture, and lifestyle. Third, socioeconomic position is a measure of position in the social hierarchy, which is related to **power relationships**. People higher in the hierarchy have more control over their own, and other people's, lives. These power relations operate in the workplace, but not exclusively so.

Figure 1 shows standardized mortality ratios from ischemic heart disease (IHD) by Registrar General's social classes in England and Wales.[56] Focusing on the 1991–93 period, we see that IHD is markedly higher among men in social class V, unskilled manual workers. The gradient is shown clearly. Men in social class I have a mortality ratio about 35% lower than the England and Wales average, and men in social class IV

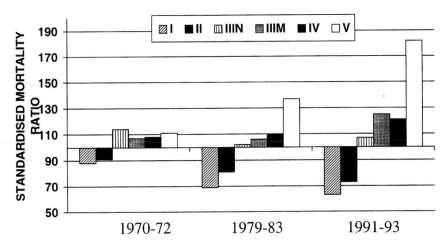

FIGURE 1. Ischemic heart disease by social class in England and Wales, males 1970–93. (Data from Drever F, Whitehead M, Roden M: Current patterns and trends in male mortality by social class (based on occupation). Popul Trends 86:15–20, 1996; with permission.)

have mortality 25% higher. The high mortality of men in the lowest social class could be attributed, in part, to the effect of absolute deprivation. It is difficult to attribute the rest of the gradient to differing degrees of material deprivation. In contemporary Britain, the overwhelming majority of these men in classes I to IV are adequately housed, nourished, and clothed, with adequate provision of safe water and food, and safe handling of sewage. In addition, the steepening of the gradient over the 20-year period shown occurred at a time when material prosperity was increasing for the top 80% of the population. Absolute deprivation does not, therefore, provide a ready explanation for the gradient in IHD mortality. Using data on U.S. counties grouped according to the proportion in white-collar occupations, Wing, et al. showed that the inverse social gradient in CHD mortality has become progressively steeper between 1968 and 1982.[290]

The other two concepts of social stratification are more likely to provide explanations for the gradient. The research task is to distinguish influences associated with power relations that are linked to work from influences related to general social standing that are linked more to lifestyle. Neither of the other two models alone gives a fully adequate accounting of the changing social class relations of IHD. Extending the comparisons in Figure 1, there is evidence from England, Wales, and the Netherlands that in the 1950s and earlier, heart disease mortality may have been more common in people of higher socioeconomic position.[146] Lifestyle may play some role in this; there is evidence that when the smoking epidemic first hit, it was at least as common among people of higher status but, with time, higher status people gave up smoking or declined to take up the habit to a greater degree than people of lower status. Physical activity may have followed a similar course. With the decline of physical activity in the workplace, the greater tendency for high-status people to be physically active in leisure time may have conferred increasing protection on them. One particular feature of diet—consumption of fresh fruit and vegetables that contain antioxidants and other protective nutrients—also may be related to the lower rate of heart disease in people of higher status.

The evidence from the Whitehall and Whitehall II studies is that these lifestyle factors may account for some, but by no means all, of the social gradient in CVD. In the Whitehall studies there was a social gradient in smoking, consumption of fruit

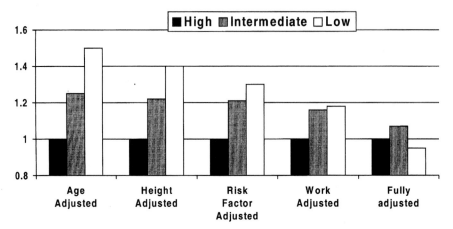

FIGURE 2. Odds ratio for new coronary heart disease in Whitehall II by employment grade, males. (From Marmot MG, Bosma H, Hemingway H, et al: Contribution of job control and other risk factors to social variations in coronary heart disease incidence. Lancet 350:235–239, 1997.)

and vegetables, and sedentary lifestyle, but only for a limited extent in obesity and blood pressure level, and not at all in plasma cholesterol. In Whitehall I (CHD mortality) and Whitehall II (CHD incidence), adjusting for coronary risk factors related to lifestyle accounted for about a third of the social gradient.[169,170] Among nonsmokers the social gradient in CHD incidence and mortality was similar to the gradient in smokers. In Whitehall II, low control in the workplace was related to CHD incidence[29] and accounted for about half the social gradient[169] (Fig. 2).

In seeking to interpret this finding of the importance of the psychosocial work environment, consider two related questions: Did low control appear to be associated with CHD because low control is associated with low socioeconomic status, and *other* factors account for the association of low socioeconomic status with disease; in other words was there confounding? Did low control appear to be an important mediator of the relation between social position and CHD because low control is simply a measure of low socioeconomic position? Several convincing lines of argument indicate that these results were not simply the result of problems of confounding and/or measurement.

In the Whitehall II study and in a Czech case-control study, the relation between low control and CHD was not removed by adjusting for socioeconomic status.[24,29] This finding implies that within a particular employment level, those with more control over their work have lower incidence of CHD than those with less control.

In separate studies in Sweden, first Johnson and Hall and then Hallqvist showed that job strain according to the demand/control model (DCM) was more strongly related to CHD in blue-collar than in white-collar workers.[87,114] Of course, it could be argued that manual workers with more control, and lower coronary risk, are of higher status compared to manual workers with less control. This, however, is not an argument against the importance of low control in the workplace because it may be precisely this particular feature of low social status that is responsible for part of the social gradient in disease. One approach to deciding if it is low control or other characteristics associated with low social status that are related to CHD is multivariate analyses. In the Whitehall II study, multivariate analysis showed an independent effect of low control. The second approach is to explore biological markers, such as plasma fibrinogen, which is a risk factor for coronary disease. In Whitehall II, smoking, obesity, and lack of exercise were associated with plasma fibrinogen level. Independent of this finding, low control at work also was associated with plasma fibrinogen level.[36]

In the Whitehall II study and the Czech case-control study, high demand was not associated with coronary risk. The fact that these civil servants were office-based workers may be relevant. In Sweden, the DCM was related to disease more strongly in manual than in nonmanual workers. Thus, the degree to which the full DCM predicts disease may be influenced by the nature of employment in different settings.

These findings do suggest that low control in the workplace is independently related to CHD and makes an important contribution to the social gradient in CHD, along with other risk factors, including those related to lifestyle and early life. There still is a problem, however. A social gradient in CHD exists in people who are not working in formal employment: homemakers, the unemployed, and retired people. Low control *in the workplace* does not apply to them, but they may be affected by power relations that apply throughout society. High-status people among these groups who are "not working" may have power, control, and mastery that derives from their general position in the social hierarchy, rather than the workplace. This is in accord with the results of studies in nonhuman primates that show high-status animals to have less atherosclerosis and less activation of stress hormones.[232]

Kawachi and Kennedy and others have shown a relation between income inequality and mortality internationally; in the U.S., the relation was shown at the state level. Their interpretation of this finding is that income inequality is a marker for the quality of the social environment which, in turn, affects disease risk.[128,129,289] One reason for focusing on the role of work as one of the causes of the social gradient is that redesign of the workplace is more feasible than redesign of society, and may have other beneficial consequences.

WOMEN, WORK, AND CVD *by Chantal Brisson, PhD*

In several industrialized countries, CVDs are the leading cause of death in women, as they are in men, and generate an equal amount of heart disease expenditure in both groups.[60,224a] CHD, the largest component of CVD, shows a lower rate in women than in men in younger age groups, but approaches similar rates for women and men in older groups.[73] Therefore, the study of CHD in women of working age is more difficult than the study of men of similar age because larger populations of working women have to be enrolled to obtain a sufficient number of CHD events. Over the last two decades, CVD mortality rates have shown consistent decreases.[15,266] However, in several countries there has been no decrease in women[69,216,278] or the decrease has been less marked than in men.[102,278] This difference could be due to changes that have occurred in women's lives since the 1970s—such as paid employment.[193] It is estimated that the proportion of women aged 25–49 involved in paid work will be 82% in the year 2000 in countries of the European Union.[177]

Gender Differences in Work and Home Exposures

Most women and men are employed in jobs where their own gender has a large majority.[12,177,194] Jobs held predominantly by women are concentrated in the services.[177] In countries participating in the Organisation de Coopération et de Développement Économiques, four service industries contained half of working women: office work, sales, health care, and teaching.[194]

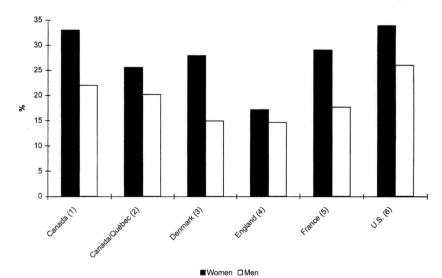

■Women □Men

Notes: Prevalences cannot be compared between countries because different methods were used to categorize exposure groups.

(1) Random population sample—3847 male and 2587 female workers. Psychological demands and decision latitude assessed with 7 items from Job Content Questionnaire (JCQ). Median splits used to define high job strain.[34]

(2) Stratified random population sample—721 male and 389 female workers. Psychological demands and decision latitude assessed with full JCQ. Median splits used to define high job strain.[156]

(3) 748 male and 756 female white- and blue-collar workers living in 11 municipalities in Copenhagen County. Psychological demands and decision latitude assessed with 2 and 7 items. Job strain defined as combination of low degree of decision latitude (score ≥ 3) and high work pace (work pace reported too high or time pressure).[186]

(4) 6895 male and 3413 female London civil servants. Psychological demands and decision latitude assessed respectively with 4 and 9 items. Medians splits used to define high job strain.[30]

(5) 8277 male and 3170 female workers from the Gazel cohort. Psychological demands and decision latitude assessed with full JCQ. Median splits used to define high job strain.[188]

(6) 4018 mailhandlers from U.S. Postal Service. Psychological demands and decision latitude assessed respectively with 5 and 9 items from JCQ. Median splits used to define high job strain.[39]

FIGURE 3. Prevalence (%) of high job strain by gender in six populations from five countries.

Given this gender division of jobs it is expected that job characteristics potentially related to CV diseases also will differ. This clearly is the case regarding high job strain, defined as the combination of high psychological demands and low job decision latitude.[122] Indeed, studies conducted in Canada, Denmark, England, France, and the U.S. all found a higher prevalence of job strain in women than in men (Fig. 3).[30,34,39,156,186,188] It is particularly the level of control that is lower in women's jobs.[29,39,82,84,122,156,188] In some studies, higher psychological demands were observed in women,[39,82,156] but other studies found little difference between women and men on this factor.[85,131]

Potentially stressful exposures related to family responsibilities are also more prevalent in women than in men. Indeed, despite their increasing involvement in paid work, women spend more hours than men in child caring and housework.[20,157,160,293] For example, in countries of western Europe women spent an average of 35 hours/week in child caring and housework before 1975, and 31 hours/week after 1975. Men spent 8 and 11 hours, respectively during the same periods.[94]

Job Strain

JOB STRAIN AND CARDIOVASCULAR DISEASES

High job strain has been defined by Karasek as the combination of high psychological demands and low decision latitude.[122] *Psychological demands* refers to the quantity of work, the mental requirements, and the time constraints. *Decision latitude* refers to the ability to make decisions about one's own work and the possibility of being creative and using and developing skills. The Job Strain Model emphasizes that high psychological demands are not, in themselves, a great source of strain if they are combined with decision latitude, i.e., influence on one's own work, since this influence enables a person to adequately meet the demands to which he or she is subject.

From 1981 on, a number of studies investigated the effect of job strain on CHD risk.[6,7,9,29,30,83,86,88,103,114–116,119,124,148,218,247,260,265] In the area of stress at work and CHD, these studies constitute the largest group using a common conceptual model.[125,144,226] Some recent studies found a high CHD risk mainly in workers exposed to low decision latitude.[29,30,86,116,247,265] Others found little effect.[9,103,218] Some studies also found that low social support at work had a main effect on CHD and could amplify the effect of job strain on CHD risk.[114,115]

Few of the previous studies were conducted among women. Table 7 shows studies using a prospective cohort or case-control design in women. A majority (five) of these studies found that women exposed to high job strain or one of its components had significant increases in CHD risk. Three evaluated job strain using the job title method,[7,86,88] which relies on the attribution of an inferred mean score to all women having the same job title.[229] This method may lead to misclassification of exposure in that it does not take into account the within-occupational variance that can be important in many occupations.[124,229] Misclassification may lead to an underestimation of the true effect, and may explain why studies using the job title method tended to show lower relative risk (1.3–1.6) than other studies (2.5–5.0).

In two of the four studies using the individual method (reporting by the subject of her job characteristics), the measure of psychological demands[83] or decision latitude[148] was a proxy of the original job strain measure.[120] In a third study these measures were taken after the occurrence of the myocardial infarction.[197] Therefore, the

TABLE 7. Effect of Job Strain on CHD Risk in Women

Author	Year	Country	Study Design	Number of Subjects	Job Strain Evaluation Method	RR (95% CI or p Value)	
Lacroix	1984	U.S.	Cohort	389	Individual	2.9 (p ≤ .01)	(1)
Alfredsson	1985	Sweden	Cohort	319,365	Job title	1.6 (1.1–2.3)	
Haan	1988	Finland	Cohort	902	Individual	5.0 (p = .03)	(2)
Hall	1993	Sweden	Cohort	5921	Job title	1.3 (0.9–1.8)	(3)
Hammar	1994	Sweden	Case-control	4667	Job title	1.3 (1.1–1.6)	
Bosma	1997–98	England	Cohort	3413	Individual	1.7 (1.1–2.6)	(4)
Orth-Gomer	1998	Sweden	Case-control	584	Individual	2.5 (1.2–5.3)	

(1) In the subsample of clerical women, the RR was 5.2 (p < .001).
(2) The study population includes both men (N = 603) and women (N = 299).
(3) RR for women exposed to low decision latitude only. The RR for women exposed to low work social support was of similar magnitude.
(4) RR observed for women exposed to low decision latitude only. The RR for job strain exposure was 1.1 (0.8–1.7).[30]

high risk found in these studies must be interpreted with caution. In Bosma's study, the population was very specific (London civil servants); therefore the absence of an effect of job strain could be specific to this population.[30] Similar limitations, and others not mentioned here,[125,144,226] also are present in studies conducted in men.

In two studies, an elevated risk was observed only for women exposed to low decision latitude,[29,86] which parallels what has been noted previously in some studies of men. In the Hall, et al. study the combination of low decision latitude and low work social support seemed to be associated with higher risk.[86] In several studies including both women and men, the effect of job strain on CHD risk tended to be of similar magnitude in both groups.[7,30,83,88]

Job Strain and Blood Pressure

A number of studies have reported that workers exposed to high job strain had increased blood pressure.[23,130,149,159,227,228,258,259,263,276] However, null results also have been found.[4,32a,43,82,91,186,209,249,262] Studies conducted among women are presented in Table 8. Four out of six studies that used ambulatory measures of BP found an effect of job strain.[23,149,258,276] Two studies that did not were conducted on very small samples of 64[159] and 22[263] women, and the percentage of participants was either not provided[159] or very low (22%).[263] Five of six studies using casual measures of BP at rest did not find an effect of job strain.[32a,43,52,82,186] These findings demonstrate that the *type* of BP measure is an important factor explaining the discrepancy in the results. Ambulatory BP measures: (1) take into consideration the normal BP level at work and outside work rather than the level measured in a clinic-type situation; (2) control for BP variability related to the observer or to the presence of medical personnel; and (3) may have about twice the precision of a single measure. In studies using ambulatory measures, women exposed to high job strain had increases in BP of 4–7 mmHg. A similar pattern of results has been observed in studies using ambulatory BP measures in men.[149]

There is evidence that the effect of job strain on BP is persistent beyond working hours. For example, in the study by Laflamme, et al. among women holding a university degree, those exposed to high job strain had an average of 6 mmHg (p = .012) higher systolic BP than nonexposed women over the 24 hours of a working day (Fig. 4).[149] The difference was, on average, 5.5 mmHg (p < 0.05) in the morning, 10.5 mmHg (p < 0.001) in the afternoon, and 8.5 mmHg (p = .005) in the evening.

There is also some evidence of a stronger effect when duration of exposure increases. Indeed, Laflamme, et al. measured job strain at two different times (T1 and T2) with a median of 14.4 months between the two measures. Among women holding a university degree, those with high strain at both T1 and T2 had a significant elevation in systolic BP of 7.7 mmHg (p = .001), on average, over the 24 hours when compared to women unexposed at both T1 and T2 (Fig. 5). Women exposed only at T1 and women exposed only at T2 had a slight but nonsignificant elevation in BP when compared to women unexposed at both times. These findings are consistent with a larger effect on BP when duration of exposure is prolonged, and with an effect that diminishes when exposure ceases. Such findings are consistent with those observed in a 3-year longitudinal study conducted in men.[227]

Most available studies on job strain and BP are cross-sectional. The cross-sectional design is subject to differential selection and information bias.[45] For example, it is plausible that individuals employed in high-strain jobs will tend to move, in time, to a low-strain job. Evidence of such a selection effect has been found.[149]

TABLE 8. Effect of Job Strain on Blood Pressure in Women

Author	Year	Country	Study Design	Number of Subjects	BP Evaluation Method	Differences in BP Between Exposed and Nonexposed (mmHg)		
						Diastolic (95% CI or p value)	*Systolic (95% CI or p value)*	
Theorell	1988	Sweden	Cohort	22	Ambulatory	N.S.	4 (N.S.)	(1)
Chapman	1990	Australia	Cohort	534	Casual	N.S.	N.S.	
Netterstrom	1991	Denmark	Cross-sectional	1209	Casual	–.4 (N.S.)	1.7 (N.S.)	(2)
Van Egeren	1992	U.S.	Cross-sectional	37	Ambulatory	4.0 (p = .04)	12.0 (p = .001)	(3)
Light	1992	U.S.	Cross-sectional	64	Ambulatory	–2.2 (N.S.)	–1 (N.S.)	
Theorell	1993	Sweden	Cross-sectional	56	Ambulatory	3.7 (p < .05)	4.4 (p < .05)	(4)
Blumenthal	1995	U.S.	Cross-sectional	38	Ambulatory	N.S.	5.0 (N.A.)	
Greenlund	1995	U.S.	Cross-sectional	601	Casual	0.2 (N.S.)	1.0 (N.S.)	(5)
Curtis	1997	U.S.	Cross-sectional	453	Casual	0.7 (–2.0–3.4)	–0.4 (–4.1–3.4)	
Laflamme	1998	Canada	Cross-sectional	71	Ambulatory	6.4 (p = .01)	8.0 (p = .005)	(6)
Brisson	1999a	Canada	Cross-sectional	212	Casual	6.5 (1.1–11.9)	N.S.	(7)
Brisson	1999c	Canada	Cross-sectional	3864	Casual	0.2 (N.S.)	0.4 (N.S.)	

N.S. = nonsignificant, N.A. = unavailable

(1) Differences between occasion with highest and lowest strain on four assessments during a 1-year followup.

(2) Study population includes both men (N = 664) and women (N = 545). Job strain evaluation based on job title yielded comparable estimates.

(3) Study population includes both men and women.

(4) Differences estimated from published article using corresponding multiple regression coefficients. Differences corresponded to an increase of 0.15 on job strain score as observed between female physicians (low) and waitresses (high) in a previous study.[260]

(5) Results observed among black women. Similarly, no effect observed among white women.

(6) Results observed among university-educated women (N = 71). No effect observed among women without a university degree (N = 139).

(7) Results observed in women who had children (N = 212). No effect observed in women without children (N = 150). For all women (N = 362), the difference was 4.1 (0.6–7.6) for diastolic BP. Similar trends observed for systolic BP, although not statistically significant.

Indeed, in that study, twice as many women moved to another job among women exposed to high strain (23.8%) as among those exposed to low strain (12.4%) at T1 (p = .003). If job strain is related to higher BP, this selection effect may lead to an underestimation of the true association in cross-sectional studies. The absence of an association among less-educated women also could be due to selection.

The increases in BP observed in women exposed to high job strain are clinically significant. Indeed, it has been demonstrated in a meta-analysis of nine prospective studies conducted among women and men that a persistent elevation of 5 mmHg of diastolic BP increases the risk of strokes by 34% and the risk of coronary heart disease by 21%.[166] The association between daytime ambulatory BP and these disease endpoints is stronger than that of casual BP.[201]

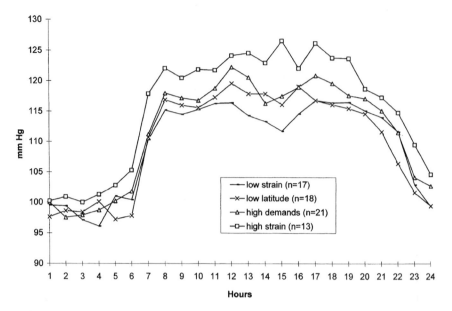

FIGURE 4.   Hourly mean systolic blood pressure by current job strain exposure among white-collar women holding a university degree (1 mmHg ≈ 0.133 kPa). (From Laflamme N, Brisson C, Moisan J, et al: Job strain and ambulatory blood pressure among female white-collar workers. Scand J Work Environ Health 24(5):334–343, 1998; with permission.)

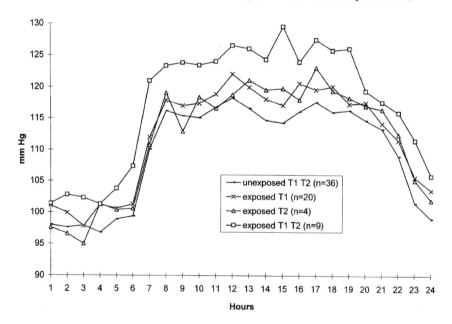

FIGURE 5.   Hourly mean systolic BP by cumulative job strain exposure among white-collar women holding a university degree (T1 = 1991–1993, T2 = 1993–1994, 1 mmHg ≈ 0.133 kPa). (From Laflamme N, Brisson C, Moisan J, et al: Job strain and ambulatory blood pressure among female white-collar workers. Scand J Work Environ Health 24(5):334–343, 1998; with permission.)

Little is known about the long-term effect of job strain on BP in women or men. Indeed, very few of the previous studies used a prospective design or evaluated the effect of exposure duration. Well-designed prospective studies are needed to evaluate the effect of prolonged exposure to job strain and the effect of exposure withdrawal on BP. The issue of exposure withdrawal is particularly relevant for assessing the potential benefits of intervention studies aimed at reducing job strain in the workplace.

JOB STRAIN AND OTHER CARDIOVASCULAR RISK FACTORS

Psychosocial factors at work may contribute to the risk of CVD by the adoption of unhealthy behaviors (e.g., smoking, sedentary activity, high fat intake).[226] A number of studies found that some psychosocial factors at work were associated with the prevalence[9,98,113,121] or the intensity[81,98,176,283] of smoking; the prevalence of sedentary behavior[98,113]; and obesity.[78,98] However, null results also have been observed.[107,151,176,186,209] Studies largely are conducted among men. Only one previous study used a prospective design.[151]

In studies conducted among women, job strain was not consistently associated with CVD risk factors. None of the four studies on the association with smoking found an effect.[31,82,98,186] However, the prevalence of smoking was associated with psychological demands in two studies.[31,98] Two studies observed that women with high job strain had a higher BMI than nonexposed women.[98,186] However, other studies failed to find an association.[31,280] Job strain was not associated with cholesterol (total and HDL)[186] or high fat intake.[98] Brisson[31] found an association between job strain and sedentary behavior, but Hellerstedt[98] did not. Sedentary behavior was associated with lower decision latitude[98,113] and with psychological demands.[113] The two studies on plasma fibrinogen observed an association with high job strain[186] and with low job control.[36]

TABLE 9.   Effect of Job Strain and Family Load in White-Collar Women

Time Period	High FL	High Job Strain	n	Systolic BP (mmHg)	Diastolic BP (mmHg)
Work 9h–16th	no	no	42	116.3 ± 1.2	74.3 ± 1.0
	no	yes	7	119.7 ± 3.0	77.8 ± 2.4
	yes	no	14	119.9 ± 2.1	76.3 ± 1.7
	yes	yes	6	127.3 ± 3.2**	80.6 ± 2.6*
Evening 17h–21h	no	no	42	116.7 ± 1.2	74.4 ±1.0
	no	yes	7	119.1 ± 3.0	76.5 ± 2.4
	yes	no	14	119.1 ± 2.1	74.9 ± 1.7
	yes	yes	6	128.6 ± 3.3***	81.2 ± 2.6*
Night 0h–6h	no	no	42	98.6 ±1.0	57.8 ± 0.9
	no	yes	7	98.8 ± 2.5	58.0 ± 2.1
	yes	no	14	100.2 ± 1.8	58.7 ± 1.5
	yes	yes	6	105.4 ± 2.7*	63.4 ± 2.3*
All day (24 hours)	no	no	42	110.0 ± 1.0	68.4 ± 0.8
	no	yes	7	112.5 ± 2.4	71.0 ± 2.0
	yes	no	14	113.0 ± 1.7	69.9 ± 1.4
	yes	yes	6	119.7 ± 2.6***	74.7 ± 2.2**

* $p \leq .05$; ** $p \leq .01$; *** $p \leq .001$; FL = family load.
Values are means ± standard errors adjusted for age, smoking, and use of oral contraceptives. Exposed categories are compared with the reference category (first category of each variable). Significance of the differences is estimated by Student's t test.
From Brisson C, Laflamme N, Moisan J, et al: Effect of family responsibilities and job strain on ambulatory blood pressure among white-collar women. Psychosom Med 61(2):205–213, 1999; with permission.

JOB STRAIN AND FAMILY RESPONSIBILITIES

Several authors have reported that the high prevalence of job strain in women and its combination with large-family responsibilities may lead to high CV risk.[72,85,96,117,153,163,226] In the Framingham study, employed women who had three or more children had a higher incidence of CV diseases than employed women who had no children or than housewives with three or more children.[97] Frankenhaeuser has shown that among women managers, BP remained elevated in the evening after work, unlike men managers, who showed a decrease.[72] Brisson, et al. found that, among women having children, those exposed to high strain had a significant increase in diastolic BP, while among women without children, little effect was observed.[33]

In another study, Brisson, et al. investigated specifically the combined effect of high job strain and large-family responsibilities on ambulatory BP.[32] Significant effects were found among white-collar women holding a university degree (Table 9). The combined exposure of large-family responsibilities and high job strain tended to have a greater effect on BP than the exposure to either one of these factors. The combination of large-family responsibilities and high job strain was associated with higher systolic and diastolic BPs for all three periods (work, evening, and night), which also suggests a persistent effect beyond the work setting. Family responsibilities were measured with a composite index taking into account the presence of children, their age, and the proportion of domestic work performed. Further studies are needed to evaluate the combined effect of large-family responsibilities and high job strain on BP and the possible modifying effect of education on these associations.

Effort-Reward Imbalance at Work and Cardiovascular Outcomes

The Effort-Reward Imbalance Model was developed by Siegrist to explore adverse health effects of psychosocial factors at work. This model defines stressful experience at work as an imbalance between high effort spent and low reward received.[233] Effort comes from two sources: an extrinsic source (the demands of the job) and an intrinsic source (the motivation of the individual worker). Rewards at work are distributed in money, esteem, and status control.[233]

In the Whitehall study, Bosma, et al. have observed that this model and the decision latitude dimension from Karasek's model had independent effects,[30] suggesting the complementarity of the two models. The Swedish WOLF Study found that women who exercised high effort at work but received not enough reward had a higher prevalence of hypertension than other women (adjusted OR 1.6, 95% CI, 0.9–2.7).[202] This study also found that high intrinsic effort (overcommitment) was related to increased LDL-cholesterol in women (POR 1.4, 95% CI, 1.1–1.8).

Other Job Conditions and Cardiovascular Diseases

Shiftwork[47,256,270] and long working hours[64,95,274] have been associated with CVD in studies conducted among men. Few studies were conducted in women. In a case-control study, Knutsson, et al. found that women exposed to shiftwork had higher risk of MI than unexposed women (OR 1.3, 95% CI, 0.9–1.8 for women aged 45–70 and OR 3, 95% CI, 1.4–6.5 for women aged 45–55).[134] Alfredsson, et al. reported that at 1-year followup, the SMR for hospitalization for MI was 131 (95% CI, 105–162) for women working in occupations with long working hours and 152 (95% CI, 119–191) for women in occupations with irregular working hours.[7] For men, moderate overtime was a protective factor against hospitalization for MI. This gender difference could be explained by the fact that it may be more difficult for women to combine their family responsibilities with overtime.[161,179]

In another prospective study, the age-adjusted relative risk of CHD was 1.4 (95% CI, 1.1–1.8) in nurses who reported ever doing shiftwork. This excess risk persisted after adjustment for smoking and other CV risk factors. Among nurses reporting 6 or more years of shiftwork, the adjusted relative risk was 1.5 (95% CI, 1.1–2.0).[127] Brugère, et al. have observed no association between shiftwork and the prevalence of hypertension among 8928 women followed by occupational medicine specialists.[35]

HIGH-RISK OCCUPATIONS FOR CARDIOVASCULAR DISEASE
by Finn Tüchsen, MSc

The burden of CVD is unequally distributed across various occupations. The identification of occupational groups at high cardiac risk can be extremely helpful in generating etiologic hypotheses. Culpable single factors, e.g., exposure to carbon disulfide, and more complex psychosocial exposures, e.g., work comprising high psychological demand and low decision latitude, might be identified. However, combined exposures or some measure of total occupational burden (see Chapter 3) may best explain why certain occupations consistently show high risk of CVD.

Knowledge about occupational exposures and CVDs can be obtained from studies within a single occupation, insofar as there is sufficient variance, as well as from studies comparing one occupation with a reference occupation and studies comparing all occupations with a common standard. Each of these designs has strengths and weaknesses. The following pages focus on the latter study design.

Mortality and Morbidity Studies of "All" Occupations

Early Studies Using Proportional Mortality Ratios

Information from the Great Britain decennial census has been used together with national death registration data to study socioeconomic differences in mortality.[184] The first study of disease-specific mortality by occupation was published in 1851, and since then updates have been published every 10 years.[196] This design is not very reliable for CVD, however, because the proportional mortality ratio (PMR) measure should only be used for rare diseases. Another serious problem is that the occupational title is taken from the death certificate, and the title might be a consequence of the disease rather than a valid proxy measure for the occupational exposure. The most recent update illustrates clearly these methodological problems. For men, the occupation with the highest PMR was clergymen (PMR 120). The authors concluded: "The ranking of PMRs did not point to any obvious occupational hazards, and the jobs at the top of the ranking were not those that would be considered unusually stressful. Nor were they sedentary occupations." The problem with this design is that CVD accounts for one third of the mortality of the men and 23% for the women. As expected, the differentiation in PMR was low among men and higher among women. The highest PMR found was 178 among female railway signal workers. Larger differentials were observed for rarer diseases, like stroke.

A New Generation of Studies Based on Census Data

A new generation of mortality and/or morbidity studies based on census data in Denmark,[53,272] Norway,[28] Finland,[167,191,225] and Sweden[7,88,89] has successfully overcome the aforementioned shortcomings. Additional studies come from West

Germany[27] and Western Australia.[279] Information on occupation is collected prior to and independently of followup for death, and there is practically no loss to followup. While the Nordic studies followed the entire population, a comparable longitudinal study covering England and Wales was based on a 1% sample.[79] These cohort studies with a 5-year and later a 10-, 15- and 20-year followup may control well for the "healthy worker" effect. Furthermore, some of them use the economically active and not the entire population as their standard population. This is especially important when studying CVD because of the very strong selection effect of these diseases.

Data from all five Nordic countries also have been pooled into one data set.[190] The occupations had to be aggregated to 55 broad occupations because there were some differences in the detailed classifications between the countries. In Italy, a cross-sectional mortality study was published in 1995, together with a followup study of morbidity.[49,271] Recently, Danish and Swedish data were pooled to obtain better estimates for occupations with few employees.[5] The study supported the hypothesis that working in a brewery, cannery, slaughterhouse, or dairy, or in the chemical, paper, or rubber and plastics industries may lead to increased risk of MI. Alfredsson, et al. also draw our attention to the large differences among occupational groups. In a case control study including most of the Swedish population, they found a nine-fold higher risk in metal process workers (RR 2.8) than judges (R 0.3).[145]

All these studies may produce positive findings due to chance and multiple comparisons. One way to avoid such misinterpretations is to focus on the occupations found to be at high risk in more than one country or study (Table 10).

Professional Drivers: The Most Consistent Evidence of Elevated Risk. In these studies, professional drivers, particularly urban transport operators, emerge as the workers with the most consistent evidence of elevated risk. The high risk in bus drivers has been known for several decades. A recent review cites 34 of 40 studies as confirming the increased risk of ischemic heart disease and hypertension among professional drivers.[16] These authors conclude: "Such a consistent and large body of data concerning cardiac risk does not appear to exist for any other specific occupational group." One particularly well-controlled study revealed that, after a mean of 11.8 years of followup, 103 middle-aged male mass-transit drivers in Gothenberg had an OR 3.0 (95% CI, 1.8–5.2) for incident CHD compared to 6596 men from other occupational groups, after adjusting for age, serum cholesterol, BP, smoking, body mass index (BMI), diabetes, positive family history of CHD, leisure and occupational physical activity, and sociodemographic factors.[223] Another study reported that the risk of hospitalization for stroke is also increased among professional drivers in Denmark.[269] Compared to employed referents, the age-specific standardized hospitalization ratio was 114 (95% CI, 108.2–120.4) among men and 130 (100–168) among women. Furthermore, there was a gradient of risk within the occupation that appeared to be stress-related. Netterstrom and Juel found that objective workload based on traffic intensity was a significant, independent predictor of acute MI incidence among bus drivers in Denmark.[185] For high versus low traffic intensity, the RR was 2.7 (95% CI, 0.9–7.6) in Copenhagen, and 3.4 (1.2–9.5) in the province.

Methodologic Issues

For some occupations there is conflicting or weak evidence about high risk. These null or negative studies underscore the need for more and better designed research. For example, there are conflicting findings concerning the risk in police. According to a study by Tüchsen and colleagues, it may only be higher ranking policemen who are at elevated risk for CVD.[271] It is also helpful to detect low-risk

TABLE 10. Occupations at Increased Risk of Either Acute Myocardial Infarction or Ischemic Heart Disease Mortality or Morbidity in More than One Study

Men		Women
Air traffic controllers	Lorry drivers	Bus drivers
Bakers	Paper industry workers	Cleaners
Bus drivers	Police	Home help
Butchers	Prison wardens	Rubber and plastics workers
Cannery workers	Rubber and plastics workers	Paper workers
Cooks	Ship's deck officers and	Self-employed in hotel and catering
Fire fighters	sea pilots	Taxi drivers
Fishermen	Taxi drivers	Unskilled worker in tube,
Foundry workers	Waiters	sheet, and steel construction
Hairdressers	Warehousemen, storekeepers	Waitresses

Lower limit of the 95% confidence intervals must have been > 1 for each study considered to be positive. Cohort studies: references 28, 49, 79, 167, 191, 271, 279. Case control studies: references 5, 27, 89.

groups, to maximize the risk differences among occupational groups.[5,145] Note, however, that the magnitude of the risk in such studies is not necessarily representative for the groups as a whole, because it depends on the precise definition of both the index group and the standard group.

The need for improved design also includes conducting quantitative studies of the various occupational exposures with variable degrees of exposure. There are few studies in this field that take exposure intensity and peak values into consideration. However, length of exposure has been a valuable variable in some studies. For example, the prevalence of hypertension among San Francisco Municipal Transit vehicle operators was found to increase "in a step-wise fashion" with length of exposure to that job.[214] The increase from one category to the next (pre-employment, < 10 years, 10–20 years, > 20 years) controlling for age, race, gender, BMI, and alcohol

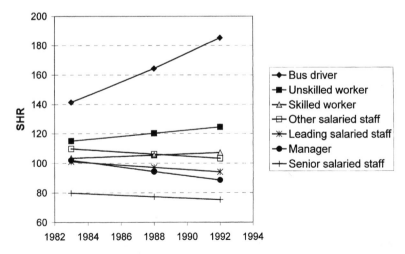

FIGURE 6. Time trend in predicted standardized hospitalization ratios due to ischemic heart disease among male employment status groups and single occupations in Denmark, 1981–1993. (From Tüchsen F, Endahl LA: Increasing inequality in ischaemic heart disease morbidity among employed men in Denmark 1981–1993: The need for a new preventive policy. Int J Epidemiol 28:640–644, 1999; with permission.

consumption showed OR 1.19 (95% CI, 1.0–1.41) for mild hypertension and OR 1.25 (1.03–1.52) for moderate to severe hypertension.

Future Analysis

One may expect that the next generation of occupational mortality and morbidity studies will focus on changes in relative risk over time. A recent study from Denmark demonstrates the potential in such analyses.[273] An unexpected increase in inequality of CHD risk over time was found (Fig. 6). Bus drivers not only had a high risk, but the risk was increasing. These results convinced Danish authorities that a large-scale workplace health promotion program among bus drivers had to be initiated; such a program is now in progress in Copenhagen.

REFERENCES

1. The world's women 1970–1990: Trends and statistics. New York, United Nations, 1991.
2. Akerstedt T, Knutsson A, Alfredsson L, Theorell T: Shift work and cardiovascular disease. Scand J Work Environ Health 10:409–414, 1984.
3. Akhtar MJ, al-Nozha M, Al-Harthi S, Nouh M: Electrocardiographic abnormalities in patients with heat stroke. Chest 104:411–414, 1993.
4. Albright CL, Winkleby MA, Ragland DR, et al: Job strain and prevalence of hypertension in a biracial population of urban bus drivers. Am J Public Health 82:984–989, 1992.
5. Alfredsson L, Bach E, Hammar N, Tuchsen F: Acute myocardial infarction in selected occupations in Denmark and Sweden. Copenhagen, Nordic Council of Ministers. TemaNord: 507, 1996.
6. Alfredsson L, Karasek R, Theorell T: Myocardial infarction risk and psychosocial work environment: An analysis of the male Swedish working force. Soc Sci Med 16:463–467, 1982.
7. Alfredsson L, Spetz C, Theorell T: Type of occupation and near-future hospitalization for myocardial infarction and some other diagnoses. International Journal of Epidemiology 14:378–388, 1985.
8. Alfredsson L, Theorell T: Job characteristics of occupations and myocardial infarction risk: Effect of possible confounding factors. Soc Sci Med 17:1497–1503, 1983.
8a. Al-Nashash H, Qassem W, Zabin A, Othman M: ECG response of the human body subject to vibrations. J Med Eng Technol 20:2–10, 1996.
9. Alterman T, Shekelle RB, Vernon SW, Burau KD: Decision latitude, psychologic demand, job strain and coronary heart disease in the Western Electric Study. Am J Epidemiol 139:620–627, 1994.
10. American Heart Association: Job strain not a predictor of heart attack in patients. NR:95-4308, 1995.
11. Angersbach D, Knauth P, Loskant H, et al: A retrospective cohort study comparing complaints and diseases in day and shift workers. Int Arch Occup Environ Health 45:127–140, 1980.
12. Anker R: Gender and jobs: Sex segregation of occupations in the world. Geneva, International Labour Office, 1998.
13. Axelson O, Seleden A, Andersson K, Hogstedt C: Updated and expanded Swedish cohort study on trichloroethylene and cancer risk. JOM 36:556–562, 1994.
14. Baumgart P, Walger P, Fuchs G, et al: Diurnal variations of blood pressure in shift workers during day and night shifts. Int Arch Occup Environ Health 61:463–466, 1989.
15. Beaglehole R, Stewart AW, Jackson R, et al: Declining rates of coronary heart disease in New Zealand and Australia, 1983–1993. Am J Epidemiol 145:707–713, 1997.
16. Belkic K, Emdad R, Theorell T: Occupational profile and cardiac risk: Possible mechanisms and implications for professional drivers. Int J Occup Med Environ Health 11:37–57, 1998.
17. Belkic K, Savic C, Theorell T, et al: Mechanisms of cardiac risk among professional drivers. Scand J Work Environ Health 20:73–86, 1994.
18. Ben-David A: Cardiac arrest in an explosives factory worker due to withdrawal from nitroglycerin exposure. Am J Ind Med 15:719–722, 1989.
19. Beniamini Y, Rubenstein JJ, Faigenbaum AD, et al: High-intensity strength training of patients enrolled in an outpatient cardiac rehabilitation program. J Cardiopulm Rehabil 19:8–17, 1998.
20. Biernat M, Wortman CB: Sharing of home responsibilities between professionally employed women and their husbands. J Pers Soc Psychol 60:844–860, 1991.
21. Billing E, Hjemdahl P, Rehnqvist N: Psychosocial variables in female vs male patients with stable angina pectoris and matched healthy controls. Eur Heart J 18:911–918, 1997.
22. Blair A, Hartge P, Stewart PA, et al: Mortality and cancer incidence of aircraft maintenance workers exposed to trichloroethylene and other organic solvents and chemicals: Extended follow up. Occup Environ Med 55:161–171, 1998.
23. Blumenthal JA, Thyrum TE, Siegel WC: Contribution of job strain, job status and marital status to laboratory and ambulatory blood pressure in patients with mild hypertension. J Psychosom Res 39:133–144, 1995.
24. Bobak M, Hertzman C, Skodova Z, Marmot M: Association between psychosocial factors at work and nonfatal MI in a population based case-control study in Czech men. Epidemiology 9:43–47, 1998.
25. Bøggild H, Knutsson A: Shift work, risk factors, and cardiovascular disease. Scand J Work Environ Health 25:85–89, 1999.
26. Bøggild H, Suadicaui P, Hein J, Gyntelberg F: Shift-work, social class, and ischemic heart disease in middle-aged and elderly men: A 22-year follow-up in the Copenhagen Male Study. (In press), 1999.

27. Bolm-Audorff U, Siegrist J: Occupational morbidity data in myocardial infarction. A case-referent study in West Germany. J Occup Med 25:367–371, 1983.
28. Borgan J-K, Kristoffersen LB: Dodelighet i yrker og sociookonomiske grupper 1970–1980. Oslo, Statistick sentralbyra, 1986.
29. Bosma H, Marmot MG, Hemingway H, et al: Low job control and risk of coronary heart disease in Whitehall II (prospective cohort) study. Br Med J 314:558–565, 1997.
30. Bosma H, Peter R, Siegrist J, Marmot M: Two alternative job stress models and the risk of coronary heart disease. Am J Public Health 88:68–74, 1998.
31. Brisson C, Larocque B, Moisan J, et al: Psychosocial constraints at work, smoking, sedentary behavior and body mass index: A prevalence study among 8,000 white collar workers. J Occup Environ Med (accepted), 1999c.
32. Brisson C, Laflamme N, Moisan J, et al: Effect of family responsibilities and job strain on ambulatory blood pressure among white-collar women. Psychosomatic Medicine 61:205–213, 1999d.
32a. Brisson C, Laflamme N, Moisan J, et al: Job strain and blood pressure at rest: A cross-sectional study among 4000 white-collar women (submitted) 1999e.
33. Brisson C, Laflamme N, Vezina M: Job strain and blood pressure in a random population sample of women. Am J Industr Med (accepted), 1999a.
34. Brisson C, Larocque B, Laflamme N, et al: Les contraintes psychosociales chez les Canadiennes et les Canadiens. (submitted), 1999b.
35. Brugere D, Barrit J, Butat C, et al: Shiftwork, age, and health, an epidemiologic investigation. In J Occup Environ Health 3(Suppl 2):S15–S19, 1997.
36. Brunner EJ, Smith GD, Marmot MG, et al: Childhood social circumstances and psychosocial and behavioral factors as determinants of plasma fibrinogen. Lancet 347:1008–1013, 1996.
37. Buell P, Breslow L: Mortality from CHD in California men who work long hours. J Chron Dis 11:615–625, 1960.
38. Bursey R: A cardiovascular study of shift workers with respect to coronary artery disease risk factor prevalence. J Soc Occup Med 40:65–67, 1990.
39. Cahill J, Landsbergis PA: Job strain among post office mailhandlers. Int J Health Serv 26:731–750, 1996.
40. Carrere S, Evans GW, Palsane MN, Rivas M: Job strain and occupational stress among urban public transit operators. J Occup Psychol 64:305–316, 1991.
41. Cesana G, Ferrario M, Sega R, et al: Job strain and ambulatory blood pressure levels in a population-based employed sample of men from northern Italy. Scand J Work Environ Health 22:294–305, 1996.
42. Channer KS, Papouchado M, James MA, Rees JR: Anxiety and depression in patients with chest pain referred for exercise testing. Lancet 2:818–823, 1985.
43. Chapman A, Mandryk JA, Frommer MS, et al: Chronic perceived work stress and blood pressure among Australian government employees. Scand J Work Environ Health 16:258–269, 1990.
44. Chau N, Mallion J, de Gaudemaris R, et al: Twenty-four-hour ambulatory blood pressure in shift workers. Circulation 80:341–347, 1989.
45. Checkoway H, Pearce NE, Crawford-Brown DJ: Research Methods in Occupational Epidemiology. New York, Oxford University Press, 1989.
45a. Chen CJ, Chiou HY, Chiang MH, et al: Dose-response relationship between ischemic heart disease mortality and long-term arsenic exposure. Arterioscler Thromb Vasc Biol 16:504–510, 1996.
46. Corley KC, O'Shiel F, Mauck HP: Myocardial degeneration and cardiac arrest in squirrel monkeys. Physiologic and psychologic correlates. Psychophysiology 14:322–328, 1977.
47. Costa G: The problem: Shiftwork. Chronobiology International 14:89–98, 1997.
48. Costa G, Betta A, Uber D, Alexopoulos C: Estimate of coronary risk in a group of Italian shiftworkers. In Costa G, Cesana G, Kogi K, Wedderburn A (eds): Shiftwork: Health, Sleep, and Performance. New York, Peter Lang, 1990, pp 363–369.
49. Costa G, Lagorio S, Faggiano F: Mortalita per professione in Italia negli anni '80. Roma, ISPELS (Collana Quademi ISPELS no. 2), 1995.
50. Costrini AM, Pitt HA, Gustafson AB, Uddin DE: Cardiovascular and metabolic manifestations of heat stroke and severe heat exhaustion. Am J Med 66:296–302, 1979.
51. Cunningham SR, Dalzell GWN, McGirr P, Khan MM: Myocardial infarction and primary ventricular fibrillation after glue sniffing. Brit Med J 294:739, 1987.
52. Curtis AB, James SA, Raghunathan TE, Alcser KH: Job strain and blood pressure in African Americans: The Pitt County Study. Am J Public Health 97:1297–1302, 1997.
53. Danmarks Statistick: Dodelighed og erhverv 1970–75. Copenhagen, Danmarks Statistik, 1979.
54. Donaldson GC, Ermakov SP, Komarov YM, et al: Cold related mortalities and protection against cold in Yakutsk, eastern Siberia: Observation and interview study. BMJ 317:978–982, 1998.
55. Donaldson GC, Robinson D, Allaway SL: An analysis of arterial disease mortality and BUPA health screening data in men, in relation to outdoor temperature. Clin Sci (Colch) 92:261–268, 1997.
56. Drever F, Whitehead M, Roden M: Current patterns and trends in male mortality by social class (based on occupation). Population Trends 86:15–20, 1996.
57. Drexler H, Ulm K, Hardt R, et al: Carbon disulphide. IV. Cardiovascular function in workers in the viscose industry. Int Arch Occup Environ Health 69:27–32, 1996.
58. Dwyer EM, Turino GM: Carbon monoxide and cardiovascular disease. N Engl J Med 21:1474, 1989.
59. Eaker ED: Myocardial infarction and coronary death among women: Psychosocial predictors from a 20-years follow-up of women in the Framingham study. Am J Epidemiol 135:854–864, 1992.
60. Eaker ED: Psychosocial risk factors for coronary heart disease in women. Cardiology Clinics 16:103–111, 1998.
61. Edling C, Ohlson C-G, Ljungkvist G, et al: Cardiac arrhythmia in refrigerator repairmen exposed to fluorocarbons. Brit J Ind Med 47:207, 1990.

61a. Egan CE, Espie BH, McGrann S, et al: Acute effects of vibration on peripheral blood flow in healthy subjects. Occup Environ Med 53:663–669, 1996.

62. Egeland GM, Bloom TF, Schnorr TM, et al: Fluorocarbon 113 exposure and cardiac dysrhythmias among aerospace workers. AJIM 22:851–857, 1992.

63. Emdad R, Belkic K, Theorell T, Cizinsky S: What prevents professional drivers from following physicians' cardiologic advice? Psychoth Psychosom 67:226–240, 1998.

64. Emdad R, Belkic K, Theorell T, et al: Work environment, neurophysiologic and psychophysiologic models among professional drivers with and without cardiovascular disease: Seeking an integrative neurocardiologic approach. Stress Med 13:7–21, 1997.

65. European Heart Network: Social factors, work, stress and cardiovascular disease prevention in the European Union. Brussels, Belgium, The European Heart Network, 1998.

66. Eurowinter Group: Cold exposure and winter mortality from ischaemic heart, cerebrovascular disease, respiratory disease, and all causes in warm and cold regions of Europe. Lancet 349:1341–1346, 1997.

67. Everson SA, Lynch JW, Chesney MA, et al: Interaction of workplace demands and cardiovascular reactivity in progression of carotid atherosclerosis: Population based study. British Medical J 314:553–558, 1997.

68. Falger PRJ, Schouten EGW: Exhaustion, psychologic stress in the work environment and acute myocardial infarction in adult men. J Psychosom Res 36:777–786, 1992.

69. Falkeborn M, Persson I, Terent A, et al: Long-term trends in incidence and mortality from acute myocardial infarction and stroke in women: Analyses of total first events and of deaths in the Uppsala Health Care Region, Sweden. Epidemiology 7:67–74, 1996.

70. Fogari R, Zoppi A, Vanasia A, et al: Occupational noise exposure and blood pressure. J Hypertens 12:475–479, 1994.

71. Forsman L: Individual and group differences in psychophysiological responses to stress with emphasis on sympathetic-adrenal medullary and pituitary-adrenal cortical responses. Department of Psychology. Stockholm, University of Stockholm, 1983.

72. Frankenhaeuser M, Lundberg U, Fredriskson M, et al: Stress on and off the job as related to sex and occupational status in white-collar workers. J Organizational Behav 10:321–346, 1989.

73. Fraser GE: Preventive Cardiology. New York, Oxford University Press, 1986.

74. Fredriksson M, Sundin O, Frankenhaeuser M: Cortisol excretion during the defence reaction in humans. Psychosom Med 47:313–319, 1985.

75. Friedlander BR, Hearne FT: Epidemiological investigation of employees chronically exposed to methylene chloride. J Occup Med 20:657, 1978.

76. Friedman M, Rosenman RH, Carroll V: Changes in the serum cholesterol and blood clotting time in men subjected to cyclic variations of occupational stress. Circulation 17:852–861, 1958.

77. Garcia-Rubira JC, Aguilar J, Romero D: Acute myocardial infarction in a young man after heat exhaustion. Int J Cardiol 47:297–300, 1995.

78. Georges E, Wear ML, Mueller WH: Body fat distribution and job stress in Mexican-American men of the Hispanic Health and Nutrition Examination Survey. Am J Human Biol 4:657–667, 1992.

79. Goldblatt P: Longitudinal Study 1971–1981. Mortality and Social Organisation. London, Office of Population Censuses and Surveys (HMSO, Series LS no. 6), 1990.

80. Gordon N, Cleary P, Parker C, Czeisler C: The prevalence and health impact of shiftwork. Am J Pub Health 76:1225–1228, 1986.

80a. Goyer RA: Lead toxicity: Current concerns. Environ Health Perspect 100:177–187, 1993.

81. Green KL, Johnson JV: The effects of psychosocial work organization on patterns of cigarette smoking among male chemical plant employees. Am J Public Health 80:1368–1371, 1990.

82. Greenlund KJ, Liu K, Knox S, et al: Psychosocial work characteristics and cardiovascular disease risk factors in young adults: The CARDIA study. Coronary Artery Risk Disease in Young Adults. Soc Sci Med 41:717–723, 1995.

83. Haan MN: Job strain and ischaemic heart disease: An epidemiologic study of metal workers. Ann Clin Res 20:143–145, 1988.

84. Hall EM: Gender, work control and stress: A theoretical discussion and an empirical test. Int J Health Sci 19:725–745, 1989.

85. Hall EM: Double exposure: The combined impact of the home and work environments on psychosomatic strain in Swedish women and men. Int J Health Services 22:239–260, 1992.

86. Hall EM, Johnson JV, Tsou TS: Women, occupation, and risk of cardiovascular morbidity and mortality. Occup Med 8:709–719, 1993.

87. Hallqvist J, Diderichsen F, Theorell T, et al: The SHEEP Study Group: Is the effect of job strain on myocardial infarction due to interaction between high psychological demands and low decision latitude? Results from Stockholm Heart Epidemiology Program (SHEEP). Soc Sci Med 46:1405–1415, 1998.

88. Hammar M, Alfredsson L, Theorell T: Job characteristics and the incidence of myocardial infarction: A study of men and women in Sweden, with particular reference to job strain. Int J Epidemiol 23:277–284, 1994.

89. Hammar N, Alfredsson L, Smedberg M, Ahlbom A: Differences in the incidence of myocardial infarction among occupational groups. Scand J Work Environ Health 18:178–185, 1992.

90. Hansen ES: A cohort study on the mortality of firefighters. Brit J Ind Med 47:805, 1990.

91. Harenstam A, Theorell T: Work conditions and urinary excretion of catecholamines: A study of prison staff in Sweden. Scand J Work Environ Health 14:257–264, 1988.

92. Harma M: New work times are here—are we ready (editorial). Scand J Work Environ Health 24 Suppl 3:3–6, 1998.

93. Harma M: Individual differences in tolerance to shiftwork: A review. Ergonomics 35:101–109, 1993.

94. Hatt S: Gender, work and labour markets. Suffolk, Ipswich Book, 1997.

95. Hayashi T, Kobayashi Y, Yamaoka K, Yano E: Effect of overtime work on 24-hour ambulatory blood pressure. J Occup Environ Med 38:1007–1011, 1996.

96. Haynes SG: The effect of job demands, job control, and new technologies on the health of employed women. A review. In Frankenhaeuser M (ed): Women, Work, and Health: Stress and Opportunities. New York, Plenum Press, 1991, pp 157–169.

97. Haynes SG, Feinleib M: Women, work and coronary heart disease: Prospective findings from the Framingham Heart Study. Am J Public Health 70:133–141, 1980.

98. Hellerstedt WL, Jeffery RW: The association of job strain and health behaviours in men and women. Int J Epidemiol 26:575–583, 1997.

99. Hermann HJ, Rohde HG, Schulze W, et al: Effects of noise stress and ethanol intake on hearts of spontaneously hypertensive rats. Basic Res Cardiol 89:510–523.

100. Hernberg S: Evaluation of epidemiologic studies in assessing the long term effects of occupational noxious agents. Scand J Work Environ Health 6:163–169, 1980.

101. Hessel PA, Sluis-Cremer GK: Occupational noise exposure and blood pressure: Longitudinal and cross-sectional observations in a group of underground miners. Arch Environ Health 49:128–134, 1994.

102. Higgins M, Thom T: Trends in CHD in the United States. International Journal of Epidemiology 18:s58–s66, 1989.

103. Hlatky MA, Lam LC, Lee KL, et al: Job strain and the prevalence and outcome of coronary artery disease. Circulation 92:327–333, 1995.

104. Hobbesland A, Kjuus H, Thelle DS: Mortality from cardiovascular diseases and sudden death in ferroalloy patients. Scand J Work Environ Health 23:334–341, 1997.

105. Hogstedt C, Andersson K: A cohort study of mortality among dynamite workers. J Occup Med 21:553, 1979.

106. Hogstedt C, Axelson O: Mortality from cardio-cerebrovascular diseases among dynamite workers—an extended case-referent study. Ann Acad Med Singapore 13(Suppl 2):399–403, 1984.

107. House JS, Strecher V, Metzner HL, Robbins CA: Occupational stress and health among men and women in the Tecumseh Community Health Study. J Health Soc Beh 27:62–77, 1986.

108. Howard G, Goff D: A call for caution in the interpretation of the observed smaller relative importance of risk factors in the elderly. Ann Epidemiol 8:411–414, 1998.

109. Hulley SB, Cummings SR: Designing Clinical Research: An Epidemiologic Approach. Baltimore, Williams & Wilkins, 1988.

110. Ishizaki M, Tsuritani I, Noborisaka Y, et al: Relationship between job stress and plasma fibrinolytic activity in male Japanese workers. Int Arch Occup Environ Health 68:315–320, 1996.

111. Iwaski K, Sasaki T, Oka T, Hisanaga N: Effect of working hours on biological functions related to cardiovascular system among salesmen in a machinery manufacturing company. Ind Health 36:361–367, 1998.

112. Jankovic J, et al: Environmental study of firefighters. Ann Occup Hyg 35:581–602.

113. Johansson G, Johnson JV, Hall EM: Smoking and sedentary behavior as related to work organization. Soc Sci Med 32:837–846, 1991.

114. Johnson JV, Hall EM: Job strain, workplace social support, and cardiovascular disease: A cross-sectional study of a random sample of the Swedish working population. Am J Public Health 78:1336–1342, 1988.

115. Johnson JV, Hall EM, Theorell T: Combined effects of job strain and social isolation on cardiovascular disease morbidity and mortality in a random sample of the Swedish male working population. Scand J Work Environ Health 15:271–279, 1989.

116. Johnson JV, Stewart W, Hall EM, et al: Long-term psychosocial work environment and cardiovascular mortality among Swedish men. Am J Public Health 86:324–331, 1996.

117. Jones F, Bright JEH, Searle B, Cooper L: Modelling occupational stress and health: The impact of the demand-control model on academic research and on workplace practice. Stress Med 14:231–236, 1998.

118. Kaplan GA, Keil JE: Socioeconomic factors and CVD: A review of the literature. Circulation 88:1973–1998, 1993.

119. Karasek R, Baker D, Marxer F, Ahlbom A, Theorell T: Job decision latitude, job demands, and cardiovascular disease: A prospective study of Swedish men. Am J Public Health 71:694–705, 1981.

120. Karasek R, Brisson C, Kawakami N, et al: The Job Content Questionnaire (JCQ): An instrument for internationally comparative assessments of psychosocial job characteristics. J Occup Health Psychology 3:322–355, 1998.

121. Karasek R, Gardell B, Lindell J: Work and nonwork correlates of illness and behaviour in male and female Swedish white collar workers. J Occup Behav 8:187–207, 1987.

122. Karasek R, Theorell T: Healthy Work: Stress, Productivity, and the Reconstruction of Working Life. New York, Basic Books, 1990.

123. Karasek RA: Job demands, job decision latitude and mental strain: Implications for job redesign. Adm Sci Q 24:285–308, 1979.

124. Karasek RA, Theorell T, Schwartz JE, et al: Job characteristics in relation to the prevalence of myocardial infarction in the U.S. Health Examination Survey and the Health and Nutrition Examination Survey. Am J Public Health 78:910–918, 1988.

124a. Kaski JC, Crea F, Meran D, et al: Local coronary supersensitivity to diverse vasoconstrictive stimuli in patients with variant angina. Circulation 74:1255–1265, 1986.

125. Kasl SV: The influence of the work environment on cardiovascular health: A historical, conceptual, and methodological perspective. J Occup Health Psychol 1:42–56, 1996.

126. Kaufman JD, Silverstein MA, Moure-Eraso R: Atrial fibrillation and sudden death related to occupational solvent exposure. Am J Ind Med 25:731–735, 1994.

127. Kawachi I, Colditz G, Stampfer M, et al: Prospective study of shift work and risk of coronary heart disease in women. Circulation 92:3178–3183, 1995.

128. Kawachi I, Kennedy BP: Health and social cohesion: Why care about income inequality? Br Med J 314:1037–1040, 1997.

129. Kawachi I, Kennedy BP, Lochner K, Prothrow-Stith D: Social capital, income inequality, and mortality. Am J Public Health 87:1491–1498, 1997.

130. Kawakami N, Haratani T, Araki S: Job strain and arterial blood pressure, serum cholesterol, and smoking as risk factors for coronary heart disease in Japan. Int Arch Occup Environ Health 71:429–432, 1998.

131. Kawakami N, Kobayahi F, Araki S, et al: Assessment of job stress dimensions based on the job demands—Control model of employees of telecommunications and electric power companies in Japan: Reliability and validity of the Japanese version of the Job Content Questionnaire. Int J Behav Med 2:358–375, 1995.

132. Kleinman MT, Leaf DA, Kelly E, et al: Urban angina in the mountains: Effects of carbon monoxide and mild hypoxemia on subjects with chronic stable angina. Arch Environ Health 53:388–397, 1998.

133. Knox S, Theorell T, Svensson J, Waller D: The relation of social support and working environment to medical variables associated with elevated BP in young males: A structural model. Soc Sci Med 21:525–531, 1985.

134. Knutsson A, et al: Shiftwork and myocardial infarction: A case-control study. Occup Environ Med 56:46–50, 1999.

135. Knutsson A, Akerstedt T: The healthy-worker effect: Self-selection among Swedish shift workers. Work and Stress 6:163–167, 1992.

136. Knutsson A, Akerstedt T, Jonsson BG, Orth-Gomer K: Increased risk of ischaemic heart disease in shift workers. Lancet 8498:89–92, 1986.

137. Knutsson A, Akerstedt T, Jonsson B: Prevalence of risk factors for coronary artery disease among day and shift workers. Scand J Work Environ Health 14:317–321, 1988.

138. Knutsson A, Andersson H, Berglund U: Serum lipoprotein in day and shift workers: A prospective study. Br J Ind Med 47:132–134, 1990.

139. Knutsson A, Nilsson T: Tobacco use and exposure to environmental tobacco smoke in relation to certain work characteristics. Scand J Soc Med 26:183–189, 1998.

140. Koller M: Health risks related to shift work. An example of time-contingent effects of long-term stress. Int Arch Occup Environ Health 53:59–75, 1983.

141. Koskela RS: Cardiovascular diseases among foundry workers exposed to carbon monoxide. Scand J Work Environ Health 20:286–293, 1994.

142. Kosteva K: Study of the cardiovascular effects of occupational exposure to organic solvents. Int Arch Occup Environ Health 71(Suppl):S87–91, 1998.

143. Kristensen TS: The demand-control-support model: Methodological challenges for future research. Stress Medicine 11:17–26, 1995.

144. Kristensen TS: Job stress and CVD: A theoretic critical review. J Occup Health Psychol 1:246–260, 1996.

145. Kristensen TS, Kronitzer M, Alfredsson L: Social factors, work, stress and cardiovascular disease prevention. Brussels, The European Heart Network, 1998.

146. Kunst AE, Looman CWN, Mackenbach JP: Socioeconomic mortality differences in the Netherlands in 1950–1984: A regional study of cause specific mortality. Soc Sci Med 31:141–152, 1990.

147. Kuo HW, Lai JA, Lin M, Su ES: Effects of exposure to carbon disulfide (CS2) on electrocardiographic features of ischemic heart disease among viscose rayon factory workers. Int Arch Occup Environ Health 70:61–66, 1997.

148. LaCroix A, Haynes SG: Occupational exposure to high demand/low control work and coronary heart disease incidence in the Framingham cohort. Am J Epidemiol 120:481, 1984.

149. Laflamme N, Brisson C, Moisan J, et al: Job strain and ambulatory blood pressure among female white-collar workers. Scand J Work Environ Health 24:334–343, 1998.

150. Landrigan PJ: Toxicity of lead at low dose. Brit J Ind Med 46:593, 1989.

151. Landsbergis PA, Schnall PL, Deitz DK, et al: Job strain and health behaviors: Resuls of a prospective study. Am J Health Promo 12:237–245, 1998.

152. Landsbergis PA, Schnall PL, Warren K, et al: Association between ambulatory blood pressure and alternative formulations of job strain. Scand J Work Environ Health 20:349–363, 1994.

153. Landsbergis PA, Schurman SJ, Israel BA, et al: Job stress and heart disease: Evidence and strategies for prevention. New Solutions Summer:42–58, 1993.

154. Lantigna LJ, Sprafkin RP, Mc Croskery JH, et al: One-year psychosocial follow-up of patients with chest pain and angiographically normal coronary arteries. Am J Cardiol 62:209–213, 1988.

155. Larfargues G, Sylvaine V, Caces B, et al: Relations among night work, dietary habits, biological measures, and health status. Int J Behav Med 3:123–134, 1996.

156. Larocque B, Brisson C, Blanchette C: Coherence interne, validite factorielle et validite discriminante de la traduction francaise des echelles de demande psychologique et de latitude decisionnelle de "Job Content Questionnaire" de Karasek. Revue d'epidemiologie et de sante publique 46:371–381, 1998.

157. Le Bourdais C, Hamel PJ, Bernard P: Le travail et l'ouvrage. Charge et partage des taches domestiques chez les couples quebecois. Sociologie et Societes 19:37–55, 1987.

158. Lee IM, Paffenbarger RS Jr, Hennenkens CH: Pysical activity, physical fitness, and longevity. Aging (Milano) 9:2–11, 1997.

159. Light KC, Turner JR, Hinderliter AL: Job strain and ambulatory work blood pressure in healthy young men and women. Hypertension 20:214–218, 1992.

160. Lundberg U, Mardberg B, Frankenhaeuser M: The total workload of male and female white-collar workers as related to age, occupational level, and number of children. Scand J Psychol 35:315–317, 1994.

161. Loudoun RJ, Bohle PL: Work/non-work conflict and health in shiftwork: Relationships with family status and social support. Int J Occup Environ Health 3(Suppl 2):S71–S77, 1997.

162. Lown B: Role of higher nervous activity in sudden cardiac death. Jpn Circ J 54:581–602, 1990.

163. Lundberg U: Work and stress in women. In Orth-Gomer K, Chesney M, Wenger N (eds): Women, Stress, and Heart Disease. Mahwah, NJ, Lawrence Erlbaum Associates, 1998, pp 41–56.

164. Lynch J, Krause N, Kaplan GA, et al: Workplace demands, economic reward and progression of carotid atherosclerosis. Circulation 96:302–307, 1997a.

165. Lynch J, Krause N, Kaplan GA, et al: Work place conditions, socioeconomic status, and the risk of mortality and acute myocardial infarction: The Kuopio Ischemic Heart Disease Risk Factor Study. Am J Public Health 87:617–622, 1997b.

166. MacMahon S, Peto R, Cutler J, et al: Blood pressure, stroke, and CHD. Part 1, Prolonged differences in blood pressure: Prospective observational studies corrected for the regression dilution. Lancet 335:765–774, 1990.

167. Marin R: Occupational Mortality 1971–80. Helsinki, Tilastokeskus, 1986.

168. Mark DB, Lam LC, Lee KL, et al: Identification of patients with coronary disease at high risk for loss of employment. A prospective validation study. Circulation 86:1485–1494, 1992.

169. Marmot MG, Bosma H, Hemingway H, et al: Contribution of job control and other risk factors to social variations in coronary heart disease incidence. Lancet 350:235–239, 1997.

170. Marmot MG, Shipley MJ, Rose G: Inequalities in death—specific explanations of a general pattern. Lancet i:1003–1006, 1984.

171. McCammon CS, Wells VE, Glaser RA, et al: Worker exposure to methylene chloride during furniture stripping as determined by air, breath and blood samples. J Applied Ind Hyg, 1991.

172. McNamee R, Binks K, Jones S, et al: Shiftwork and mortality from ischaemic heart disease. Occ Env Med 53:367–373, 1996.

173. Melamed S, Ben-Avi I, Luz J, Green MS: Repetitive work, work underload and coronary heart disease risk factors among blue-collar workers—the CORDIS Study. Cardiovascular Occupational Risk Factors Determination in Israel. J Psychosomatic Research 39:19–29, 1995.

174. Melamed S, Froom P, Kristal-Boneh E, et al: Industrial noise exposure, noise annoyance, and serum lipid levels in blue-collar workers—the CORDIS Study. Arch Environ Health 52:292–298, 1997.

175. Menotti A, Seccareccia F: Physical activity at work and job responsibility as risk factors for fatal coronary heart disease and other causes of death. J Epidemiol Commun Health 39:325–329, 1985.

176. Mensch BS, Kandel DB: Do job conditions influence the use of drugs? J Health Soc Behav 29:169–184, 1988.

177. Meulders D, Plasman R, Vander Stricht V: Position of women in the labour market in the European community. Aldershot, Darmouth Publishing Company, 1998.

178. Moller L, Kristensen TS: Plasma fibrinogen and ischaemic heart disease risk factors. Arteriosclerosis and Thrombosis 11:344–350, 1991.

179. Morehouse RL: Shiftwork: The special challenges for women. AAOHN J 43:532–535, 1995.

180. Muntaner C, Nieto FJ, Cooper L, et al: Work organization and atherosclerosis: Findings from the ARIC study. Artherosclerosis Risk in Communities. Am J Prev Med 14:9–18, 1998.

181. Murphy LR: Job dimensions associated with severe disability due to CVD. J Clin Epidemiol 44:155–166, 1991.

182. Nachreimer F: Individual and social determinants of shiftwork tolerance. Scand J Work Environ Health 24 Suppl 3:35–42, 1998.

183. Nakamura K, Shimai S, Kikuchi S, et al: Shift work and risk factors for coronary heart disease in Japanese blue-collar workers: Serum lipids and anthropometric characteristics. Occup Med 47:142–146, 1999.

184. National Health Statistics: Occupational Health Decennial Supplement, series DS no. 10. London, Her Majesty's Stationary Office, 1995.

185. Netterstrom B, Juel K: Impact of work-related and psychosocial factors on the development of ischemic heart disease among urban bus drivers in Denmark. Scand J Work Environ Health 14:231–238, 1988.

186. Netterstrom B, Kristensen TS, Damsgaard MT, et al: Job strain and cardiovascular risk factors: A cross-sectional study of employed Danish men and women. Br J Ind Med 48:684–689, 1991.

187. Netterstrom B, Suadicani P: Self-assessed job satisfaction and ischemic heart disease mortality: A 10-year follow-up of urban bus drivers. Int J Epidemiol 22:51–56, 1993.

188. Niedhammer I, Bugel I, Goldberg M, et al: Psychosocial factors at work and sickness absence in the Gazel cohort: A prospective study. Occup Environ Med 55:735–741, 1998.

189. NIOSH: NIOSH Alert Request for Assistance in Preventing Death from Excessive Exposure to Chlorofluorocarbon 113 (CFC-113). Cincinnati, OH, U.S. Department of Health and Human Services, Public Health Service, Centers for Disease and Prevention Control, National Institute for Occupational Safety and Health, Publication No. 89-109, 1989.

190. Nordic Statistical Secretariat: Occupational Mortality in the Nordic Countries 1971–1980. Copenhagen, Statistical Reports of the Nordic Countries, 1988.

191. Notkola V, Pajunene A, Leino-Arjas P: Occupational mortality by cause in Finland 1971–1991 and occupational mobility. Helsinki, Statistics Finland, Health:1, 1997.

192. Nurminen M, Hernberg S: Effects of intervention on the cardiovascular mortality of workers exposed to carbon disulfide: A 15 year follow up. Brit J Ind Med 42:32–35, 1985.

193. OCDE (Organization de cooperation et de developpement economiques): Eco-Sante, version 1.5., 1993.

194. OCDE (Organization de cooperation et de la developpement economiques): L'avenir des professions a predominance feminine. Paris, Organisation de cooperation et de developpement economiques, 1998.

195. Ockene IS, Shaw MJ, Alpert JS, et al: Unexplained chest pain in patients with normal coronary arteriograms. N Engl J Med 303:1249–1252, 1980.

196. Office of Population Censuses and Surveys: Occupational mortality 1979–80, 1982–83. Great Britain. Decennial Supplement. London, Her Majesty's Stationary Office, 1986.

196a. Omae K, Takebayashi T, Nomiyama T, et al: Cross-sectional observation of the effects of carbon disulphide on artriosclerosis in rayon manufacturing workers. Occup Environ Med 55: 1998.

197. Orth-Gomer K: Psychosocial risk factor profile in women with CHD. In Orth-Gomer K, Chesney M, Wenger N (eds): Women, Stress, and Heart Disease. Mahwah, NJ, Lawrence Erlbaum Associates, 1998, pp 25–38.

198. Ott MG, Skory LK, Holder BB, et al: Health evaluation of employees occupationally exposed to methylene chloride: Mortality. Scand J Work Environ Health 9(Suppl 8), 1983.

199. Pasceri V, Lanza GA, Buffon A, et al: Role of abnormal pain sensitivity and behavioral factors in determining chest pain in Syndrome X. J Am Coll Cardiol 31:62–66, 1998.

200. Pasternak RC, Thibault GE, Svoia M, et al: Chest pain with angiographically insignificant coronary arterial obstruction. Clinical presentation and long-term follow-up. Am J Med 68:813–817, 1980.
201. Perloff D, Sokolow M, Cowan RM, Juster RP: Prognostic value of ambulatory blood pressure measurements: Further analyses. J Hypertens 7 Suppl 3:S3–S10, 1989.
202. Peter R, Alfredsson L, Hammar N, et al: High effort, low reward and cardiovascular risk factors in employed Swedish men and women: Baseline results from the WOLF study. J Epidemiol Community Health 52:540–547, 1998.
203. Peter R, Alfredsson L, Knutsson A, et al: Is a stressful psychosocial work environment mediating the effects of shiftwork on cardiovascular risk factors in men? Scand J Work Environ Health (accepted for publication), 1999a.
204. Peter R, Hallqvist J, Reuterwall C, et al: The SHEEP Study Group: Psychosocial work environment and myocardial infarction: Improving risk prediction by combining two alternative job stress models in the SHEEP Study. (Submitted), 1999b.
205. Peter R, Siegrist J: Chronic work stress, sickness absence, and hypertension in middle managers: General and specific sociological explanations? Social Sci Med 45:1111–1120, 1997.
206. Pickering TG: Job strain and the prevalence and outcome of coronary artery disease [letter; comment]. Circulation 94:1138–1139, 1996.
207. Pickering TG: White coat hypertension. In Laragh JH, Brenner BM (eds): Hypertension: Pathophysiology, Diagnosis, and Management. New York, Raven Press, Ltd., 1995, pp 1913–1927.
208. Pickering TG: Should studies of patients undergoing coronary angiography be used to evaluate the role of behavioral risk factors for coronary heart disease? J Behav Med 8:203–213, 1985.
209. Pieper C, LaCroix AZ, Karasek RA: The relation of psychosocial dimensions of work with coronary heart disease risk factors: A meta-analysis of five United States data bases. Am J Epidemiol 129:483–494, 1989.
210. Pieper C, Warren K, Pickering TG: A comparison of ambulatory blood pressure and heart rate at home and work on work and non-work days. J Hypertens 11:177–183, 1993.
211. Price B, Bergman TS, Rodriguez M, et al: A review of carbon disulfide exposure data and the association between carbon disulfide exposure and ischemic heart disease mortality. Reg Toxicol Pharmacol 26:119–128, 1997.
212. Reference deleted.
213. Prunier-Poulmaire S, Gadbois C, Volkoff S: Combined effects of shift systems and work requirements on customs officers. Scand J Work Environ Health 24 suppl 3:134–140, 1998.
214. Ragland DR, Greiner BA, Holman BL, Fisher JM: Hypertension and years of driving in transit vehicle operators. Scand J Soc Med 25:271–279, 1997.
215. Ragland DR, Helmer DC, Seeman TE: Patient selection factors in angiographic studies: A conceptual formulation and empirical test. J Behav Med 14:541–553, 1991.
216. Rasnsson V: Mortality from ischemic heart disease in Iceland, 1951–1985. Ann Epidemiol 1:493–503, 1991.
217. Redmond CK, Gustin J, Kamon E: Long-term mortality experience of steelworkers. VIII. Mortality patterns of open hearth steelworkers (a preliminary report). J Occup Med 17:40–43, 1975.
218. Reed DM, LaCroix AZ, Karasek RA, et al: Occupational strain and the incidence of coronary heart disease. Am J Epidemiol 129:495–502, 1989.
219. Reeder BA, Lui L, Horlick L: Sociodemographic variation in the prevalence of cardiovascular disease in Saskatchewan: Results from the Saskatchewan Heart Health Survey. Can J Cardiol 12:271–277, 1996.
220. Reinhardt CF, et al: Cardiac arrhythmias and aerosol sniffing. Arch Environ Health 22:265, 1971.
221. Repace JL, Jinot J, Bayard S, Emmons K, Hammond SK: Air nicotin and saliva cotinine as indicators of workplace passive smoking exposure and risk. Risk Anal 18:71–83, 1998.
221a. Rodger JC, Railton R, Parekh P, Newman P: Effects of cold stimulation on myocardial perfusion: An investigation using thallium-201 scintigraphy. Br Heart J 52:57–62, 1984.
222. Romon M, Nuttens M, Fievet C, et al: Increased triglyceride levels in shift workers. Am J Med 93:259–262, 1992.
223. Rosengren A, Anderson K, Wilhelmsen L: Risk of coronary heart disease in middle-aged male bus and tram drivers compared to men in other occupations: A prospective study. Int J Epidemiol 20:82–87, 1991.
224. Russek HI, Zohman BL: Relative significance of heredity, diet, and occupational stress in coronary heart disease of young adults. Am J Med Sci 235:266–275, 1958.
224a. Santé Canada: Les maladies cardio-vasculaires et les accidents vasculaires cérébraux au Canada. Santé Canada, Direction générale de la protection de la santé-Laboratoire de lutte contre la maladie, 1997.
225. Sauli H: Occupational Mortality 1971–75. Helsinki, Tilastokeskus, 1979.
226. Schnall PL, Landsbergis PA, Baker D: Job strain and CVD. Annu Rev Public Health 15:381–411, 1994.
227. Schnall PL, Landsbergis PA, Schwartz J, et al: A longitudinal study of job strain and ambulatory blood pressure: Results from a 3-year follow-up. Psychosom Med 60:697–706, 1998.
228. Schnall PL, Pieper C, Schwartz JE, et al: The relationship between "job strain," workplace diastolic blood pressure, and left ventricular mass index. Results of a case-control study [published erratum appears in JAMA 1992 Mar 4;267(9):1209]. JAMA 263:1929–1935, 1990.
228a. Schnall PL, et al: Relation between job strain, alcohol, and ambulatory BP. Hypertension 19:488–494, 1992.
229. Schwartz JE, Pieper C, Karasek RA: A procedure for linking psychosocial job characteristic data to health surveys. Am J Public Health 78:904–909, 1988.
230. Sheldahl LM, Wilke NA, Sougherty S, Tristani FE: Cardiac responses to combined moderate heat and exercise in men with coronary artery disease. Am J Cardiol 70:186–191, 1992.
231. Reference deleted.
232. Shively CA, Clarkson TB: Social status and coronary artery atherosclerosis in female monkeys. Arterioscler Thromb 14:721–726, 1994.
233. Siegrist J: Adverse health effects of high-effort/low-reward conditions. J Occup Health Psychol 1:27–41, 1996.
234. Siegrist J: Threat to social status and cardiovascular risk. Psychotherapy and Psychosomatics 42:90–96, 1984.

235. Siegrist J, Matschinger H, Cremer P, Seidel D: Atherogenic risk in men suffering from occupational stress. Atherosclerosis 69:211–218, 1988.
236. Siegrist J, Peter R: Job stressors and coping characteristics in work-related disease: Issues of validity. Work & Stress 8:130–140, 1994.
237. Siegrist J, Peter R, Cremer P, Seidel D: Chronic work stress is associated with atherogenic lipids and elevated fibrinogens in middle aged men. Journal of Internal Medicine 242:149–156, 1997.
238. Siegrist J, Peter R, Georg W, et al: Psychosocial and biobehavioral characteristics of hypertensive men with elevated atherogenic lipids. Atherosclerosis 86:211–218, 1991.
239. Siegrist J, Peter R, Junge A, et al: Low status control, high effort at work and ischaemic heart disease: Prospective evidence from blue collar men. Social Science & Medicine 31:1127–1134, 1990.
240. Siegrist J, Peter R, Motz W, Strauer BE: The role of hypertension, left ventricular hypertrophy and psychosocial risks in cardiovascular disease: Prospective evidence from blue-collar men. Eur Heart J 13 Suppl D:89–95, 1992.
240a. Sierra Pajares Ortiz M, Diaz Jimenez H, Montero Rubio JC, et al: Daily mortality in the Madrid community during 1986–1991 for 45- to 64-year-olds: Relationship to air temperature. Rev Esp Salud Publica 2:149–160, 1997.
241. Sihm I, Delholm G, Hansen ES, et al: The psychosocial work environment of younger men surviving acute myocardial infarction. European Heart Journal 12:203–209, 1991.
242. Skipper J, Jung F, Coffey L: Nurses and shiftwork: Effects on physical health and mental depression. J Advanced Nursing 15:835–842, 1990.
243. Sokejima S, Kagamimori S: Working hours as a risk factor for acute myocardial infarction in Japan: Case-control study. Brit Med J 317:775–780, 1998.
244. Speizer FE, Wegman DH, Ramirez A: Palpitation rates associated with fluorocarbon exposure in a hospital setting. N Engl J Med 292:624, 1975.
244a. Stayner LT, A.L. D, Thun M, et al: Cardiovascular mortality among workers exposed to nitroglycerin and dinitrotoluene. Scand J Work Environ Health 18:34–43, 1992.
245. Steenland K, Deddens J, Salvan A, Stayner L: Negative bias in exposure-response trends in occupational studies: Modeling the healthy worker survivor effect. Am J Epidemiol 143:202–210, 1996.
246. Steenland K, Fine L: Shift work, shift change, and risk of death from heart disease at work. Am J Ind Med 29:278–281, 1996.
247. Steenland K, Johnson J, Nowlin S: A follow-up study of job strain and heart disease among males in the NHANES1 population. Am J Ind Med 31:256–259, 1997.
247a. Steenland K, Piacitelli L, Deddens J, et al: Cancer, heart disease, and diabetes in workers exposed to 2,3,7,8-tetrochlorodibenzo-p-dioxin. J Nat Cancer Inst 91:779–786, 1999.
248. Steptoe A, Cropley M, Joekes K: Job strain, blood pressure and response to uncontrollable stress. J Hypertens 17:193–200, 1999.
249. Steptoe A, Roy MP, Evans O, Snashall D: Cardiovascular stress reactivity and job strain as determinants of ambulatory blood pressure at work. J Hypertension 13:201–210, 1995.
249a. Stern FB, Halperin WE, Hornung RW, et al: Heart disease mortality among bridge and tunnel officers exposed to carbon monoxide. Am J Epidemiol 128:1276–1288, 1988.
249b. Staessen JA, Roels S, Lauwerys RR, Amery A: Low-level lead exposure and blood pressure. J Hum Hypertens 9:303–328, 1995.
250. Sternberg H, Rosenthal T, Shamiss A, Green M: Altered circadian rhythm of blood pressure in shift workers. J Hum Hypertens 9:349–353, 1995.
251. Suurnakki T, Ilmarinen J, Wagar G, et al: Municipal employees' cardiovascular diseases and occupational stress factors in Finland. Int Arch Occup Environ Health 59:107–114, 1987.
251a. Swaen GM, Braun C, Slangen JJ: Mortality of Dutch workers exposed to carbon disulfide. Int Arch Occup Environ Health 66:103–110, 1994.
251b. Sweetnam PM, Taylor SW, Elwood PS: Exposure to carbon disulphide and ischaemic heart disease in a viscose rayon factory. Br J Ind Med 44:220–227, 1987.
251c. Taggart P, et al: Cardiac responses to thermal, physical, and emotional stress. Br Med J 3:71–76, 1972.
252. Tarumi K, Hagihara A, Morimoto K: An inquiry into the relationship between job strain and blood pressure in male white-collar workers. Jpn J Ind Health 35:269–276, 1993.
253. Taylor P: A comparison of sickness absence, lateness, and other absence behavior in an oil refinery from 1962–1965. Brit J Ind Med 24:93–102, 1967.
254. Taylor P, Pocock S: Mortality of shift and day workers 1956–1968. Brit J Ind Med 29:201–207, 1972.
255. Tenkanen L, Sjoblom T, Harma M: Joint effect of shift work and adverse life-style factors on the risk of coronary heart disease. Scand J Work Environ Health 24:351–357, 1998.
256. Tenkanen L, Sjoblom T, Kalimo R, et al: Shift work, occupation, and coronary heart disease over 6 years of follow-up in the Helsinki Heart Study. Scand J Work Environ Health 23:257–265, 1997.
257. Theorell T: Family history of hypertension—an individual trait interacting with spontaneously occuring job stressors. Scand J Work Environ Health 16 Suppl 1:74–79, 1990.
258. Theorell T, Ahlberg-Hulten G, Jodko M, et al: Influence of job strain and emotion on blood pressure in female hospital personnel during work hours. Scand J Work Environ Health 19:313–318, 1993.
259. Theorell T, de Faire U, Johnson J, et al: Job strain and ambulatory blood pressure profiles. Scand J Work Environ Health 17:380–385, 1991b.
259a. Theorell J, et al: The effects of the strain of returning to work on the risk of cardiac death after an MI before age 45. Int J Cardiol 30:61–67, 1991.
260. Theorell T, Hamsten A, de Faire U, et al: Psychosocial work conditions before myocardial infarction in young men. International Journal of Cardiology 15:33–46, 1987.

261. Theorell T, Karasek R: Current issues relating to psychosocial job strain and cardiovascular disease research. Journal of Occupational Health Psychology 1:9–26, 1996.
262. Theorell T, Knox S, Svensson J, Waller D: Blood pressure variation during a working day at age 28: Effects of different types of work on blood pressure level at age 18. J Human Stress 2:36–41, 1985.
263. Theorell T, Perski A, Akerstedt T, et al: Changes in job strain in relation to changes in physiological states—a longitudinal study. Scand J Work Environ Health 14:189–196, 1988.
264. Theorell T, Rahe RH: Behavior and life satisfactions of Swedish subjects with myocardial infarction. J Chron Dis 25:139–147, 1972.
265. Theorell T, Tsutsumi A, Hallqvist J, et al: SHEEP Study Group. Decision latitude, job strain and myocardial infarction. Am J Public Health 88:382–388, 1998.
266. Thomas JT, Epstein FH: Heart disease, cancer, and stroke mortality trends and their interrelations. An international perspective. Circulation 90:574–582, 1994.
267. Thompson SJ: Review: Extraaural health effects of chronic noise exposure in humans. Schriftenr Ver Wasser Boden Lufthyg 88:91–117.
268. Trout D, Decker J, Mueller C, et al: Exposure of casino employees to environmental tobacco smoke. J Occup Environ Med 40:270–276, 1998.
269. Tüchsen F: Stroke morbidity in professional drivers in Denmark 1981–1990. Int J Epidemiol 26:989–994, 1997.
270. Tüchsen F: Working hours and ischaemic heart disease in Danish men: A 4-year cohort study of hospitalization. Int J Epidemiol 22:215–221, 1993.
271. Tüchsen F, Andersen O, Costa G, et al: Occupation and ischemic heart disease in the European Community: A comparative study of occupations at potential high risk. Am J Ind Med 30:407–414, 1996.
272. Tüchsen F, Bach E, Marmot M: Occupation and hospitalization with ischaemic heart disease: A new nation wide surveillance system based on hospital admissions. Int J Epidemiol 21:450–459, 1992.
273. Tüchsen F, Endahl LA: Increasing inequality in ischaemic heart disease morbidity among employed men in Denmark 1981–1993: The need for a new preventive policy. Int J Epidemiol 28:640–644, 1999.
274. Uehata T: Long working hours and occupational stress-related cardiovascular attacks among middle-aged workers in Japan. J Human Ergol 20:147–153, 1991.
275. van Amelsvoort LGPM: Coronary heart disease among truck drivers. Report of the International Workshop on the Epidemiology of CHD among European Truck Drivers. Bilthoven, European Commission, 1995.
276. van Egeren LF: The relationship between job strain and blood pressure at work, at home, and during sleep. Psychosom Med 54:337–343, 1992.
277. Vanhoorne M, De Bacquer D, De Backer G: Epidemiological study of the cardiovascular effects of carbon disulphide. Int J Epidemiol 21:745–752, 1992.
278. Volmink JA, Newton JN, Hicks NR, et al: Coronary event and case fatality rates in an English population: Results of the Oxford myocardial infarction incidence study. Heart 80:40–44, 1998.
279. Waddell VP, Holman CD, Armstrong BK, et al: Variation in hospital morbidity in the male workforce of Western Australia. Br J Ind Med 45:139–147, 1988.
280. Wamala SP, Wolk A, Orth-Gomer K: Determinants of obesity in relation to socioeconomic status among middle-aged Swedish women. Preventive Med 26:734–744, 1997.
281. Weinberg C: Toward a clearer definition of confounding. Am J Epidemiol 137:1–8, 1993.
282. Wenger NK: Cardiovascular disease in the elderly and in women. In Goldman L, Braunwald E (eds): Primary Cardiology. Philadelphia, WB Saunders, Co., 1998, pp 70–81.
283. Westman M, Eden D, Shirom A: Job stress, cigarette smoking and cessation: The conditioning effects of peer support. Soc Sci Med 20:637–644, 1985.
284. Whaley MH, Blair SN: Epidemiology of physical activity, physical fitness, and coronary heart disease. J Cardiovasc Risk 2:289–295, 1995.
285. Wickramatillake HD, Gun RT, Ryan P: Carbon monoxide exposures in Australian workplaces could precipitate myocardial ischaemia in smoking workers with coronary artery disease. Aust N Z Public Health 22 (Suppl 3):389–393, 1998.
286. Wilcosky TC, Simonsen NR: Solvent exposure and cardiovascular disease. Am J Ind Med 19:569–586, 1991.
287. Wilcosky TC, Tyroler HA: Mortality from heart disease among workers exposed to solvents. J Occup Med 25:879, 1983.
288. Wild P, Moulin JJ, Ley FX, Schaffer P: Mortality from cardiovascular diseases among potash miners exposed to heat. Epidemiology 6:243–247, 1995.
289. Wilkinson R: How can secular improvements in life expectancy be explained? In Blane D, Brunner E, Wilkinson R (eds): Health and Social Organization. London, Routledge, 1996, pp 109–122.
289a. Willich SN, Lewis M, Lowel H, et al: Physical exertion as a trigger of myocardial infarction. Triggers and mechanisms of myocardial infarction study group. N Engl J Med 329:1684–1690, 1993.
290. Wing S, Dargent-Molina P, Casper M, et al: Changing association between community structure and ischaemic heart disease mortality in the United States. Lancet 2:1067–1070, 1987.
291. Winkleby MA, Ragland DR, Fisher JM, Syme SL: Excess risk of sickness and disease in bus drivers: A review and synthesis of epidemiological studies. Int J Epidemiol 17:255–262, 1988.
292. Winkleby MA, Ragland DR, Syme SL: Self-reported stressors and hypertension: Evidence of an inverse association. Am J Epidemiol 127:124–134, 1988.
293. Wright EO, Shire K, Hwang S-L, et al: The non-effects of class on the gender division of labor in the home: A comparative study of Sweden and the United States. Gender & Society 6:252–282, 1992.
294. Yamasaki F, Schwartz JE, Gerber LM, et al: Impact of shift work and race/ethnicity on the diurnal rhythm of blood pressure and catecholamines. Hypertension 32:417–423, 1998.
295. Zhao YM, Zhang SZ, Selvin S, Spear RC: A dose response relation for noise induced hypertension. Br J Ind Med 48:179–184.

STRESSORS AT THE WORKPLACE: THEORETICAL MODELS

A HISTORICAL OVERVIEW   *by Lennart Levi, MD, PhD*

To create knowledge about occupational stressors, stress, and health, we need to study: the stressors (at the workplace and elsewhere); the way they are experienced, interpreted, and appraised by the exposed person; the way he or she is "programmed" by genetic factors and earlier environmental influences; resulting pathogenic reactions; various (e.g., cardiovascular) outcomes of these reactions, in terms of morbidity, and their interaction with and feedback to other components of the system; and interacting variables (e.g., coping repertoire, social support) that could modify these processes.

Briefly, then, we need to study over time the whole person interacting with his or her whole environment. A conceptual model of such a worker-workplace ecosystem can serve as a basis for research approaches as well as for therapeutic and preventive interventions[108,137,143] (Fig. 1).

The phenomenon of psychosocially mediated, stress-related ill health is, of course, in no way new to humankind.[264] Our early ancestors no doubt confronted acute and chronic physical and other stressors and attracted some of the diseases we know today. Theological explanations frequently were invoked, such as possession by evil spirits. Rituals were used to rid the body of evil influences.

However, nearly two and a half millennia ago, Socrates came back from army service to report to his Greek countrymen that in one respect the Thracians were ahead of Greek civilization: they knew that the body could not be cured without the mind. "This," he continued, "is the reason why the cure of many diseases is unknown to the physicians of Hellas, because they are ignorant of the whole."[45] And his contemporary Hippocrates, one of the Fathers of Medicine, believed that many diseases were caused by emotions, or passions as they were known, and theorized a mind-body physiology based on combinations of four basic humors (yellow bile, black bile, phlegm, and blood) with the four basic elements (air, earth, fire, and water), i.e., with environmental influences. Various combinations of these building blocks produced different mental states and diseases. To cope with such a complexity and to cure the human body, "it is necessary to have a knowledge of the whole of things."[264] About one millennium later Paracelsus emphasized that "true medicine only arises from the creative knowledge of the last and deepest powers of the whole universe." Perhaps these assertions represent an early, intuitive understanding of what we today refer to as a cybernetic or systems approach.

OCCUPATIONAL MEDICINE: State of the Art Reviews—
Vol. 15, No. 1, January–March 2000. Philadelphia, Hanley & Belfus, Inc.   **69**

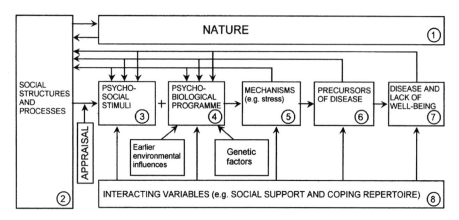

FIGURE 1. A theoretical model for psychosocially mediated disease. (Adapted from Kagan AR, Levi L: Health and environment—Psychosocial stimuli. A review. In Levi L (ed): Society, Stress, and Disease. Vol. II: Childhood and Adolescence. New York, Oxford University Press, 1975, pp 241–260; with permission.)

During our own century, we often have relinquished as an ideal the mastery of the whole realm of human knowledge by one person, and our training as specialists has made it difficult for us to accept the ideal of intelligent cooperation.[45] This training has tended to keep each of us so closely limited by our own field that we have remained ignorant even of the fundamental principles in the fields outside our own.

Ecological and Systems Approaches

How is the organism related to itself and to its environment? This is a fundamental problem presenting diverse facets to various specialists. The physician interested in either the maintenance and promotion of health or the cure of illness is working in the dark and by rule of thumb, as a mere technician, unless he or she has grappled with this problem and reviewed his or her practice in terms of it.[45]

IMPORTANT STEPS

Work-related stress and stress of other origin and their combined effects on cardiovascular and other morbidity and mortality have been approached by a number of eminent scientists. One of the early pioneers in this field was Bernhardi Ramazzini (1633–1714), Professor of Medicine at the University of Padua. Although his *De morbis artificum diatriba* is more intuitive and impressionistic than scientific, it is a systematic discourse on the maladies of those who practice some 40 different professions, covering possible causes and proposals for ways to prevent or cure them. He exhibited an intuitive understanding of the relationship between conditions of living and working of the poor and the risk of developing a number of work-related diseases.[203]

Alice Hamilton was the first American physician to devote her life to the practice of industrial medicine.[207] She wrote *Industrial Poisons in the United States* in 1925 and *Exploring the Dangerous Trades*, her autobiography, in 1943. In the latter, she lamented the status of occupational medicine in the United States:

"American medical authorities have never taken industrial diseases seriously, the American Medical Association has never held a meeting on the subject, and while European journals were full of articles on industrial poisonings, the number published in American medical journals up to 1910 could be counted on one's fingers . . . The employers could, if they wished, shut their eyes to the dangers their workmen faced, for nobody held them responsible, while the workers accepted the risks with fatalistic submissiveness as a part of the price one must pay for being poor."[80]

Crucially important contributions to our knowledge of the impact of psychosocially induced psychophysiological reactions were made by Walter Cannon, whose animal studies demonstrated the existence of a complex pattern of bodily reactions preparing the organism for fight or flight under environmental conditions causing pain, hunger, fear, and rage.[30] Ivan P. Pavlov's studies on dogs demonstrated a remarkable ability of the central nervous system to modulate neuroendocrine responses[184] (see Fig. 1, boxes 2–5). Another important contribution to this research field was made by Hans Selye, who demonstrated that a wide variety of physical, chemical, biological, and psychosocial stimuli elicit a reaction pattern, whose nonspecific components he termed "stress."[221–223] If prolonged, frequent, or intensive, stress increased "the rate of wear and tear" in the organism and accordingly was of pathogenic significance (see Fig. 1, boxes 2–7).

Franz Alexander presented some evidence indicating that psychosocially induced stress could not only influence but actually produce specific physical diseases.[3] He formulated a "specificity theory," which related specific psychological phenomena to specific somatic diseases (see Fig. 1, boxes 4–7), but had difficulties finding empirical support for it. Harold G. Wolff and Stewart Wolf, in their carefully conducted experiments on human subjects, demonstrated that a variety of bodily functions could be influenced psychosocially (see Fig. 1, boxes 2–5), offering important clues to etiology and pathogenesis of several important somatic diseases.[280,281] Thomas H. Holmes and Richard H. Rahe developed a method for quantifying "life changes," based on the assumption that every such change (e.g., death of a spouse, losing one's job, experiencing marital conflicts) taxed the organism and increased the wear and tear on it, leading to an increased risk of developing a wide variety of diseases, both physical and mental[91] (see Fig. 1, boxes 2–7).

Another important contribution came from Ray H. Rosenman and M. Friedman, based on their observations that many of their upper middle class cardiovascular patients exhibited a behavior pattern (Type A) characterized by a sense of urgency, competition, and hostility.[63] This pattern could be assumed to be accompanied by frequent, pronounced, and prolonged sympathoadrenomedullary responses, secondarily increasing the risk for subsequent ischemic heart disease (IHD). Another reasonable pathogenic mechanism was that such behaviors were causing frequent, prolonged, and/or intensive conflicts with fellow human beings that secondarily led to increases in sympathoadrenomedullary activity and, in a third step, to increased IHD morbidity and mortality (see Fig. 1, boxes 3–7). Although subsequent studies have failed to confirm the pathogenetic significance of the entire Type A behavior pattern, the pathogenic importance of one of its key components, hostility, has been supported by recent evidence.[126]

Richard S. Lazarus added to our knowledge by demonstrating the importance of "appraisal" and "coping" (see Fig. 1, boxes 2, 3, and 7) for the subsequent links in the chain of pathogenic events,[132,133] and James P. Henry and P.M. Stephens demonstrated the importance of subjective and objective control over a noxious situation for the neuroendocrine reaction triggered by the exposure and for subsequent morbidity and mortality.[55,86] Another modifier of the stressor-stress-disease chain of events was described by James S. House, who demonstrated the importance of social networks (see Fig. 1, box 7) offering emotional, practical, and/or economic support, thereby counteracting morbidity and mortality.[93,94]

I remember Hans Selye once commenting on the abundance of "manufacturers of bricks"—bits and pieces of important information—and the lack of "builders and architects" who were able and willing to put the "bricks" together to produce "buildings." One builder was George L. Engel, who proposed a "biopsychosocial" model of etiology, pathogenesis, therapy, and prevention, as a timely and necessary challenge for biomedicine.[52,53,108,136–139,141,144] This biopsychosocial concept brings us back to the "wholistic" approaches recommended by the ancient Greeks. However, since the times of Socrates and Hippocrates, the amount of knowledge in biology, psychology, and sociology has increased exponentially, making such an approach rather difficult to handle. It follows that we need to *collaborate* across scientific disciplines and societal sectors, but also *simplify*—"as much as possible, but not more." (James Grier Miller, private conversation)

MODELS

As pointed out by Gardell, ill effects of "Tayloristic" mass-production methods include *alienation* of the worker, not only during working hours, but with a spillover to leisure time as well.[66] An increase in fatigue, passivity, or apathy may grow out of this disaffection, leading to a decreased willingness of the worker to help change working conditions as well as participate in activities outside work. Further, it seems reasonable that the speed with which a person "unwinds" after work could influence the magnitude of the physiological and psychosocial effects, as well as affect the extent to which stress at work is carried over into leisure time.[56–58]

Promising attempts to include all of these theories have been made by Robert Karasek, Töres Theorell, and Jeffrey V. Johnson in their three-dimensional model of psychosocially induced morbidity and mortality.[99,117] The three dimensions are: environmental demands (Fig. 1, boxes 2 and 3), individual control (boxes 2 and 3), and social support (box 8). The most noxious combination is high demands + low control + low support. This model has been the basis of much research and has found considerable support in empirical studies.

Another basic model is based on the notion of person-environment fit (Fig. 1, boxes 2–4), according to which a misfit in a number of respects acts as a stressor.[61,81] A type of misfit is the basis for a third model by Johannes Siegrist, with his evidence-supported hypothesis of the pathogenic significance of high effort but low reward[228] (Fig. 1, boxes 4–6).

Until recently, virtually all research has focused on pathogenesis. Against this background, Aron Antonovsky asked why we don't all become ill, exposed as we are to "the slings and arrows of outrageous fortune."[6] He formulated his hypothesis about *salutogenesis* and "sense of coherence," with its three dimensions of comprehensibility, manageability, and meaningfulness. High scores in these three respects seem to exercise a protective or even health-promoting influence (Fig. 1, boxes 4–7).

During recent decades, increasing attention has been paid to psychosocially induced, potentially pathogenic *behaviors*, such as alcohol, tobacco, and other substance abuse, risk taking, and other self-destructive behaviors. There is some evidence that work-related stress is one of their determinants. Although not included in Selye's original stress concept, they are probably at least as important for human morbidity and mortality as the more direct psychoneuroendocrinoimmunologic mechanisms. An excellent review of the present state-of-the art is found in a recent paper commissioned by the European Heart Network.[48]

Needless to say, the early approaches to stress and health were purely speculative. Subsequent ones were based on scattered clinical observations and anecdotal evidence. The next step comprised studies on mice, rats, and other animals under laboratory conditions and in real life.[55] Subsequently, the favorite experimental animal increasingly chosen was the medical student. Descriptive and observational studies were gradually complemented by hypotheses testing and interventional studies, and experimental studies were used together with epidemiological ones, in "package" approaches. Simple stimulus-response approaches, initially unifactorial, gradually became multifactorial, ecological and, eventually, *systems* oriented.[213] The focus on the individual patient gradually broadened to a *community* approach.[273] There has been a parallel development from therapy to primary and secondary prevention and health promotion.[140,144-146]

SOCIAL CLASS AND POWER RELATIONS AT THE WORKPLACE *by Mel Bartley, PhD and Michael Marmot, FFPHM—*

MB gratefully acknowledges the support of the U.K. Medical Research Council, grant no. G8802774. MM is supported by an MRC Research Professorship.

Classical social theories did not concentrate on the effects of the workplace on the individual (in contrast to occupational psychology) but on how the organization of production affects stability and change in norms, values, and other social institutions such as the family and the economy. Social psychology and epidemiology have built on these insights to ask how the position of each individual within the structure of economic relations may influence their psychological makeup and, ultimately, mental and physical health.

Contemporary epidemiologic theories relating work relations and conditions to health have focused on the amount of control exercised over the work process,[84,103] variety and the scope for use of initiative and skill,[156,177] excessive work pressure, and the mismatch between effort and rewards.[191,233,235] All of these concerns have a basis in social theory.[226,227,233]

The classical theories from which our present day approaches to power in the workplace are derived were formulated at a time of great turbulence and change. In Marx's words the new industrialists had "put an end to all feudal, patriarchal, idyllic relations. . . . pitilessly torn asunder the motley feudal ties that bound man to his 'natural superiors' . . . resolved personal worth into exchange value . . . Constant revolutionizing of production, uninterrupted disturbance of all social conditions, everlasting uncertainty and agitation distinguish the bourgeois epoch from all earlier ones."[160]

At this time, the very nature of social and economic relationships was in flux. Old certainties based on fixed statuses and associated obligations were being torn down, and it was not at all clear what would take their place. From the perspective of the present day, it is surprising how relevant this work now appears, if we substitute for questions regarding the relationship between lord and serf the more contemporary questions about the relationship between men and women, or parents and children.

Divisions of Labor, Anomie, and Alienation

Marx and Durkheim shared a concern about the changing nature of social bonds that accompanied the development of a modern industrial economy and its "division of labour," or separation of increasing numbers of different types of work. Although they agreed that the decline of feudal traditions increased the productive capacity of societies and the scope for individual action, their views on the nature of what had replaced these traditions, and of future directions for society, were different. However, for our present purposes, their commonality is more important than their differences, because while each perspective focused on different aspects of the question, both had a major influence on the ways in which we think about the relationship between employment and health.

Durkheim regarded increasing division of labor as a normal phase in the development of societies. "Social pathologies" such as economic crises, mass unemployment, and conflict between factory owners and workers were ascribed to *abnormal forms of the division of labor*. He characterized the course of normal development, as territories became more densely populated and urbanized, as a change from "mechanical" to "organic" forms of solidarity.[46] The ideas behind the different forms of social solidarity are still relevant to social and political debates today. **Mechanical solidarity** is present where collective rules and sanctions are mainly religious in nature, and powerful beliefs tie individuals together so strongly that the idea of the individual is itself problematic. In the mechanically solidaristic society, social bonds are of obligation rather than contract; there is little specialization of work tasks, low levels of individual autonomy, and swift and severely repressive punishment for deviant behavior. As populations grow and come together in larger towns and cities, however, new social divisions arise, based more on the necessary organization of work tasks than on family, tribal, or religious allegiances. Tolerance of differences in beliefs and behavior increases. Social bonds become increasingly a matter of mutually satisfactory arrangements to ensure that productive activity can proceed. In these societies of **organic solidarity**, social relations are based on contracts and agreements rather than religion or sentiment; occupations rather than kinship defines social position. However, in the absence of abnormalities of development, the *conscience collective* ensures that a set of agreed norms underlie the more complex set of social relations.[46,171]

Durkheim did not regard hierarchical differentiation between groups who carry out different tasks within a division of labor as necessary or desirable.[68,154] If one social class becomes too powerful and is in a position to enforce a division of labor on other groups, this results in **anomie**, that is, an enforced specialization that is meaningless and purposeless to those who carry out the specialized tasks. The common values involved in the various branches of the division of labor are lost. Social groups lose track of the larger picture—that all of their different functions are intended to bring about the welfare of the society as a whole. Coordination of different types of work breaks down. Financial crises and industrial conflicts were, for Durkheim, failures of mutual understanding and shared purpose. The welfare of the individual worker and the quality of his or her relations at work were, therefore, central to society's ability to function.

Durkheim's ideas have had a profound influence on the study of social factors in disease. He carried out a study of regional variations in suicide, showing that it was more common in more anomic sections of society where shared norms and social ties were looser.[47] More recently, this finding has been extended to the investigation of the effect of social support and social cohesion on disease.[152,156,200,242] Durkheim's conviction that a society based solely on market relationships was impossible has been carried forward into the investigation of the relationship of social and economic inequality to measures of population health.[121,276–278]

Marx's focus on and concern to explain the social changes of the 18th and 19th centuries was in many respects similar to that of Durkheim. Where Durkheim is relatively vague in dealing with the causes of the social changes he describes as the division of labor, Marx is more explicit in attempting to explain these changes. He attributes them to advances in technology and associated changes in the ownership of a society's most important productive resources. Marx accordingly devoted more attention to the economic aspects of social relations. In feudal societies (which would be regarded as relatively mechanical according to Durkheim's classification), traditional social and legal norms defined legitimate social relationships. The work of producing consumer goods was also heavily regulated by custom and tradition, presided over by the guilds.[95] Land owners also owed certain duties of protection to their serfs, and master craftsmen similarly owed duties to their apprentices. Agriculture and craft were the main forms of work.

During the 18th century, new agricultural and industrial technologies arose that changed the nature of production, both of food and goods. Skilled crafts declined and began to be replaced by fragmented forms of production in factories.[161] During this time, profound legal and political changes took place, including the right to buy and sell land and to lend money at interest. Once this happened, two types of control were lost: (1) Manufacturing workers lost control of the production process when they no longer owned their own tools. (2) Families lost control of the provision of food after the enclosures of common land, when even the most basic foods had to be bought with wages from employment rather than produced at home. We see the importance of this second control today in the former Soviet Union, where access to produce of the land (in the form of extended family members still living in rural areas) can make a major difference in the living conditions of workers who find themselves suddenly in a modern, free-labor market.[32] It also has been pointed out by Amartya Sen that, paradoxically, in the Indian sub continent, the landless laborer is most in need of work and yet least attractive to employers because he starves in between jobs, whereas the laborer with a little land is able to remain fitter and healthier.[43,224]

Whereas Durkheim's central interests have made his work helpful to the study of psychological health and illness, Marx's emphasis on production processes and economic forces are more relevant to the study of industrial causes of disease, the effects of economic deprivation, and issues of control over the work process. We inherit from Durkheim the concept of anomie, the loss of the sense of belonging to a community with common values. Marx's development of the **concept of alienation** is a more economic and less psychological process.[159] All workers are alienated from the things they produce when they have done so under an "over-segmented" and forced division of labor, in a situation where they have no voice in the organization of production. The prices of the goods produced are partly determined by the level of supply: once the market is saturated, demand disappears. Under this division of labor, the harder the worker works, the greater the risk of a glut, with resulting unemployment. As a result: "With the increasing value of the world of things proceeds in direct proportion the devaluation of the world of men. . . . the more objects the worker produces the fewer he can possess."[159] Even a worker who responds to a questionnaire by reporting a high level of work satisfaction may therefore be alienated in this objective sense, if his or her high productivity potentially threatens employment prospects.

Alienation has another meaning in Marx's analysis: that of humankind alienated from its "species-being." What distinguishes person from animal is that men and women produce creatively, from previously imagined ideas rather than from instinct, and they produce far more and far different things than that which is necessary for mere survival. Therefore, to place human beings in a situation where their acts of production are constrained by the will of a controlling group or class, and are undertaken purely for survival, is to deny—or alienate people from—human nature itself.[159,266]

Bureaucracy, Hierarchy, and Lifestyle

Like Durkheim and Marx, Weber was concerned to understand the conflict and change of 19th century Europe. Like Marx, he discussed the role of property ownership in creating wealth and advantage. He differed in four major ways: First, his model of social change put *ideas and beliefs* in the driving seat as the causes rather than the consequences of technological change.[267] Second, he defined a dimension of social division he termed *status*, which is based not on work, production, and the social relationships at work, but on patterns of consumption and lifestyle.[268] The "status group" was defined as a group of individuals who share the same level of prestige or esteem. They express their shared status in terms of common forms of consumption and lifestyle and by limiting their interactions with members of other groups. Third, Weber stressed the role of both status group membership and education in giving a person a better or worse *market position* according to the demand for these attributes. Fourth, Weber paid more attention to the large *bureaucracies* that increasingly presided over both industrial production and government by the time he was writing his major works.

It was not, for Weber, either the forms of material production or of group solidarity that determined individuals' actions, but individual beliefs themselves, as exemplified in perhaps his best known work on the genesis of capitalism in the religious beliefs of Protestantism.[267] The most important aspect of belief was acceptance of the legitimacy of the prevailing rules of behavior. This aspect is, of course, quite similar to the shared norms of Durkheim's conscience collective.

Weber's major contribution to present-day research on the relationship between work and health is his analysis of the labor market, in particular of the differentiation within the newly growing (at the time he was writing, and again today) white-collar labor force of managers, professionals, technicians, supervisors, and clerks. He did not explicitly link labor market position to individual well-being. However, the Austrian sociologist Renner developed the concept of the "service class," a form of employment characterized by the necessity for the employer to place trust in the employee and to organize the relations of employment to produce loyalty. There is a strong connection between the characteristics of Renner's "service relationship" between employer and employee, and the concerns of Durkheim and Marx with anomie and alienation. In order to ensure loyalty and the conscientious performance of intricate tasks, the working conditions of professional, managerial, and technical workers developed in a way that minimized feelings of anomie and alienation and maximized perceptions of just reward and of being personally valued. Not least, in Renner's words, "The payment of a salary is not meant to provide food and shelter from week to week, but to establish a lifestyle . . . which improves as the individual becomes older."[205] The loyal service worker from a more humble background could therefore be expected, over time, to move into higher-status groups.

Relation of Classical Theories to Modern Research on Work and Health

There are at present two leading alternative interpretations of the relationship of the psychosocial conditions of work to disease risk. The demand-control model seems to be related more closely to Marx's concept of alienation, and the Effort-Reward Imbalance (ERI) Model to Weber's analysis of the need to regulate and motivate the new service class in emerging large organizations and government bureaucracies. Industrial capitalism resulted in a situation where employees had no control over what they would produce, how they would produce it, or what happened to the goods they made. Continued involvement in work was motivated purely by the need to earn money to be exchanged for food and shelter—devoid of autonomy or creativity. The increasing sophistication of industry gave rise to a need for well-educated workers who could be entrusted with responsibility in large and complex private and public organizations. These workers had to be persuaded of the legitimacy of their employers' demands: mere surveillance was not a guarantee of performance. The solution that developed was that key workers were given more autonomy within the organization and the resources to develop and sustain an elite lifestyle. They acquired power over their status in the wider society: this was accomplished by various combinations of increased pay, incremental pay scales, and conferring of symbolic signs of status as rewards. Taken singly, none of the classical social theories gives us a full picture, but combining them reveals a social structure in which one section of the working population, due to their value on the labor market bestowed by the social status of their families and by their level of education and skills, has access to a form of employment in which anomie and alienation are relatively attenuated.

An example of how the concept of social stratification and its possible effects on health are being operationalized and tested in epidemiologic study can be taken from the Whitehall study of health differences between different levels of a hierarchical organization: the British Civil Service.[157] This research has included measures of psychosocial conditions and relationships at work from its inception. Empirically, as one might expect, work control and ERI have been found to constitute independent dimensions of psychosocial risk.[24] In the "more alienated" groups with low work control, ERI had a large effect on CVD incidence, whereas in those with "less alienated" work (higher levels of job control), the effect of ERI was less strong.

Recent economic developments in some countries have eroded the privileged position of professional and managerial workers. Epidemiologic studies so far have not revealed any narrowing tendency of morbidity or mortality differentials between the service (managerial and professional) and working classes in the U.S.[198,199,279] nor in some European countries.[21,42] However, it may be too soon to see the effects on health of recent deteriorations in the working conditions of white-collar workers.

Conclusion

The classical theorists were not concerned primarily with the physical well-being of individuals, although it would certainly not have surprised Marx or Durkheim to find that the psychosocial consequences of occupying different positions in society could influence rates of disease and mortality. The points upon which there was broad agreement between the different schools of thought focused on the importance of social relationships, of which employment was the most important. It is possible to trace this theme forward to see the ways in which concepts of anomie, alienation, and status have been used in various combinations to illuminate the processes underlying inequalities in health.

The relationship between work characteristics and health is an example of the unintended consequences of structured social action. In the presence of class division and private ownership of the means of production, much work is undertaken for financial reasons only, and is neither creative nor self-motivated. Control and autonomy at work vary between occupations and between occupational settings, and have been shown to be associated with CVD[23] and its precursors.[216] Employers offer rewards in terms of material goods and status to ensure the conduct of necessarily self-monitored, highly skilled and responsible work involved in many (mostly white-collar) forms of employment. As well as providing work incentives, these forms of reward also appear to have beneficial effects on health.[120,147] There appears also to be a process that relates the degree of work effort and the perceived fairness and appropriateness of financial and/or status rewards, to the risk of CVD.[189] In these ways the operationalization and measurement of concepts derived from theories of social structures and dynamics have contributed to epidemiologic research.

THE DEMAND-CONTROL-SUPPORT MODEL AND CVD
by Robert Karasek, PhD and Töres Theorell, MD, PhD

The demand-control model (DCM) was introduced by Karasek in his doctoral thesis.[114] It was developed for work environments where stressors are chronic, not initially life threatening, and the product of sophisticated human organizational decision making. In decision making the controllability of the stressor is critical, and it becomes more important as increasingly complex and integrated social organizations develop, with ever more complex limitations on individual behavior. The model is based on psychosocial characteristics of work. It has two components: **psychological demands**, and a combined measure of task control and skill use, or **decision latitude**. The model predicts (1) stress-related illness risk and (2) active/passive behavioral correlates of jobs. It has been used mainly in epidemiologic studies of chronic disease, such as coronary heart disease.

The health outcome measures in the original studies were mental health variables. The first article with this perspective in an international journal appeared in 1979, on epidemiologic studies of working Swedes.[118] The cardiovascular perspective was introduced in the late 1970s, and the first prospective study appeared in 1981.[115] The latter was based on randomly selected working men in Sweden who were surveyed initially in 1968 and then followed up in 1974. The outcome measures were cardiovascular mortality and a composite measure of cardiovascular symptoms. The study showed a significant association between working in jobs that were psychologically demanding and uncontrollable, and increased likelihood of subsequent development of heart disease symptoms and/or cardiovascular mortality.

The DCM is useful educationally when a worksite is being explored. The model has great face value, and the employees immediately grasp the importance of it in the practical exploration of the psychosocial work environment.

Historical Context
Kornitzer and his collaborators observed in the 1970s in a retrospective study of two bank groups in Belgium, one private and one state-owned, that employees in the private banks had a higher incidence of myocardial infarction (MI) than employees in the state-owned banks. This study was one of the first to indicate a possible relationship between psychological work demands (which were higher in the private banks) and risk of MI. In the 1960s, an important prospective study demonstrated a higher incidence of MI among lower-level than among higher-level employees in large companies.[187] For the first time, suspicion arose that psychosocial stress may

not be a problem only for people with a lot of responsibility, as researchers had tended to believe previously (see Chapter 2).

The environment's impact on the cardiovascular system via the CNS has been well-appreciated empirically since ancient times. Currently, sociologists and social psychologists have helped to apply theoretically-based models of this dynamic to cardiovascular research.

The Demand-Control Model

Several theoretical models, for instance those of the Michigan school of sociology (Person-Environment Fit)[119] and Cooper's comprehensive model,[36] describe the psychosocial aspects of white-collar work. Karasek's DCM was a synthesis of the *demand* (psychological stress) and the *lack of control* (sociological) research.[118] In generating the concept of lack of control, or "lack of decision latitude" as Karasek labeled it, he had been following sociological traditions on alienation and organizational behavior.

According to the model, there is interaction between high psychological demands and low decision latitude. If demands are regarded as the x-axis and decision latitude as the y-axis in a two-dimensional system, four combinations are recognized (Fig. 2). The high demand–low decision latitude combination is labeled *job strain* (high strain); the high demand–high decision situation *active work*; the low demand–low decision latitude combination *passive work*; and the ideal low demand–high decision latitude combination *low strain work*.

JOB STRAIN HYPOTHESIS

The first hypothesis is that the most adverse reactions of psychological strain (fatigue, anxiety, depression, and physical illness) occur when the psychological demands of the job are high and the worker's decision latitude in the task is low. For example, the assembly-line worker has almost every behavior rigidly constrained. In a situation of increased demands ("speed-up"), more than just the constructive response of arousal, the often helpless, long-lasting, and negatively experienced response of residual psychological strain occurs. During a restaurant's lunch-time rush, it is the waiter or waitress who does not know how to "control" the customer's

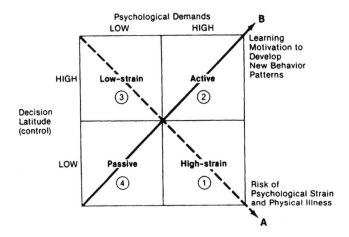

FIGURE 2. Psychological demand/decision latitude model. (From Karasek R, Theorell T: Healthy Work. New York, Basic Books, 1990; with permission.)

behavior ("get the jump on the customer") who experiences the greatest strain on the job.[274] Kerckhoff and Back have described garment workers under heavy deadline pressure and the subsequent threat of layoff.[122] They concluded that when the actions normally needed to cope with job pressures cannot be taken, the most severe behavioral symptoms of strain occur (fainting, hysteria, social contagion).

It is not only the freedom to determine how the formal work task is accomplished that relieves strain, but also the freedom to engage in informal rituals such as the coffee break or fidgeting, which serve as supplementary "tension release" mechanisms during the workday.[40] These mechanisms often are social activities with other workers—precisely those activities eliminated as "wasted motions" and "soldiering" by Frederick Taylor's methods from 1911.[249] Thus, the DCM must expand to include social relations and social support for strain relief. According to the theory, prolonged and repeated job strain increases sympathoadrenal arousal and decreases anabolism, the body's ability to restore and repair tissues.

In the DCM, decision latitude refers to the worker's ability to control his or her own activities and skill usage, not to control others. Decision latitude scales have two components: **task authority**—a socially predetermined control over detailed aspects of task performance (also called autonomy), and **skill discretion**—control over use of skills by the individual, also socially determined at work (and often called variety or substantive complexity).[77,123] In modern organizational hierarchies, the highest level of knowledge legitimizes the exercise of the highest levels of authority, and workers undertaking limited, specialized tasks are coordinated by managers with higher authority levels. Skill discretion and authority over decisions are so closely related theoretically and empirically that they often are combined.

Examples of work's psychological demands—"how hard you work"—include the presence of deadlines, the mental arousal or stimulation necessary to accomplish the task, and coordination burdens. The physical demands are not included, although psychological arousal comes with physical exertion, and for some groups of workers responses to questions about working hard may include physical aspects of work.[106] The assessment of psychological job demands has turned out to be methodologically more difficult than was hitherto believed. In particular, the interpretation of questions regarding psychological demands may differ between different groups, e.g., white-collar and blue-collar workers, and men and women. Furthermore, psychological demands may change in nature as information technology and other ongoing working life changes affect working conditions. Assessment difficulties may explain why the psychological demands part of the DCM has less empirical support than the control part.

ACTIVE LEARNING HYPOTHESIS

When control on the job is high and psychological demands are also high but not overwhelming, learning and growth are the predicted behavioral outcomes. The combination of high psychological demands–high decision latitude is defined as the active situation; workers experiencing this combination of work environment factors are the most active group outside of work, in leisure and political activities, despite heavy work demands.[117] Only average psychological strain is predicted for the active job because much of the energy mobilized by the job's many stressors ("challenges") are translated into direct action—effective problem solving—with little residual strain to cause disturbance. This hypothesis parallels White's "concept of competence," an environment-based theory of motivation: the psychological state of individuals in challenging circumstances is enhanced by increasing demands. The model also predicts that the growth and learning stimuli of these settings, when they occur in a job context, are conducive to high productivity. According to the DCM, learning occurs in situations that require both individual psychological energy expenditure and the exercise of decision-making capability.

In an active environment, the worker can cope with high psychological demands because he/she can make relevant decisions, such as planning working hours according to personal biological rhythm and the naturally optimal use of internal physiologic resources. In addition, the worker can improve coping strategies and thereby facilitate a feeling of knowledge and authority, as well as improve access to information in unforeseen situations. These possibilities correspond to psychological growth.

PASSIVE WORK AND LOW-STRAIN WORK

The DCM predicts that situations of low demand–low decision latitude (the passive combination) cause an unmotivating job setting that leads to "negative learning," gradual loss of previously acquired skills. Evidence shows that disengagement from leisure and political activity outside the job appear to increase over time in such jobs.[117] This atrophication may represent "learned helplessness"[220] and may be the result of a sequence of job situations that reject workers' initiatives. The low demand–high decision latitude situation—low strain—is theoretically ideal from the strain perspective. Low demand in the modern working environment really means no *excessive* demands; it should not be perceived literally, since low demands may be problematic from the perspective of social engagement.[114,117]

DYNAMIC DEMAND/CONTROL HYPOTHESES

Figure 3 shows the dynamic version of the DCM, which integrates environment and personality orientations over the long term. Active learning in the active situation stimulates feelings of mastery. This high mastery personality orientation, in turn, allows more successful coping with the inevitable job stressors, reduces residual job strain, and leaves the individual with extra energy to engage in the challenges of further active learning situations. Overall, this is a feedback spiral with positive consequences, but a "negative" spiral is also possible. High-strain situations lead to withdrawal, reduced mastery, and further reduced coping effectiveness.

Environmental demands can be conceptualized in both positive and negative terms, congruent with the common understanding that there is both "good" and "bad" stress. However, the DCM is not congruent with a model of "demands and resources," allowing a simple fit with currently common cost-benefit thinking, in which the positive benefits of resources are subtracted from the negative costs of demands. The logic of the DCM cannot be collapsed into a unidimensional form. The distinction between decision latitude and psychological demands must be retained because the model predicts both job strain and active learning associated with psychological demands, depending on the level of control.

The Demand-Control-Support Model

It soon became evident that a third component was needed in the DCM: social support. Johnson has pointed out that collective support may be difficult to separate theoretically from collective control.[99] Workers who are exposed to adverse working conditions may join forces and increase their control over the working conditions. The worst hypothesized situation is **iso-strain**—job strain and lack of social support.[100] Several different aspects of social support are relevant. At work the *source* of support is important; the supervisor and colleagues are the main sources for most employees. Customers or patients also can be important sources of social support.

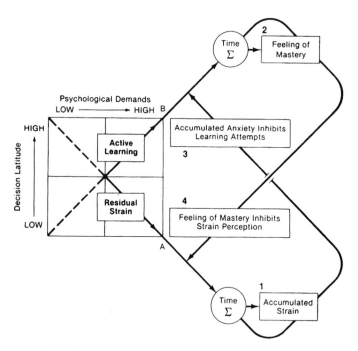

FIGURE 3. Dynamic associations linking environmental strain and learning to evolution of personality. (From Karasek R, Theorell T: Healthy Work. New York, Basic Books, 1990; with permission.)

Two of the most important types of support are *instrumental* (when there is a lack of material resources, someone should be available to help) and *emotional* (someone to share inner feelings with about job problems).

Social support buffering of psychological strain may depend on the degree of social and emotional integration and trust between coworkers and supervisors, i.e., **socio-emotional support**. Addition of social support also makes the demand-control perspective more useful in job redesigning. Changes in social relations between workers (e.g., autonomous work groups) and changes in decision latitude are almost inseparable in job redesign processes, particularly "participatory" processes.[93]

Occupation and Psychosocial Job Characteristics

The relationship between occupations and job characteristics has been described by means of national surveys, for instance in Sweden and the U.S. Maps have been published that illustrate the relative positions of different occupations in relation to decision latitude and psychological demands. Typical active jobs are lawyers, judges, engineers, nurses, and managers of all kinds. Examples of passive jobs are clerical workers, such as stock and billing clerks, and service personnel, such as janitors. In the job strain groups, typical occupations are machine-paced, including assemblers, inspectors, and freight handlers, as well as service-based, including waiters and cooks. Examples of low strain jobs are self-paced occupations such as repairmen, foresters, linemen, and natural scientists.

Note, however, that the labor market is changing. In Sweden, for instance, national surveys indicate that there was a long period during the 1970s and 1980s when the psychosocial job characteristics of most jobs were improving with regard to intellectual discretion and authority over decisions.[214] During the 1990s, risk of unemployment and demands for effectiveness have increased, while decision latitude has decreased markedly for certain groups. One clear example of this labor market evolution is that physicians who belonged to the active group in the late 1970s and early 1980s now belong to the job strain category, according to national surveys.[214] On the whole, workers in the healthcare sector have been disfavored in the societal financial crisis in Sweden. Decision latitude was reported as lower in this sector than in other branches in the Stockholm labor market, and the differences between physicians and others were not as pronounced as expected.[214a]

Aggregation of individual job scores within a work group or occupation is a method for counteracting potential self-report bias in job assessment. This is the basis for the much used occupation-based linkage system. However, subgroups with significantly differing job experiences can be aggregated, leading also to misclassification problems. Thus, adequate operationalization of constructs or objective assessments may be additionally needed. For example, professional bus drivers from inner city areas have a high risk of developing MI in detailed studies, but when all bus drivers (urban and rural) are grouped together and simple questionnaire responses are used, this distinctive inner city bus driving risk is lost.

According to occupational studies, executives and professionals do not belong to the job strain group and, accordingly, they do not record the highest level of stress, as popular belief often holds. While managerial stress certainly exists because of the high psychological demands that come with these jobs, it appears that the frequent occasions for decision making and deciding how to do the job are a significant stress moderator. Of course, at the highest status levels, decision making is the primary psychological demand, and then the demand-control model fails. The implication here is that executives could reduce their stress if they made fewer decisions, and lower-status workers would be better off with a more equal share of decision power. Interestingly, managed care often severely compromises control as well as increases demand among physicians and other healthcare professionals.

Men are more likely than women to have high control over their work process at the task level.[117] Another major gender difference in some U.S. and Swedish samples is the negative correlation between decision latitude and demands for women: women with low control also have higher job demands. This means that women are several times more likely than men to hold high-strain jobs in the general working population. By contrast, men's high-demand jobs generally are accompanied by somewhat higher decision latitude.

THE EFFORT-REWARD IMBALANCE MODEL
by Johannes Siegrist, PhD and Richard Peter, PhD

Theoretical work in the field of occupational stress and health is faced with two challenges. A first challenge is defined by scientists who maintain that stressful experience at work is essentially an individual phenomenon determined by a person's psychobiological program, learning history, appraisal, and coping resources, thus precluding any generalization beyond the level of individual variation.[37] Opposite to this approach is a position claiming that the notion of stressful experience at work is amenable to scientific generalization, but that any generalization must reflect the complexity of a dynamic person-environment transaction operating at the macro-, the meso-, and the micro-social level.[107] In an analytical perspective, the challenge of this latter position consists in a meaningful reduction of complexity, that is in a theory-driven selective emphasis on specific situational and personal characteristics that elicit or enhance stressful experience at work.

The model of effort-reward imbalance (ERI) defines one such theory-driven selective approach. It has been developed to answer the following three questions: (1) Is it possible to identify those dimensions of stressful experience at work that are *typical* for a wide variety of occupations both in the industrial and in the service sector? (2) Can we identify work-related conditions that are likely to elicit recurrent, *chronically stressful* experience? (3) To what extent can we distinguish *situation-specific* versus *person-specific* components of stressful experience at work? Answers to these questions were not obvious from the very beginning.[225] Rather, the theoretical formulations and their adequate operational measurement were elaborated over the years.[228] The following pages summarize what we consider a most updated and valid account of the theoretical model and its contribution toward explaining links between work and cardiovascular (CV) disease.

Theory and Description of the ERI Model

To determine what kind of stressful experience might be typical for a broad variety of occupations, the focus is put on the centrality of paid employment in adult life. Obviously, having a job is a principal prerequisite for continuous income opportunities and an important means of acquiring social status and social identity. In particular, the **work role** defines a crucial link between self-regulatory needs of a person (e.g., self-esteem, self-efficacy) and the social opportunity structure. Conferment of occupational status is associated with recurrent options of contributing and performing, of being rewarded or esteemed, and of belonging to some significant group (work colleagues). Yet these potentially beneficial effects are contingent on a basic prerequisite of exchange in social life, that is, **reciprocity**. Effort at work is spent as part of a socially organized exchange process to which society at large contributes in terms of rewards. Rewards are distributed by **three transmitter systems:** money, esteem, and career opportunities, including job security.

The ERI model claims that lack of reciprocity between "costs" and "gains" (i.e., high cost/low gain conditions) defines a state of emotional distress that can lead to the arousal of the autonomic nervous system and associated strain reactions. For instance, having a demanding but unstable job or achieving at a high level without being offered any promotion prospects are examples of high cost/low gain conditions at work. In terms of current developments of the labor market in a global economy, the emphasis on occupational rewards reflects the growing importance of fragmented careers, job instability, under-employment, redundancy, and forced occupational mobility, including their financial consequences. The ERI model applies to a wide range of occupational settings, most markedly to groups that suffer from a growing segmentation of the labor market and are exposed to structural unemployment and rapid socioeconomic change. Experience of ERI at work is frequent among service occupations and professions, in particular the ones dealing with client interaction.

But how can we make sure that these widely prevalent high cost/low gain conditions at work elicit chronically stressful experience? The expectancy-value theory of motivation asserts that workers exposed to high effort/low reward conditions escape the situation, or if that is not feasible, reduce their efforts to minimize negative outcome.[219] Conversely, the ERI model predicts continued high effort and, thus, chronically stressful experience, under the following conditions: (1) **lack of alternative choice** in the labor market may prevent people from giving up even unfavorable jobs, as the anticipated costs of disengagement (e.g., the risk of being laid off or of facing downward mobility) outweigh costs of accepting inadequate benefits; (2) unfair job arrangements may be accepted for a certain period of one's occupational trajectory for **strategic reasons**, perhaps to improve chances for career promotion and related rewards at a later stage; (3) a specific **personal pattern of coping** with demands and of eliciting rewards characterized by *overcommitment* may prevent people from accurately assessing cost-gain relations.[228] "Overcommitment" defines a set of attitudes, behaviors, and emotions reflecting excessive striving in combination with a strong desire of being approved and esteemed. People characterized by overcommitment are exaggerating their efforts beyond levels usually considered appropriate. There is evidence that excessive efforts result from perceptual distortion (in particular an underestimation of challenges and an overestimation of one's coping resources), which in turn may be triggered by an underlying motivation of experiencing recurrent esteem and approval.[162,228] This latter argument points to the third question asked on page 84: it defines a *person-specific component* of the model (overcommitment) in addition to the *situation-specific component* of high extrinsic effort and low reward.

In summary, the model claims that stressful experience is most likely to result from an imbalance between (high) extrinsic effort and (low) extrinsic reward in combination with a high level of overcommitment. But even in the absence of the intrinsic component, high cost/low gain conditions at work evoke stressful experience, given the significance of unmet reciprocity in social exchange. Alternatively, continued excessive efforts in combination with disappointed reward expectancy that is attributable to a high level of overcommitment may produce stressful experience even in the absence of the situation-specific component. Thus, a comprehensive test of the model covers all three conditions mentioned (Fig. 4).

Two final comments on the model are needed. First, while we make a conceptual and methodological distinction between the situation-specific and the person-specific components of the model, we do not claim that overcommitment is considered a personality trait that remains unaffected by social contexts. Rather, this personal pattern of coping with demands and reward expectancies may be reinforced to some extent by specific circumstances in occupational life, most likely at early

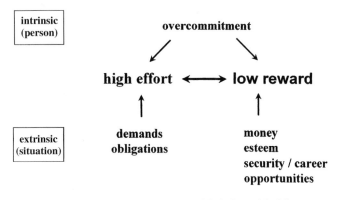

FIGURE 4.　The Effort-Reward Imbalance Model

career stages. Although overcommitment was found to be rather stable over time, more research is needed to explore this question. A second comment concerns the significance of the reward dimension. As stated, emphasis in stress-theoretical terms is put on violations of expectancies of reciprocity and fairness underlying exchange in significant social roles (here: the work role). Unmet reward expectancy following effort is likely to provoke strong negative emotional reactions, as this conflicts with a taken-for-granted basic "grammar" of social exchange.[39] All three reward dimensions contribute to this negative experience, although most powerful effects may result from poor rewards related to labor market conditions, such as inadequate wages and salaries, lack of promotion prospects, forced downward mobility, and job loss. In view of this latter observation, ERI at work is likely to be more prevalent among lower socioeconomic status groups.

Policy Implications

So far, ERI at work was found to predict *new manifestations* of CHD[24,152,236] and to contribute to the explanation of CV risk factors, such as hypertension,[190,193] elevated atherogenic lipids,[229,231] and elevated fibrinogen.[105,234] Further validation of the model is provided by studies that document adverse health effects (e.g., gastrointestinal disorders,[209] psychiatric disorders,[243] poor subjective health[191,242]).

Policy implications of these results in terms of stress prevention and health promotion at work are far-reaching, following the theoretical argument presented on page 84, and they affect both situational and person-specific activities. At the **individual (or interpersonal) level**, specific measures of stress management can be applied, aiming at a reduction of excessive overcommitment and an enhancement of esteem and positive feedback from superiors and work colleagues. One such approach, although supplemented by distinct organizational changes, has been developed and successfully applied in a group of highly stressed, inner-city bus drivers.[12] At the **structural level** of organizational development and, if feasible, of trade union and labor market policy, adequate terms of exchange between extrinsic efforts and rewards should be established. Examples of such measures include developing compensatory wage systems, providing models of gain sharing, and strengthening non-monetary gratifications. Investment in continued training and reskilling programs and collective bargaining over job security and promotional opportunities are important measures in this regard. Clearly, the power structure of economic life and the far-reaching transformations of current work limit the options and impact of workplace health promotion programs that transcend individual risk factor change.

The Demand-Control-Support Model

Analytical models selectively emphasize specific aspects of the complex psychosocial work environment, thereby enabling us to create new knowledge. At the same time, they point to obvious limitations. The analytical approach underlying the ERI model is based on the stress-theoretical paradigm of social reward.[39] A different analytical approach, the demand-control-support (DCS) model, is mainly based on the stress-theoretical paradigm of personal control.[117] The notions of control and reward may overlap to some extent, but in terms of psychological theory of self, control is more closely related to the notion of self-efficacy,[241] whereas reward is more closely associated with self-esteem.[186] In sociological terms, control is associated with power,[101] and reward points to a basic grammar of social exchange, i.e., reciprocity and fairness.[39]

At the conceptual level, the two models differ in several regards: (1) The DCS model has been introduced and measured as a concept that is restricted to the extrinsic or situational aspects of the psychosocial work environment, whereas the ERI model includes both extrinsic and intrinsic components; (2) The DCS model offers a broader approach, as its bidirectional conceptualization includes a stress dimension with relevance to health and a skill dimension with relevance to personal growth and development.[251] In this regard, the ERI model is more narrowly focused on the biopsychosocial determinants of health and well-being; (3) Components of the ERI model (salaries, career opportunities/job security) are linked to more distant macro-economic conditions, while the DCS model's major focus is on workplace characteristics.

Future Directions

Despite these differences, there is promise in studying the combined effects of the two models in future research.[251] Preliminary evidence comes from currently unpublished findings of a Swedish case-control study and a British prospective study, indicating that combined effects on CV health are considerably stronger compared to the separate effects of each model.[24,192] A second promising future direction of research concerns the study of combined effects of psychosocial work stress and traditional occupational hazards and stressors. For instance, psychosocial work stress as measured by the ERI and DCS models may mediate effects of shiftwork on CV health.[190]

Much remains to be done concerning an adequate conceptualization of the cumulative effects of ERI over time. For instance, elderly workers may be unable to maintain high effort on the job because after many years of exposure their resources are exhausted. If this situation is not reflected in compensatory wage differentials, the stressful effects of imbalance are expected to be much worse than those experienced by younger workers. The dynamic, time-sensitive aspects of the intrinsic part of the model (the coping pattern of overcommitment) has been discussed in more detail elsewhere.[162,228]

Finally, adverse health effects of ERI generated in social roles other than work (e.g., marriage, family, neighborhood, civic life) need to be explored to learn how they compensate or aggravate the afflictions produced by chronically stressful work conditions.

DEHUMANIZATION VERSUS HUMANIZATION OF WORK:
Insights From Cognitive Ergonomics and Brain Research
by Karen Belkić, MD, PhD and Čedo Savić, MD, PhD

Spectacular advances have been made in our understanding of how the human being—via the central nervous system (CNS)—handles information, transforming it into productive output of various kinds. How can that knowledge be harnessed to inform us in our quest to organize work so that it harmonizes better with human needs and capacities? How is this endeavor relevant to the cardiovascular (CV) system? Mentally stressful work has been associated with a panoply of untoward CV changes, including elevations in blood pressure and rate pressure product, myocardial ischemia, metabolic and coagulation abnormalities, and possibly even cardiac electrical instability (see Chapters 2 and 5). These processes may result in acute cardiac events, which are potentially life-threatening and, at the very least, profoundly debilitating. Thus, it does appear that we can justify our exploration of human cognitive ergonomic process from a clinical–public health perspective.

One particularly salient example concerns the way in which branches of research have developed with respect to heart rate variability (HRV). It was cognitive ergonomists who first described the relation between loss of HRV or respiratory sinus arrhythmia, and mental burden.[25,110,113,149,172] Although there was also some recognition by clinical investigators that diminished HRV was associated with cardiac dysfunction[270] and with sudden arrhythmic cardiac death in infants[92] and in adults,[218,280] nearly two decades elapsed before the clinical importance of HRV became broadly apparent, with the confirmation that HRV is a strong, independent predictor of mortality in post-acute MI patients.[248]

Obviously, there is still a great deal to be elucidated concerning causal webs linking mentally stressful work, the CNS and CV markers such as HRV, and CVD outcomes. It is an intriguing line of inquiry: the more insight we gain into what mental burden actually means, and the better we implement this knowledge to humanize work, the better the CV system might be protected. The emotional dimensions of human labor also need to be interwoven into these considerations. Some principles of cognitive ergonomics and results of advanced neurophysiologic methods allow us to explore these hypotheses, which are broadly coherent with postulations from the Tokyo Declaration:

> *The growth of neuroscience and stress science has allowed elucidation of the links between social structures and processes (at work and outside it), the way in which these are perceived and appraised and the resulting interaction between the central nervous system and other organ systems to promote or counteract workers' health, based on a bio-psychosocial ecosystem and its dynamics. These dynamics include organization restructuring, mergers, acquisitions and downsizing, the frantic pace of work and life, the erosion of leisure time and/or the blending of work and home time. Most of these developments are driven by economic and technological changes aiming at short-term productivity and profit gain.[256]*

A Model of Mental Burden on The Human Operator

COGNITIVE ERGONOMICS

The domain of cognitive ergonomics encompasses questions about how the human being processes information, makes decisions, and then carries out actions.[238] Examinations of these "levels of information transmission"[269] provides a useful framework both for work simulation studies[148] and on-site, independent-observer job analysis. Work tasks then can be defined in terms of their "mental structure" and, according to "action regulation theory," be viewed within the context of a dynamic interaction between the person and his or her environment vis-à-vis the achievement of defined goals.[62,72,76,261]

Gaillard incorporates the concept of "energy regulation" into cognitive ergonomics.[65] This energy is derived from arousal mechanisms, and when mental processing demands increase, energy resources are mobilized. However, these cognitive energy reserves have their limitations, a fact often ignored, especially in "developments . . . driven by economic and technological changes aiming at short-term productivity and profit gain."[256]

The relative mental burden of a given task can be considered quantitatively: for example, by the number of signals to be processed; the complexity, dynamics, clarity, and congruence of the signals; the nature of the decision[148]; and the type of action taken. The additional burden created by stressors such as time pressure, adverse physical conditions, and barriers that hinder task performance also can be assessed.[71]

Quantitization Using the Time Dimension. Allocation of mental resources is a key concept, for which the time dimension represents one means of measurement. In field studies, Greiner and colleagues demonstrated that each of a number of barriers—such as unruly passengers, obstructions, or vehicular problems—substantially prolonged the average work time of urban transit drivers, and often required intensified concentration and split attention[70,72] (see Chapter 6).

In the laboratory, one way to temporally quantitate the relative burden of various tasks is by examining the reaction time (RT). In the last century it was already known that the mean RT increases curvilinearly with the number of alternatives.[167] Thus, with only one alternative, e.g., a clearly visible red traffic light, the normal simple RT is about 200 milliseconds (ms). It rises to over 300 ms with two equiprobable choices, e.g., a red and a green light, and the target being the latter. With nine alternatives, the RT increases to 600 ms or more.[134] Besides the number of alternatives to be sorted out, many other characteristics of the incoming signal affect RT. If, in a two-choice RT task, the signals are both subtly different shades of green and/or visibility is poor, the signal detection process becomes more difficult, leading to longer RT due to impaired discrimination.[165]

Overload Versus Underload. The dynamics of signal flow and the length of the task also affect performance. Overly rapid as well as exceedingly slow rate of incoming signals, especially if of prolonged duration, impair correct and timely action. This finding coincides with the well-known U-shaped curve, showing optimal performance associated with moderate arousal levels, and a performance decrement with heightened catecholamine excretion associated with over- and understimulation.[59,83] Molloy and Parasuraman corroborate this data by demonstrating that accurate and quick detection of a single (i.e., rare) event during a simulated flight paradigm deteriorated over time during highly complex but also during overly simple visual task performance.

Underload or monotony is characteristic of many branches of automatic production as well as long-haul transport operation, in which a high level of vigilance must be maintained to detect infrequently or irregularly occurring signals. The mental burden and safety risks of this type of work, requiring frequent rest breaks and other protective measures, have been underscored.[27,141]

Controlled Versus Automatic Processing. On the decision-making level, of critical importance is whether the process is automatic or controlled. *Controlled processing*, which also has been called "knowledge-based," requires conscious attentional resources and is called into play for decisions involving planning. Human capacity for controlled processing is limited, especially since it is performed in series. Some important examples of knowledge-based decision making include: complex human interactions, use of a new apparatus, emergency operations, apparatus failure, and dealing with irregularities. Kalsbeek has emphasized this distinction in his analysis of air traffic controllers' (ATC) task load, noting that when new, nonroutine decisions are required due to unforeseen events, the ATC must consciously intervene, thereby substantially rearranging the "brain control program."[111] According to Levi, work requiring continuous, conscious attention should only be performed for very limited periods of time.[141]

In contrast, the human capacity for *automatic processing* (also termed "skill-based") is much less limited. This type of processing involves rapid, smooth, learned, highly integrated patterns, and can be performed in parallel.[65,175] The ratio between knowledge-based and skill-based activity is extremely important, with the critical dimension being time. The former is most sensitive to time limitations, whereas a long stretch of solely skill-based processing creates underload. Neerincx and Griffioen formulated this rule of thumb: "The more actions to be executed in a period, the less knowledge-based actions are preferable."[175]

Conflict-Interference. "Task load is not a simple summation of the load of the individual processes. Interference between concurrent information processes increases task load."[175] Thus, in contrast to a normal, smooth work routine in which there is reinforcement of the correctness of work decisions and actions, conflict or uncertainty arises when untimely or inaccurate correlations disrupt work and its rhythm. Pavlov termed this the "difficult meeting of excitation and inhibition."[185] Wickens points out that the increase in task load is greatest when the interfering information impinges on the *same* processing dimension, and is much less when different processing dimensions are involved (e.g., spatial and linguistic).[275]

COGNITIVE ERGONOMICS AND BRAIN PROCESSES

An almost baffling array of paradigms has been used to model the dynamics of cognitive ergonomics. The actual brain processes occurring in relation to these dynamics can be studied in a number of ways, e.g., power spectrum analysis of the electroencephalogram (EEG), averaged electrocortical event-related potentials, and/or positron emission tomography (PET). The PET scan can reveal the involvement of various neuroanatomic structures and identify which neurochemical pathways are activated.[181] Attenuation or blocking of EEG rhythms within the alpha range, termed "event-related desynchronization," is found to occur with cognitive loading.[194,259] Conversely, occipital beta band activity increases proportionally to mental workload,[128,168] and a frontal midline beta rhythm has been recorded with performance of mental tasks and with learning.[130,173]

Event-Related Potentials: Latency and Mental Chronometry. The unique role of event-related potentials (ERP) in reflecting higher nervous system processing required by a given task, as well as the relative objectivity of ERP compared to self-perceptive methods, have been emphasized repeatedly.[35,127,197,282] Besides providing a scalp localization of higher nervous activity, ERP can be a gauge of "mental chronometry."[165] That is, using ERP we can map brain activity *over time* as it processes information, makes decisions, and lays the basis for task execution.[97] Using the concepts from cognitive ergonomics, ERP can help quantitate mental burden using the time dimension.

The following discussion concerns the P300, which is a positively-oriented, averaged electrocortical wave appearing 300–500 ms after stimulus presentation. The P300 is most commonly elicited when the subject's attention is focused on an infrequently-occurring signal, especially if this signal has some motivational or emotional significance. The P300 is produced by task-relevant stimuli that occur relatively unexpectedly, and require either some kind of motor response or cognitive decision.[206] Basic reviews of these processes have appeared elsewhere.[33,35,38]

The latency of the P300 ERP component is related to the time required to evaluate and correctly categorize a signal.[129] When detection is made more difficult, or when contrast is diminished, the latency of the P300 in the visual modality becomes prolonged.[265] The burden of adverse physical or other external conditions on brain chronometry as manifested by ERP component latencies also can be observed. In a simulated aircraft landing paradigm, adding hypoxia and turbulence during task performance was associated with a prolongation of P300 latency.[127] Exposure to noise and to sleep deprivation also increases P300 latency.[73,195]

Subcomponents of the ERP waves can be even more illustrative of how these exacerbating stressors deleteriously affect mental processes. Hohnsbein and colleagues found that when the subject was placed under time pressure to perform two-choice reactions, the choice reaction subcomponent of the P300 shortened, even though the stimulus assessment time remained unchanged.[90] The consequence was a greater number of performance errors. This electrophysiologic data provides insight into the brain mechanisms that may mediate the compromise of safe performance, including the observed increase in accident rate, associated with high levels of time pressure.[67,69,70]

Allocation of Mental Resources and ERP Amplitude. The amplitude of ERP components, notably the P300 wave, can reflect allocation of mental resources to a given task.[41] As the complexity of a primary task increases, the amplitude of the P300 as well as some other ERP components is often found to rise.[164,239,258] However, in dual task performance the P300 amplitude to a subsidiary task diminishes as the primary task becomes more difficult. These findings demonstrate the withdrawal of processing resources from a lower priority task as the primary one consumes progressively more of the subject's mental energy.[96,239] Also, as the load upon memory increases, P300 amplitude falls, even with single task performance. This dynamic may similarly reflect competing demands on mental resources; there also may be more uncertainty or equivocation with increasing memory load.[124]

The effect of exacerbating stressors also is observable in the amplitude of the P300. Acute experimental exposures to noise and to sleep deprivation are associated with attenuation of P300 amplitude.[73,195] Among professional drivers, an inverse relation has been reported between number of work hours behind the wheel and the P300 amplitude to a visual, odd-ball, reaction-time task. This finding was considered to be related to fatigue,[16] which is known to attenuate P300 amplitude and prolong its latency.[195]

IMPLICATIONS

Approaches to quantitizing the mental burden of occupational endeavor using objective means can help circumvent some of the difficulties inherent in self-report methods.[29,70,211,215] Ideally, this information would complement the worker's own perceptions of his or her occupational tasks and in that way help guide participatory intervention strategies. Such an approach is being applied, e.g., among San Francisco transport operators.[70,201,257] Nachreiner describes a "credo," still far from being fully implemented, but which can serve as a goal or guideline: "Applying ergonomics knowledge in the light of practical experience shall provide for optimal working conditions with regard to health and safety and unimpaired performance of the work, and contribute to a more reliable, effective and efficient system performance."[174] This cognitive ergonomic approach was demonstrated by Neerincx and Griffioen to be of greater utility than more traditional noncognitive methods in developing specific recommendations for harmonizing the tasks of railway traffic controllers.[175] The approach provided provisional standards for eliminating the dual risks of momentary overload and underload.

MENTAL WORKLOAD VERSUS MENTAL STRAIN: NOT SYNONYMOUS

Mental workload is not synonymous with mental strain. As formulated by Karasek and confirmed by numerous empirical studies, lack of control or decision latitude coupled to high psychological demands is of crucial importance in creating strain conditions and concomitant cardiac risk.[118] High workload alone leads to mental effort that is oriented to execution of the task, and under optimal conditions can even be associated with positive feelings of competence and accomplishment,[65,212] as is seen in the active quadrant jobs described by Karasek and Theorell.[117] With sufficient decision-latitude or control, one can modulate even a fairly onerous, though not overwhelming, psychological workload to meet moment-to-moment needs and capacities.

Another critical element of mental stress is the intervening variable of threat, meaning that one anticipates the possibility of encountering harm of some sort.[132] When the potential consequences of one's actions include disaster, work becomes a "threat-avoidant" activity with a primary goal of self-protection—inevitably associated with negative emotion and potentially with untoward CV outcomes.

Emotional Dimensions of Human Labor

EMOTIONAL REWARDS VERSUS EMOTIONAL TOLL

There is a growing appreciation of the emotional rewards, as well as the potential tolls, of human labor. These rewards, i.e., emotional gratification and a sense of meaning, may compensate to some extent for the objective difficulties of such professions as teaching, social work, and the health professions. Previous research has revealed a hierarchical distribution of emotional (as well as economic) rewards, favoring those who have greater responsibility, power, and control within the work organization.[74,196,247] However, more recent data imply that under *optimal* conditions, new technologies could offer a more egalitarian distribution of these nonmaterial rewards, related to collaboration and sharing of information.[13] Concordantly, Karasek and Theorell note that new production technologies in workers' hands could allow workers to receive direct feedback from the public concerning their contribution, and in this way promote a sense of meaningfulness in work and provide new challenges for customizing services and products to meet the public's needs.[117]

The "invisible" or unpaid labor performed at home likewise may be emotionally gratifying, but it also can represent an emotional burden. Hochschild observes that a good deal of energy is required to display the predefined emotions often demanded by a given situation, and as a consequence, to suppress expression of one's true feelings.[88] These emotional demands are particularly heavy with the double burden of performing paid as well as unpaid labor, which is a reality for an ever-increasing number of working people, particularly women. The physiological costs of this double burden have been demonstrated repeatedly (see Chapter 2).

Numerous psychometric tools have been developed to assess the emotional dimension of human labor. Neurophysiologic methods also have been used. For example, ERP responses to signals experienced as stressors, or to signals associated in other ways with emotion, can be distinguished from ERP responses to signals that are relatively neutral for an individual.[35,44,104] Motivational aspects also can be reflected in ERPs.[14]

SENSITIZATION: REPEATED EXPOSURE TO ANXIETY- OR FEAR-INDUCING STIMULI

A closely related dimension is sensitization, which is particularly important when the worker performs activity fraught with the possibility of accidents or other untoward consequences. Sensitization has been defined as an increase in behavioral or physiological responsiveness that occurs following repeated exposure to an anxiety- or fear-inducing stimulus. The brain mechanisms for this process are described as follows:

Once a fear- or anxiety-inducing sensory stimulus is related through the thalamus into neural circuits involving the cortex, hippocampus, and amygdala, relevant memory traces of past traumatic experiences are stimulated. It is likely that the potency of the cognitive and somatic response to the stimuli will be strongly correlated with prior experiences due to the strengthening of neural connections within the circuit. These functional neuroanatomical relationships can explain how a single stimulus such as a sight or sound can elicit a specific memory. Moreover, if the sight or sound was associated with a particular traumatic event, a cascade of anxiety- and fear-related symptoms will ensue.[31]

Stimuli can be sensitizing or acquire an "aversive potential" based upon their *symbolic* association with disastrous events. It is not absolutely essential that the individual has personally experienced such events. Brain mechanisms exist that focus attention on potentially dangerous phenomena in one's surroundings; neocortical pathways that respond preferentially to danger-evoking signals have been identified in primates. These pathways are of obvious survival benefit. Normal human subjects selectively attend to threatening visual stimuli such as snakes, spiders, or angry faces when presented subliminally.[180] *Visual signals* are particularly important, because of their primary consumption of attentional resources.[237] The intimate neuroanatomical connections between the visual system and cortical arousal, via the midbrain reticular formation, as well as with critical outflow tracts to the cardiovascular system have been emphasized in relation to stress-mediated CVD.[20]

THREAT-AVOIDANT VIGILANT ACTIVITY

The heaviest burden on conscious attentional resources occurs when the human operator must continuously follow a barrage of incoming, predominantly visual, signals to which he or she must be prepared to rapidly respond, whereby a momentary lapse, error, or delay could have serious, potentially fatal consequences.[17,112,141,183,245] This activity is termed threat-avoidant vigilant (TAV) activity. Epidemiologic, human laboratory, and experimental animal data directly and indirectly link prolonged exposure to this kind of activity to dangerous CV hemodynamic and electrical events, including sudden cardiac death. Professional drivers, sea pilots, air traffic controllers, and some other classes of control panel workers, all of whom perform primarily TAV work with predominantly visual signals, are found to be at high risk for hypertension and ischemic heart disease (IHD).

Driving: A Prototypic Threat-Avoidant Vigilant Activity. Evaluation of higher cortical as well as autonomic responses to stimuli that in some way are linked to TAV activity provides a means of modeling the stress response among these occupational groups. This approach, developed and applied among professional drivers and concordant with the formulation of Fuller,[64] reveals that this occupational group shows heightened electrocortical as well as CV arousal (most notably, diastolic pressor response with digital vasoconstriction and, in some cases, ventricular arrhythmias) in response to such relevant stimuli as headlight glare.[17] Using an ERP paradigm with imperative target visual stimuli that were tacitly and then explicitly linked to accident avoidance, healthy drivers manifested a large contingent negative variation (CNV) when anticipating the appearance of imperative signals,[18] consistent with heightened expenditure of processing resources.[208] Later work using a P300 ERP paradigm revealed augmented selective attention to target visual stimuli among professional drivers with borderline and essential hypertension, compared to those who were normotensive, suggesting that these hypertensive drivers had an excessive expenditure of higher cortical resources when performing TAV activity. In contrast, drivers with IHD showed attenuated selective attentional responses consistent with exhaustion.[51]

Martin, et al. provide yet another view of how TAV activity burdens higher CNS resources. Among amateur drivers they found a differentially greater P300 amplitude and latency, but shorter reaction times (actually preceding the P300), in response to slides of imminent traffic accidents compared to those showing safe scenes. The P300 to the accident slides appeared even under conditions of high signal probability (0.5) and indicates an unusually augmented level of selective attention to these threatening visual stimuli. These findings also suggest that the subjects hastened their motor response to such an extent that information processing was not yet complete.[158] This situation is similar to that described by Fuller, in which "delayed avoidance responses" occur when aversive stimuli appear suddenly and unexpectedly, leaving the driver with limited or perhaps even inadequate time to respond safely.[64] Other ERP findings indicate that under time-pressure, response selection time is accelerated, while stimulus assessment time stays unchanged; consequently, the chances for error are increased.[90,158]

Open-ended queries to workers whose jobs entail a high degree of TAV activity have revealed that it generally is the most difficult part of their work.[15,16] Furthermore, as a corroboration to the neuro- and psychophysiologic data, *progressive sensitization*—not adaptation—appears to be occurring, since this activity is more often cited as the major burden of work with greater number of years on the job.

TAV activity is a relatively fixed feature of a number of occupations. A key strategy for coping with this special exigency is **anticipatory avoidance response** whereby the experienced worker recognizes the precursors to the potentially disastrous stimulus and takes appropriate measures. For example, in traffic this would include slowing down at a blind intersection so as to circumvent a potential collision with an unseen, approaching vehicle.[64] These anticipatory avoidance responses are vital to safety, but they consume a large share of these workers' already overburdened attentional resources.

Lennart Levi has stated: "Real life conditions usually lead to a combination of many exposures. These may become superimposed on each other in an additive way, or synergistically. In this way, the straw that breaks the camel's back may be a very trivial environmental factor which, however, is added to a very considerable existing environmental load."[141] To prevent the potentially disastrous consequences of that "straw," assessment of the total burden of exposure to physical, ergonomic, and psychosocial stressors at the workplace becomes imperative.

MULTIPLE EXPOSURES: TOWARD A MODEL OF TOTAL OCCUPATIONAL BURDEN   *by Karen Belkić , MD, PhD, Peter Schnall, MD, Čedo Savić , MD, PhD, Paul Landsbergis, PhD*

Although occupational health research traditionally has relied on a deterministic approach of assessing causal relations between a given exposure and a given outcome, recognition of the complexity of the work environment has obligated a more integrative assessment of physical, ergonomic, and psychosocial stressors on the job.[26,54,78,141,153,163,166,272] Substantial empirical evidence links each of a large number of these diverse stressors to clinically important CV occurrences.

A fairly small, but emerging body of literature has dealt with combined exposure to various types of cardionoxious factors. To cite a few examples: Lercher and colleagues reported a roughly additive effect on blood pressure of exposure to noise and night shiftwork.[135] A diastolic pressor effect has been observed with laboratory exposure to heat together with 90 dB noise.[22] Noise also increases the self-reported stressfulness of muscular work and of exposure to heat and stochastic vibration.[153] The pressor effects of performing a stressful mental task increase when noise is added to the laboratory environment.[150,246]

The Occupational Stress Index

Brabant and colleagues underscore the need for assessing "the globality of the work environment," which includes physical, ergonomic, and organizational stressors.[26] Matsubara and colleagues suggest that additive models with nonspecific scales, such as a linear combination of moderate exposures and higher weight for extreme exposures, would represent an appropriate approach to combined environmental studies.[163]

One attempt to comprehensively assess the panoply of potentially cardionoxious work stressors using such an additive model is found in the Occupational Stress Index (OSI).[19] The OSI integrates several paradigms of stress-related cardiovascular dysfunction and is reflective of cognitive ergonomic and neurophysiologic findings. The OSI contains 58 equally weighted factors, and highest scores are given for extreme exposure. The factors are organized into a two-dimensional matrix (Table 1), with the stress dimensions (underload, high demand, strictness, extrinsic time pressure, noxious physical exposures, threat-avoidant characteristics, and conflict/uncertainty) forming the horizontal axis. The levels of human information transmission—sensory input, central decision-making, and task execution[269]—plus a general level are placed along the vertical axis. Thus, each factor has a set of coordinates, localizing it to the type of stress and the level at which it affects the human operator. Summations can be made by levels and by stress aspects, and a wide variety of combined effects can be assessed. For example, various manifestations of the well-known deleterious combination of underload and high demand[59] can be identified and quite precisely characterized.

The sum of the scores to all 58 factors comprises the total OSI, which represents an attempt to quantitate the overall burden upon the human operator of a given set of working conditions. Criterion validity of the total OSI has been demonstrated with respect to its ability to identify high-risk occupations. For example, professional drivers have approximately twice the total OSI scores compared to those of a heterogeneous group of building trade workers and subway guard attendants.[19,50] The authors stated: "Using the OSI, we find that driving epitomizes a stressful occupation which bears the overwhelming majority of features associated with cardiac risk."[19]

The OSI also has shown within-occupation criterion validity. The overall burden of exacerbating (i.e., nonfixed) stressors in the professional drivers' work environment, as gauged by the total OSI, independently predicts cardio-deleterious behaviors, including smoking intensity, within this group.[19,49] (See Chapter 6 for additional details.) A limitation of the current application of the OSI is the linear nature of the analyses that have been performed. There is a need to explore possibilities for multiplicative interactions and higher level terms, within the model and more generally.

The Concept of Synergy

Lercher and colleagues have emphasized that examination of only main effects may underestimate "the true public health impact" of combined exposures.[135]

TABLE 1. The Occupational Stress Index

Levels of Information Transmission	Stress Dimensions						
	Underload	*High Demand*	*Strictness*	*Extrinsic Time Pressure*	*Aversiveness (Noxious Exposures)*	*Avoidance (Symbolic Aversiveness)*	*Conflict (Uncertainty)*
Input	Homogeneous incoming signals Low frequency incoming signals Works alone	Several information sources Heterogeneous signals Visual modality primary High frequency of incoming signals Three sensory modalities Communication essential	Strict requirements for signal detection	No control over speed of incoming signals	Glare Noise	High level of attention (serious consequences of a momentary lapse)	Signal/noise conflict Signal/signal conflict
Central Decision-making	Decisions automatic from input	Complex decisions Complicated decisions Decisions affect work of others Need for rapid decision-making	Limited number of decision-making strategies Limited number of correct decisions	Decision cannot be postponed		Wrong decision can have serious (potentially fatal) consequences	Missing information needed for decision Contradictory information Unexpected events change work plan
Output/Task Execution	Homogeneous tasks Simple tasks Nothing to do	Heterogeneous tasks Simultaneous task execution Complex tasks Need for rapid task execution	Work must meet a strictly defined standard	No control over task execution rate	Vibration Isometric stress	Hazardous tasks	Conflicting tasks in space and time External factors hamper task execution
General	Fixed pay	Piece rate Overtime work Holds 2 jobs No rest breaks Night work	Fixed body position Work in confined space	Speed up Deadline pressure	Cold Heat Noxious gases/ fumes/dusts	Work accident Witness work accident	Emotionally charged work atmosphere (interpersonal conflicts)

From Belkić K, Savić Č, Theorell T, et al: Mechanisms of cardiac risk among professional drivers. Scand J Work Environ Health 20:73–86, 1994; with permission.

According to Rothman and Greenland, it is rare that the effect of exposure to a given factor is completely independent of the effect of exposure to another factor, implying that some kind of interaction is usually taking place.[210] An interaction can be demonstrated insofar as the relative risk of combined exposure to two or more factors is not equal to the sum of the relative risks of each exposure taken separately.[79,210] A greater than additive effect, i.e., synergy, is found when the combined exposure risk exceeds the latter. Various combined exposures to the psychosocial work factors of high psychological demands, low decision latitude, and/or low social support have yielded statistically significant synergistic effects with respect to risk of MI as well as self-reported CVD.[79,99]

More generically, it can be stated that with a synergistic interaction, some cases of disease would occur only if there were combined, and not just singular, exposure to noxins. This principle is illustrated in some (but not all) investigations of psychosocial factors and risk of hypertension, ischemic heart disease (IHD), and progression of carotid atherosclerotic plaque height, in which significant results have been obtained for combined exposure to high psychological demands and low decision latitude[217,254] or to high work demands and low economic rewards.[151] However, there were no significant effects for exposure to each of these stressor dimensions alone.

Rothman and Greenland present some caveats about the practical implementation of analyses for synergy. They note that tests of nonadditivity or statistical interaction of factors "may have limited utility" due to low power for usual sample sizes and low precision of the statistical tests.[210] Dose-response relationships and induction periods further complicate the issue (see Chapter 6). Notwithstanding these difficulties, there is a need for more systematic assessment of synergistic relations between and among cardionoxious factors.

The Total Burden Concept

Hockey elaborates the construct of "resources," or total burden upon the human operator, as an integrative model whose focus is not solely upon performance *per se*, but also encompasses the impact of this burden in relation to fatigue, strain, and health consequences, including those relevant to the cardiovascular system.[89] In this context, some useful inferences can be drawn from laboratory, field, and epidemiologic studies. Cognitive ergonomic and neurophysiologic data demonstrate that there is a limit to the available processing resources, and when the human being is asked to perform multiple tasks, as the primary or prioritized action becomes more difficult, less mental energy is available for subsidiary actions. Exacerbating stressors, of a physical as well as nonphysical nature, further impinge on these processing resources. With multiple exposure to work stressors, attempts to cope may include deliberate mobilization of existing mental resources, e.g., intense concentration, such that concurrent performance proceeds unimpeded. It is known that as demands increase, processing capacity can be augmented up to a certain point. This extra energy is derived from arousal mechanisms.[109] There is residuum, however, which comes after work is over, and can be reflected in difficulty or inability to unwind and/or perform subsequent mental tasks, a decreased likelihood to engage in altruistic behaviors, and delay in return to nonwork baseline of catecholamine levels.[34,54,60,72,98,204]

DURATION AND TIMING OF EXPOSURE

Perhaps the most important practical implication of the total burden concept is that related to duration and timing of exposure. Previously, we have noted that work requiring continuous mobilization of conscious attentional resources should be performed for very limited periods of time. The data linking impaired selective attention (attenuated P300 amplitude) to long work hours behind the wheel among professional drivers offers insight into the neurophysiologic consequences of prolonged exposure to this heavily burdensome activity. Our suggestion that this finding reflected driver fatigue is corroborated in more detail by Brown.[28] The "causal contributions to fatigue" among this occupational group are cited as "length of continuous work spells and daily duty periods, time available for rest and continuous sleep, and the arrangement of duty, rest, and sleep periods within each 24-hour cycle."[28] The causal relation between accidents and fatigue, particularly related to night work, among road and air transport operators as well as other classes of workers performing threat-avoidant vigilant and otherwise burdensome activity has been well documented.[2,131,169,178,179,240] There is also considerable epidemiologic evidence linking long work hours and night shiftwork to risk of IHD. Another relevant line of investigation demonstrates that extreme fatigue or "vital exhaustion" among working-aged men predicts future MI and cardiac death, after adjustment for standard cardiac risk factors.[8,9]

REFERENCES

1. Reference deleted.
2. Akerstedt T, Ficca G, Gillberg M, Kecklund G: Fatigue and irregular duty patterns: A review of causes and countermeasures. Stockholm, Statens Institut for Psycksocial Miljomedicin, 1995.
3. Alexander F: Psychosomatic Medicine. London, George Allen & Unwin, 1952.
4. Reference deleted.
5. Alfredsson L, Spetz C, Theorell T: Type of occupation and near-future hospitalization for myocardial infarction and some other diagnoses. Int J Epidemiol 14:378–388, 1985.
6. Antonovsky A: Unravelling the Mystery of Health: How People Manage Stress and Stay Well. San Fransciso, Jossey-Bass, 1987.
7. Reference deleted.
8. Appels A, Mulder P: Excess fatigue as a precursor of myocardial infarction. Eur Heart J 9:758–764, 1988.
9. Appels A, Otten F: Exhaustion as precursor of cardiac death. Br J Clin Psychol 31:351–356, 1992.
10. Reference deleted.
11. Reference deleted.
12. Aust B, Peter R, Siegrist J: Stress management in bus drivers: A pilot study based on the model of effort-reward imbalance. Int J Stress Management 4:297–305, 1997.
13. Basini SG, Hurley JJ: Hierarchy and the meaning of work. Eur Work Organizational Psychol 4:51–64, 1994.
14. Begleiter H, Porjesz B, Chou CH, Aunon JI: P3 and stimulus incentive value. Psychophysiology 20:95–101, 1983.
15. Belkic K: Field observation and semi-structured interviews among commercial pilots. Unpublished, 1995.
16. Belkic K, Emdad R, Theorell T, et al: Neurocardiac mechanisms of heart disease risk among professional drivers. Stockholm, Swedish Fund for Working Life, 1996.
17. Belkic K, Ercegovac D, Savic C, et al: EEG arousal and cardiovascular reactivity in professional drivers: The glare pressor test. Eur Heart J 13:304–309, 1992.
18. Belkic K, Savic C, Djordjevic M, et al: Event-related potentials in professional city drivers: Heightened sensitivity to cognitively relevant visual signals. Physiol Behav 52:423–427, 1992.
19. Belkic K, Savic C, Theorell T, Cizinsky S: Work Stressors and Cardiovascular Risk: Assessment for Clinical Practice. Part I. Stockholm, National Institute for Psychosocial Factors and Health, Section for Stress Research, Karolinska Institute, WHO Psychosocial Center, 1995.
20. Belkic K, Savic C, Theorell T, et al: Mechanisms of cardiac risk among professional drivers. Scand J Work Environ Health 20:73–86, 1994.
21. Borrell C, Plasencia A, Pasarin I, et al: Widening social inequalities in mortality: The case of Barcelona, a southern European city. J Epidemiol Community Health 51:659–667, 1997.
22. Borsky I, Hubacova L, Hatiar K, et al: Combined effect of physical strain, noise and hot environmental conditions on man. Arch Complex Environ Studies 5:75–83, 1993.
23. Bosma H, Marmot MG, Hemingway H, et al: Low job control and risk of coronary heart disease in Whitehall II (prospective cohort) study. Br Med J 314:558–565, 1997.
24. Bosma H, Peter R, Siegrist J, Marmot M: Two alternative job stress models and the risk of coronary heart disease. Am J Pub Health 88:68–74, 1998.
25. Boyce PPR: Sinus arrhythmias as a measure of mental load. Ergonomics 17:177–183, 1974.
26. Brabant C, Mergler D, Bedard S, Ferraris J: Exploring integrated response to ergonomic and thermal stressors: A multidimensional analytical approach. Arch Complex Environ Studies 4:35–47, 1992.
27. Braby CD, Harris D, Muir HC: A psychophysiological approach to the assessment of work underload. Ergonomics 36:1035–1042, 1993.
28. Brown ID: Driver fatigue. Human Factors 36:298–314, 1994.

29. Cacioppo JT, Tassinary LG: Psychophysiology and psychophysiological inference. In Cacioppo JT, Tassinary LG (eds): Principles of Psychophysiology—Physical, Social, and Inferential Elements. Cambridge, Cambridge University Press, 1990, pp 3–33.
30. Cannon WB: Bodily Changes in Pain, Hunger, Fear, and Rage. Boston, Branford, 1929.
31. Charney DS, Seutch AV, Southwick SM, Krystal JH: Neural circuits and mechanisms of post-traumatic stress disorder. In Friedman MJ, Charney DS, Deutch AY (eds): Neurobiological and Clinical Consequences of Stress: From Normal Adaptation to PTSD. Philadelphia, Lippincott-Raven Publishers, 1995, pp 271–287.
32. Chen LC, Wittgenstein F, Mckeon E: The upsurge of mortality in Russia—Causes and policy implications. Population and Development Review 22:517, 1996.
33. Chiappa KH: Evoked Potentials in Clinical Medicine. New York, Raven Press, 1990.
34. Cohen S: Aftereffects of stress on human performance and social behavior. Psych Bulletin 88:82–108, 1980.
35. Coles GH, Gratton G, Fabiani M: Event-related potentials. In Cacioppo JT, Tassinary LG (eds): Principles of Psychophysiology—Physical, Social, and Inferential Elements. Cambridge, Cambridge University Press, 1990, pp 413–455.
36. Cooper C, Marshal J: Occupational sources of stress: A review of the literature related to coronary heart disease and mental ill health. J Occup Psychol 49:11–28, 1976.
37. Cooper CL, Payne R: Personality and Stress: Individual Differences in the Stress Process. Chichester, Wiley, 1991.
38. Cooper R, Osselton JW, Shaw JC: EEG Technology. London, Butterworth's, 1980.
39. Cosmides L, Tooby J: Cognitive adaptations for social exchange. In Barkow JH, Cosmides L, Tooby J (eds): The Adapted Mind: Evolutionary Psychology and the Generation of Culture. New York, Oxford University Press, 1992, pp 163–228.
40. Csiksentmihalyi M: Beyond Boredom and Anxiety. San Francisco, Jossey-Bass, 1975.
41. Donchin E, Kramer AF, Wickens CD: Applications of event-related brain potentials to problems in engineering psychology. In Coles MGH, Porges SW, Donchin E (eds): Psychophysiology: System, Processes, and Applications. New York, Guilford Press, 1986, pp 26–40.
42. Drever F, Whitehead M: Health Inequalities. London, HMSA, 1997.
43. Dreze J, Sen A: Hunger and Public Action. Oxford, Oxford University Press, 1989.
44. Dubrovsky B, Solyom L, Barbas H: Characteristics of the contingent negative variation in patients suffering from specific phobias. Biol Psychiatr 13:531–540, 1978.
45. Dunbar F: Emotions and Bodily Changes. New York, Colombia University Press, 1954.
46. Durkheim E: The Division of Labour in Society. New York, Free Press, 1893 (1968).
47. Durkheim E: Suicide. New York, Free Press, 1897 (1951).
48. EHN: Social Factors, Work, Stress, and Cardiovascular Disease Prevention in the European Union. Brussels, European Heart Network, 1998.
49. Emdad R, Belkic K, Theorell T, Cizinsky S: What prevents professional drivers from following physicians' cardiologic advice? Psychoth Psychosom 67:226–240, 1998.
50. Emdad R, Belkic K, Theorell T, et al: Work environment, neurophysiologic and psychophysiologic models among professional drivers with and without cardiovascular disease: Seeking an integrative neurocardiologic approach. Stress Med 13:7–21, 1997.
51. Emdad R, Belkic K, Theorell T, et al: Electrocortical responses to ecologically relevant visual stimuli among professional drivers with and without cardiovascular disease. Integr Physiol Behav Sci 31:96–111, 1996.
52. Engel GL: The need for a new medical model: A challenge for biomedicine. Science 196:129–136, 1977.
53. Engel GL: The clinical application of the biopsychosocial model. Am J Psychiatry 137:535–544, 1980.
54. Evans GW, Carrere S, Johansson G: A multivariate perspective on environmental stress. Arch Complex Environ Studies 1:1–5, 1989.
55. Folkow B, Schmidt T, Uvnas-Moberg K: Stress, health, and the social environment—James P. Henry's ethological approach to medicine. Acta Physiologica Scandinavica 161 Suppl 640, 1997.
56. Frankenhaeuser M: Quality of life: Criteria for behavioral adjustment. Int J Psychol 12:99–110, 1977a.
57. Frankenhaeuser M: Job demands, health, and well-being. J Psychosom Res 21:313–321, 1977b.
58. Frankenhaeuser M: Psychosocial factors and occupational health. In Rantanen J, Lehtinen S, Kalimo R, et al (eds): New Epidemics in Occupational Health. Proceedings of the International Symposium on New Epidemics in Occupational Health. Helsinki, Finnish Institute of Occupational Health, 1994, pp 64–71.
59. Frankenhaeuser M, Johansson G: On the psychophysiologic consequences of understimulation and overstimulation. In Levi L (ed): Society, Stress, and Disease. Vol. 4: Working Life. New York, Oxford University Press, 1981.
60. Frankenhaeuser M, Johansson G: Stress at work: Psychobiological and psychosocial aspects. Int Rev App Psych 35:287–299, 1986.
61. French JRP Jr, Rogers W, Cobb S: A model of person-environment fit. In Levi L (ed): Society, Stress, and Disease. Vol. 4: Working Life. Oxford, Oxford University Press, 1981, pp 39–44.
62. Frese M, Zapf D: Action as the core of work psychology: A German approach. In Triandis HC, Dunette MD, Hough LM (eds): Handbook of Industrial and Organizational Psychology. Palo Alto, Consulting Psychologists Press, 1994, pp 183–224.
63. Friedman M, Rosenman RH: Association of specific overt behavior pattern with blood and cardiovascular findings. JAMA 169:1286–1296, 1959.
64. Fuller R: A conceptualization of driving behavior as threat avoidance. Ergonomics 27:1139–1155, 1984.
65. Gaillard AWK: Comparing the concepts of mental load and stress. Ergonomics 36:991–1005, 1993.
66. Gardell B: Job Content and Quality of Life (Swedish). Stockholm, Prisma, 1976.
67. Gardell B, Aronsson G, Barklof K: The Working Environment for Local Public Transport Personnel. Stockholm, The Swedish Work Environment Fund, 1983.

68. Giddens A: Capitalism and Modern Social Theory. Cambridge, Cambridge University Press, 1971.
69. Green RG, Muir H, James M, Gradwell D, Green RL: Human Factors for Pilots. Hampshire, Avebury Technical, 1991.
70. Greiner BA, Krause N, Ragland DR, Fisher J: Objective stress factors, accidents, and absenteeism in transit operators: A theoretical framework and empirical evidence. J Occup Health Psychol 3:130–146, 1998.
71. Greiner BA, Leitner K: Assessment of job stress: The RHIA instrument. In Landau K, Rohmert W (eds): Recent Developments in Work Analysis. Philadelphia, Taylor & Francis, 1989, pp 53–66.
72. Greiner BA, Ragland DR, Krause N, et al: Objective measurement of occupational stress factors—An example with San Francisco urban transit operators. J Occup Health Psychol 2:325–342, 1997.
73. Gunter TC, Van der Zande RD, Wiethoff M, et al: Visual selective attention during meaningful noise and after sleep deprivation. In Johnson R Jr, Rohrbaugh JW, Parasuraman R (eds): Current Trends in Event-Related Potential Research (EEG Supplement 40). Amsterdam, Elsevier Science Publishers B. V., 1987, pp 99–107.
74. Gurin G, Veroff H, Feld S: How Americans View their Mental Health. New York, Basic Books, 1960.
75. Reference deleted.
76. Hacker W: Activity: A fruitful concept in industrial psychology. In Frese M, Sabini J (eds): Goal-Directed Behavior: The Concept of Action in Psychology. Hillsdale, Erlbaum, 1985, pp 262–284.
77. Hackman JR, Lawler EE: Employee reactions to job characteristics. J Appl Psychol 55:259–286, 1971.
78. Haider M, Groll-Knapp E, Kundi M: Some theoretical viewpoints on combined effects of environmental factors. Arch Complex Environ Studies 1:7–13, 1989.
79. Hallqvist J, Diderichsen F, Theorell T, et al (The SHEEP Study Group): Is the effect of job strain on myocardial infarction due to interaction between high psychological demands and low decision latitude? Results from Stockholm Heart Epidemiology Program. Soc Sci Med 46:1405–1415, 1998.
80. Hamilton A: Exploring the Dangerous Trades. Boston, Little, Brown, 1943.
81. Harrison RB: Person-environment fit and job stress. In Cooper CL, Payne R (eds): Stress at Work. New York, John Wiley, 1978.
82. Reference deleted.
83. Hebb DO: Drives and the C.N.S. (conceptual nervous system). Psychological Review 62:243–254, 1955.
84. Hemingway H, Nicholson A, Stafford M, et al: The impact of socioeconomic status on health functioning as assessed by the SF-36 questionnaire: The Whitehall II study. Am J Public Health 87:1487–1490, 1997.
85. Henry JP: Culture and high blood pressure in retrospect. In Henry JP (ed): Cultural Change and High Blood Pressure. Munster, Lit-Publishing Company, 1997, pp 109–133.
86. Henry JP: Psychological and physiological responses to stress: The right hemisphere and the hypothalamo-pituitary-adrenal axis. An inquiry into problems of human bonding. Acta Physiologica Scandinavica 161:10–25, 1997.
87. Henry JP, Stephens PM: Stress, Health, and the Social Environment: A Sociobiological Approach to Medicine. New York - Heidenberg - Berlin, Springer-Verlag, 1977.
88. Hochschild A (with Machung A): The Second Shift: Working Parents and the Revolution at Home. New York, Viking Press, 1989.
89. Hockey GRL: Compensatory control in the regulation of human performance under stress and high workload: A cognitive-energetical framework. Biol Psychol 45:73–93, 1997.
90. Hohnsbein J, Falkenstein M, Hoorman J: Effects of attention and time-pressure on P300 subcomponents and implications for mental workload research. Biol Psychol 40:73–81, 1995.
91. Holmes TH, Rahe RH: The social readjustment rating scale. J Psychosomat Res 11:213–218, 1967.
92. Hon EH, Lee ST: Electronic evaluation of the fetal heart rate patterns preceding fetal death—Further observations. Am J Obstet Gynecol 87:814–826, 1965.
93. House JM: Work Stress and Social Support. Reading, MA, Addison-Wesley, 1981.
94. House JS, Landis KR, Umberson D: Social relations and health. Science 241:540–545, 1988.
95. Huberman L: Man's Worldly Goods. London, Victor Gollancz, 1937.
96. Isreal JB, Wickens CD, Donchin E: The dynamics of P300 during dual-task performance. In Kornhumber HH, Deeke L (eds): Motivation, Motor and Sensory Processes of the Brain—Electrical Potentials, Behavior, and Clinical Use. Amsterdam, North Holland, 1980, pp 416–421.
97. Ivanitsky AM: Evoked potentials and mental processes. In Lechner H, Aranibar A (eds): Electroencephaologr Clin Neurophysiol. Amsterdam, Excerpta Medica, 1980, pp 727–732.
98. Johansson G, Aronson G: Stress reactions in computerized administrative work. J Occup Behav 5:159–181, 1984.
99. Johnson JV, Hall EM: Job strain, workplace social support, and cardiovascular disease: A cross-sectional study of a random sample of the Swedish working population. Am J Public Health 78:1336–1342, 1988.
100. Johnson JV, Hall EM, Theorell T: Combined effects of job strain and social isolation on cardiovascular disease morbidity and mortality in a random sample of the Swedish male working population. Scand J Work Environ Health 15:271–279, 1989.
101. Johnson JV, Johansson G: The Psychosocial Work Environment and Health: Work Organization, Democratization, and Health. Amityville, Baywood, 1991.
102. Johnson JV, Stewart W, Fredlund P, et al: Psychosocial job exposure matrix: An occupationally aggregated attribution system for work environment exposure characteristics. Stockholm, National Institute for Psychosocial Factors and Health, 1990.
103. Johnson JV, Stewart W, Hall EM, Fredlund P, Theorell T: Long-term psychosocial work environment and cardiovascular mortality among Swedish men. Am J Public Health 86:324–331, 1996.
104. Johnston VS, Burleson MH, Miller DR: Emotional value and late positive components of ERPs. Electroencephalogr Clin Neurophysiol Suppl 40:198–203, 1987.
105. Joksimovic L, Siegrist J, Meyer-Hammer M, et al: Overcommitment predicts restenosis after successful coronary angioplasty. Int J Behav Med (in press).

106. Josephson M: Work factors and musculoskeletal disorders—An epidemiologic approach focusing on female nursing personnel. Stockholm, Karolinska Institute and National Institute for Working Life, 1998.

107. Kagan AR, Levi L: Adaptation of the psychosocial environment to man's abilities and needs. In Levi L (ed): Society, Stress, and Disease—The Psychosocial Environment and Psychosomatic Diseases. London, Oxford University Press, 1971, pp 388–404.

108. Kagan AR, Levi L: Health and environment—Psychosocial stimuli. A review. In Levi L (ed): Society, Stress, and Disease. Vol. II: Childhood and Adolescence. Oxford University Press, 1975, pp 241–260.

109. Kahneman D: Attention and Effort. Englewood Cliffs, Prentice-Hall, 1973.

110. Kalsbeek JWH: Measurement of mental work load and acceptable load, possible applications in industry. Int J Production Research 7:33–45, 1967.

111. Kalsbeek JWH: Standards of acceptable load in ATC tasks. Ergonomics 14:641–650, 1971.

112. Kalsbeek JWH: Prevention of excessive mental load, and how can the industrial engineer and the ergonomist cooperate. Laboratorium voor ergonomische psychologie van de gezondheidsarganisatie, TNO. pres., Conference of the European Federation of Productivity Service. Berlin, 1974.

113. Kalsbeek JWH, Ettema TH: Continuous recording of heart rate and the measurement of perceptual load. Ergonomics 6:306–307, 1963.

114. Karasek RA: The impact of the work environment on life outside the job. PhD dissertation, Massachusetts Institute of Technology, 1976. Distributed by National Technical Information Service. Thesis order no. PB 263-073.

115. Karasek R, Baker D, Marxer F, Ahlbom A, Theorell T: Job decision latitude, job demands, and cardiovascular disease: A prospective study of Swedish men. Am J Public Health 71:694–705, 1981.

116. Karasek R, Brisson C, Kawakami N, et al: The Job Content Questionnaire: An instrument for internationally comparative assessments of psychosocial job characteristics. J Occup Health Psychology 3:322–355, 1998.

117. Karasek R, Theorell T: Healthy Work: Stress, Productivity, and the Reconstruction of Working Life. New York, Basic Books, 1990.

118. Karasek RA: Job demands, job decision latitude, and mental strain: Implications for job redesign. Adm Sci Q 24:285–308, 1979.

119. Katz, Kahn: Social Psychology of Organizations. New York, Wiley, 1966.

120. Kaufman JS, Long AE, Liao YL, et al: The relation between income and mortality in U.S. blacks and whites. Epidemiology 9:147–155, 1998.

121. Kennedy BP, Kawachi I, Prothrow-Stith D: Income-distribution and mortality: Cross-sectional ecological study of the Robin-Hood index in the United States. Br Med J 312:1004–1007, 1996.

122. Kerckhoff A, Back B: The June Bug. New York, Appleton-Century-Croft, 1968.

123. Kohn M, Schooler C: Occupational experience and psychological functioning: An assessment of reciprocal effects. Am Sociol Rev 38:97–118, 1973.

124. Kok R: Event-related potential reflections of mental resources: A review and synthesis. Biol Psychol 45:19–56, 1997.

125. Kornitzer M: Type A behavior and coronary heart disease: An update. Nutr Metab Cardiovasc Dis 2:86–93, 1992.

126. Kornitzer M: Type A behavior and coronary heart disease: An update. Nutr Metab Cardiovasc Dis 2:86–93, 1992.

127. Kramer AF, Sirevaag E, Braune R: A psychophysiological assessment of operator workload during simulated flight missions. Human Factors 29:145–160, 1987.

128. Kurimori S, Kakizaki T: Evaluation of work stress using psychological and physiological measure of mental activity in a paced calculating task. Industrial Health 33:7–22, 1995.

129. Kutas M, McCarthy G, Donchin E: Augmenting mental chronometry: The P300 as a measure of stimulus evaluation time. Science 197:792–795, 1977.

130. Lang M, Lang W, Diekmann V, Kornhuber H: The frontal theta rhythm indicating motion and cognitive learning. Electroenceph Clin Neurophysiol Suppl 40:322–327, 1987.

131. Lauber JK, Kayten PJ: Sleepiness, circadian dysrhythmia and fatigue in transportation system accidents. Sleep 11:503–512, 1988.

132. Lazarus RS: Stress theory and psychophysiological research. In Levi L (ed): Emotional Stress. Vol. 3 Suppl 2, Forsvarsmedicin, 1967, pp 152–177.

133. Lazarus RS, Folkman S: Stress, Appraisal, and Coping. New York, Springer, 1984.

134. Legge D, Barber PJ: Information and Skill. London, Methuen, 1976.

135. Lercher P, Hortnagl J, Kofler WW: Work noise annoyance and blood pressure: Combined effects with stressful working conditions. Int Arch Occup Environ Health 65:25–28, 1993.

136. Levi L: Society, Stress, and Disease. Vol. I: The Psychosocial Environment and Psychosomatic Diseases. London - New York - Toronto, Oxford University Press, 1971.

137. Levi L: Stress and Distress in Response to Psychosocial Stimuli. New York, Pergamon Press, 1972.

138. Levi L: Society, Stress, and Disease. Vol. II: Childhood and Adolescence. London, Oxford University Press, 1975.

139. Levi L: Society, Stress, and Disease. Vol. III: The Productive and Reproductive Age—Male/Female Roles and Relationships. Oxford, Oxford University Press, 1978.

140. Levi L: Psychosocial factors in preventive medicine. In Hamburg DA, et al (eds): Healthy People—The Surgeon General's Report on Health Promotion and Disease Prevention. Background Papers. Washington DC, US Government Printing Office, DHEW (PHS) Publication No. 79-55071A, 1979, pp 207–259.

141. Levi L: Preventing Work Stress. Reading, MA, Addison-Wesley Publishing Co., 1981.

142. Levi L: Society, Stress, and Disease. Vol. IV: Working Life. Oxford, Oxford University Press, 1981.

143. Levi L: Psychosocial environmental factors and psychosocially mediated effects of physical environmental factors. Scand J Work Environ Health 23 (Suppl 3):47–52, 1997.

144. Levi L: The welfare of the future—A Swedish case study. The Verona Initiative, Arena meeting I. Copenhagen, WHO Regional Office for Europe, 1998.

145. Levi L: Stress management and prevention on a European Community level: Options and obstacles. In Kenny D (ed): Stress and Health—Research and Clinical Applications. North Ryde, Australia, Fine Arts Press, 1999, pp 279–294.
146. Levi L, Frankenhaeuser M, Gardell G: Work stress related to social structures and processes. In Elliott GR, Eisdorfer C (eds): Stress and Human Health. New York, Springer, 1982, pp 119–146.
147. Light KC, Brownley KA, Turner JR, et al: Job status and high-effort coping influence work blood pressure in women and blacks. Hypertension 25:554–559, 1995.
148. Luczak H: The use of simulators for testing individual mental working capacity. Ergonomics 14:651–660, 1971.
149. Luczak H, Lauring W: An analysis of heart rate variability. Ergonomics 16:85–97, 1973.
150. Lundberg U, Frankenhaeuser M: Psychophysiological reactions to noise as modified by personal control over noise intensive. Biol Psychol 6:51–60, 1978.
151. Lynch J, Krause N, Kaplan GA, et al: Workplace demands, economic reward and progression of carotid atherosclerosis. Circulation 96:302–307, 1997b.
152. Lynch J, Krause N, Kaplan GA, Tuomilehto J, Salonen JT: Work place conditions, socioeconomic status, and the risk of mortality and acute myocardial infarction. The Kuopio Ischemic Heart Disease Risk Factor Study. Am J Public Health 87:617–622, 1997a.
153. Manninen O: Further studies on changes in subjective stressfulness under various combinations of noise, vibration, temperature and work tasks. Arch Complex Environ Studies 2:31–39, 1990.
154. Mark N: Beyond individual differences: Social differentiation from first principles. Am Soc Review 63:309–330, 1998.
155. Marmot M: Psychosocial factors and cardiovascular disease: Epidemiological approaches. Eur Heart J 9:690–697, 1988.
156. Marmot M, Theorell T: Social class and cardiovascular disease: The contribution of work. Int J Health Services 18:659–674, 1988.
157. Marmot MG, Smith DG, Stansfeld S, et al: Health inequalities among British civil servants: The Whitehall II study. Lancet 337:1387–1393, 1991.
158. Martin F, Siddle DAT, Gourley M, et al: P300 and traffic scenes: The effect of temazepam. Biol Psychol 33:225–240, 1992.
159. Marx K: Economic and Philosophical Manuscripts of 1844. London, Lawrence and Wishart, 1844.
160. Marx K: The Communist Manifesto (1848). In Burns E (ed): A Handbook of Marxism. London, Victor Gollancz, 1935.
161. Marx K: Capital: A Critique of Political Economy. Vol. I (1867). Middlesex, UK, Penguin, 1976.
162. Matschinger H, Siegrist J, Siegrist K, Dittmann K: Type A as a coping career: Towards a conceptual and methodological re-definition. In Schmidt TH, Dembroski TM, Blumchen E (eds): Biological and Psychological Factors in Cardiovascular Disease. Berlin, Springer, 1986, pp 104–126.
163. Matsubara N, Ito K, Gassho A, Kurazumi Y: Importance of nonspecific scale and the additive model in the evaluation study of the combined environment. Arch Complex Environ Studies 7:45–53, 1995.
164. McCallum WC, Cooper R, Pocock PV: Brain slow potential and ERP changes associated with operator load in a visual tracking task. Electroencephalogr Clin Neurophysiol 69:453–468, 1988.
165. McCarthy G, Donchin E: A metric for thought: A comparison of P300 latency and reaction time. Science 211:77–80, 1981.
166. Melamed S, Luz J, Najenson T, Jucha E, Green M: Ergonomic stress levels, personal characteristics, accidence occurrence and sickness absence among factory workers. Ergonomics 32:1101–1110, 1989.
167. Merkel J: Die zeitlichen Verhaltrisse der Willenstatigkeit. Philosophie Studion 2:73–127, 1885.
168. Michel J, Koch B, Camman H, et al: System analysis of the EEG during stimulus discrimination tasks. Fiziologiya Cheloveka 8:18–25, 1982.
169. Mitler MM, Carskadon MA, Czeisler CA, et al: Catastrophies, sleep and public policy. Consensus Report. Sleep 11:100–109, 1988.
170. Molloy R, Parasuraman R: Monitoring an automatic system for a single failure: Vigilance and task complexity effects. Human Factors 38:311–322, 1996.
171. Morrison K: Marx, Durkheim, Weber: Foundations of Modern Social Thought. London, Sage, 1995.
172. Mulder G, Van Der Meulen M: Mental load and the measurement of heart rate variability. Ergonomics 16:69–83, 1973.
173. Mundy-Castle AC: Theta and beta rhythm in the electroencephalograms of normal adults. Electroenceph Clin Neurophysiol 3:477–486, 1951.
174. Nachreiner F: Standards for ergonomics principles relating to the design of work systems and to mental workload. Applied Ergonomics 26:259–263, 1995.
175. Neerincx MA, Griffioen E: Cognitive task analysis: Harmonizing tasks to human capacities. Ergonomics 39:543–561, 1996.
176. North F, Syme SL, Feeney A, et al: Explaining socioeconomic differences in sickness absence: The Whitehall II study. Br Med J 306:361–366, 1993.
177. North F, Syme SL, Feeney A, et al: Explaining socioeconomic differences in sickness absence: The Whitehall II study. Br Med J 306:361–366, 1993.
178. NTSB: Aircraft accident report. Uncontrolled collision with terrain. American International Airways flight 808. Washington D.C., National Transportation Safety Board, 1994.
179. NTSB: A review of flightcrew-involved major accidents of US Air carriers 1978 through 1990. Washington, D.C., National Transportation Safety Board, 1994.
180. Ohman A: Face the beast and fear the face: Animal and social fears as prototypes for evolutional analyses of emotion. Psychophysiology 23:123–145, 1986.

181. Orrison WW, Lewine JD, Sanders JA, Jartshorne MF: Functional Brain Imaging. St. Louis, Mosby, 1995.
182. Reference deleted.
183. Parasuraman R: Sustained attention in detection and discrimination. In Parasuraman R, Davies DR (eds): Varieties of Attention. Orlando, Academic Press, Inc., 1984, pp 243–271.
184. Pavlov IP: (1916) Refleks tseli (The Reflex of Purpose), Dvadtsatiletnii opyt objektivnovo izucheniia vysshei nervnoi deiatel'nosti (povedeniia) zhivotnykh. Uslovnye reflesksy (20 Years of Experience in the Objective Study of the Higher Nervous Activity [Behavior] of Animals. Conditioned Reflex.) Moscow, 1951.
185. Pavlov IP: Complete Collected Works. Moscow-Leningrad, 1951.
186. Pelham BW, Swann WB: From self-conceptions to self-worth: On the sources and structure of global self-esteem. J Personality Social Psychol 57:672–680, 1989.
187. Pell S, D'Alonzo CA: Acute myocardial infarction in a large employed population: Report of six-year study of 1356 cases. JAMA 185:831–841, 1963.
188. Peter R: Berufliche Belastungen, Belastungsbewaltigung und koronares Risiko bei Industriearbeitern (Chronic work stress, coping behavior, and coronary risk in blue-collar workers.) Hamburg Munster, LIT, 1991.
189. Peter R, Alfredsson L, Hammar N, et al: High effort, low reward, and cardiovascular risk factors in employed Swedish men and women: Baseline results from the WOLF study. J Epidemiol Community Health 52:540–547, 1998.
190. Peter R, Alfredsson L, Knutsson A, et al: Does a stressful psychosocial work environment mediate the effects of shiftwork on cardiovascular factors in men? Scand J Work Environ Health 25:376–381, 1999.
191. Peter R, Geissler H, Siegrist J: Associations of effort-reward imbalance at work and reported symptoms in different groups of male and female public transport workers. Stress Medicine 14:175–182, 1998.
192. Peter R, Siegrist J, Hallqvist J, et al (The SHEEP Study Group): Psychosocial work environment and myocardial infarction: Improving risk prediction by combining two alternative job stress models in the SHEEP Study. (Submitted), 1999.
193. Peter R, Siegrist J: Chronic work stress, sickness absence, and hypertension in middle managers: General or specific sociological explanations? Soc Sci Med 45:1111–1120, 1997.
194. Pfurtscheller G, Neuper C, Mohl W: Event-related desynchronization during visual processing. Int J Psychophysiol 16:147–153, 1994.
195. Polich J, Kok A: Cognitive and biological determinants of P300: An integrative review. Biol Psychol 41:103–146, 1995.
196. Porter LW: Job attitude management: Perceived deficiencies in need fulfillment as a function of job level. J Applied Psychol 66:375–384, 1962.
197. Pribram KH, McGuinness D: Attention and para-attention processing. Event related potentials as tests of a model. Ann NY Acad Sci 658:65–92, 1992.
198. Queen S, Pappas G, Hadden W, et al: The widening gap between socioeconomic status and mortality. Stat Bull Metrop Insur Co 75:31–35, 1994.
199. Quine S, Taylor R, Hayes L: Australian trends in mortality by socioeconomic status using nsw small-area data, 1970–89. J Biosoc Sci 27:409–419, 1995.
200. Rael EG, Stansfeld SA, Shipley M, et al: Sickness absence in the Whitehall II study, London: The role of social support and material problems. J Epidemiol Community Health 49:474–481, 1995.
201. Ragland DR, Bauer G, Krause N, et al: Working with a Joint Labor-Management program to develop a program for intervention. Work Stress and Health '95: Creating Healthier Workplaces. Washington, D.C., 1995.
202. Rahe RH: Subjects' recent life changes and their near-future illness suceptibility. In Reichsman F (ed): Advances in Psychosomatic Medicine. Vol. 8. Basel, 1972.
203. Ramazzini B: De morbis diatriba (Untersuchungen von den Krankheiten der Kunstler und Handwerker). Modena, 1700. Leipzig, Weidmann, 1718.
204. Razmjou S: Mental workload in heat: Toward a framework for analyses of stress states. Aviat Space Environ Med 67:530–538, 1996.
205. Renner K: Wandlungen der Modernen Gasellschaft [1953]. In Bottomore T, Goode P (eds): Austro-Marxism. Oxford, Clarendon, 1978.
206. Ritter W, Vaughan HG, Costa LD: Orienting and habituation of auditory stimuli: A study of short term changes in averaged evoked responses. Electroencephalogr Clin Neurophysiol 25:550–556, 1968.
207. Rom WN: The discipline of environmental and occupational medicine. In Rom WN (ed): Environmental and Occupational Medicine, 3rd ed. Philadelphia, Lippincott-Raven Publishers, 1998, pp 3–9.
208. Rosler F, Heil M, Roder B: Slow negative brain potentials as reflections of specific modular resources of cognition. Biol Psychol 45:109–141, 1997.
209. Rothenbacher D, Peter R, Bode G, Adler G, Brenner H: Dyspepsia in relation to *Heliobacter pylori* infection and psychosocial work stress in white collar employees. Am J Gastroenterol 93:1443–1449, 1998.
210. Rothman KJ, Greenland S: Modern Epidemiology. Philadelphia, Lippincott-Raven, 1998.
211. Sacket DL: Bias in analytic research. J Chron Dis 32:51–63, 1979.
212. Sanden P-O: Work in the Control Room: Studies of sociotechnical systems, job satisfaction, mental load and stress reactions. (Doctoral Dissertation), Department of Psychology. Stockholm, Stockholm University, 1990.
213. Sauter SL, Hurrell JJ Jr, Murphy LR, Levi L: Psychosocial and Organizational Factors. Introduction. Encyclopaedia of Occupational Health and Safety, Chapter 34.2. Geneva, International Labour Office, 1998.
214. Statistics Sweden: Valfard och jamlikhet i 10 arspespektiv 1975–1995 (Welfare and social equity in twenty years' perspective 1975–1995). Report 91. Stockholm, Statistics Sweden, 1997.
214a. Statistics Sweden: Negativ stress i arbetet. De mest utsatta yrkena (Negative stress at work. The most exposed occupations). Information om utbildning och arbetsmarknad 1997:1. Stockholm, Statistics Sweden, 1997.

215. Schnall PL, Landsbergis PA, Baker D: Job strain and cardiovascular disease. Annu Rev Public Health 15:381–411, 1994.

216. Schnall PL, Landsbergis PA, Schwartz J, et al: A longitudinal study of job strain and ambulatory blood pressure: Results from a 3-year follow-up. Psychosom Med 60:697–706, 1998.

217. Schnall PL, Pieper C, Schwartz JE, et al: The relationship between job strain, workplace diastolic blood pressure, and left ventricular mass index. Results of a case-control study [published erratum appears in JAMA 1992 Mar 4;267(9):1209]. JAMA 263:1929–1935, 1990.

218. Schneider RA, Costiloe JP, Wolf S: Arterial pressures recorded in hospital and during ordinary daily activities: Contrasting data in subjects with and without ischemic heart disease. J Chron Dis 23:647, 1971.

219. Schonpflug W, Batman W: The costs and benefits of coping. In Fisher S, Reason J (eds): Handbook of Stress, Cognition, and Health. Chichester, Wiley, 1989, pp 699–714.

220. Reference deleted.

221. Selye H: A syndrome produced by diverse noxious agents. Nature 138:32, 1936.

222. Selye H: The Physiology and Pathology of Exposure to Stress. Montreal, ACTA Press, 1950.

223. Selye H: The evolution of the stress concept—Stress and cardiovascular disease. In Levi L (ed): Society, Stress, and Disease. Vol. I: the Psychosocial Environment and Psychosomatic Diseases. London, Oxford University Press, 1971, pp 299–311.

224. Sen A: Human capital and human capability. World Development 25:1959–1961, 1997.

225. Siegrist J: Threat to social status and cardiovascular risk. Psychotherapy Psychosomatics 42:90–96, 1984.

226. Siegrist J: Contributions of sociology to the prediction of heart disease and their implications for public health. Eur Journal Public Health 1:10–21, 1991a.

227. Siegrist J: Social differentials in chronic disease: What can sociological knowledge offer to explain and possibly reduce them? Soc Sci Med 41:1603–1605, 1995.

228. Siegrist J: Adverse health effects of high-effort/low-reward conditions. J Occup Health Psychol 1:27–41, 1996.

229. Siegrist J, Bernhardt R, Feng Z, Schettler G: Socioeconomic differences in cardiovascular risk factors in China. Int J Epidemiol 19:905–910, 1990b.

230. Siegrist J, Klein D, Voight KH: Linking sociological with physiological data: The model of effort-reward imbalance at work. Acta Physiol Scand 161:112–116, 1997b.

231. Siegrist J, Matschinger H, Cremer P, Seidel D: Atherogenic risk in men suffering from occupational stress. Atherosclerosis 69:211–218, 1988.

232. Siegrist J, Peter R: Job stressors and coping characteristics in work-related disease: Issues of validity. Work Stress 8:130–140, 1994.

233. Siegrist J, Peter R: Threat to occupational status control and cardiovascular risk. Isr J Med Sci 32:179–184, 1996.

234. Siegrist J, Peter R, Cremer P, Seidel D: Chronic work stress is associated with atherogenic lipids and elevated fibrinogen in middle aged men. J Int Med 242:149–156, 1997a.

235. Siegrist J, Peter R, Georg W, Cremer P, Seidel D: Psychosocial and biobehavioral characteristics of hypertensive men with elevated atherogenic lipids. Atherosclerosis 86:211–218, 1991b.

236. Siegrist J, Peter R, Junge A, Cremer P, Seidel D: Low status control, high effort at work, and ischaemic heart disease: Prospective evidence from blue-collar men. Soc Sci Med 31:1127–1134, 1990a.

237. Singleton WT: Introduction a L'ergonomie (Introduction to ergonomics). Geneva, Organization Mondial de la Sante, 1974.

238. Singleton WT: A.T. Welford—A commemorative review. Ergonomics 40:125–140, 1997.

239. Sirevaag EJ, Kramer AF, Coles MGH, Donchin E: P300 amplitude and resource allocation (Abstract). Psychophysiology 21:598–599, 1984.

240. Smith L, Folkard S, Poole CHM: Increased injuries on night shift. Lancet 344:1137–1139, 1994.

241. Spector PE: A control theory of the job stress process. In Cooper CE (ed): Theories of Organizational Stress. Oxford, Oxford University Press, 1998, pp 153–169.

242. Stansfeld S, Bosma H, Hemingway H, Marmot M: Psychosocial work characteristics and social support as predictors of SF-36 functioning: The Whitehall II study. Psychosom Med 60:247–255, 1998.

243. Stansfeld S, Bosma H, Hemingway H, Marmot M: Work characteristics predict psychiatric disorders: Prospective results from the Whitehall II study. Occup Environ Medicine 56:302–307, 1999.

244. Stansfeld SA, Head J, Marmot MG: Explaining social class differences in depression and well-being. Soc Psychiatry Psychiatr Epidemiol 33:1–9, 1998.

245. Stroh CM: Vigilance: The Problem of Sustained Attention. Oxford, Pergamon Press, 1971.

246. Tafalla R, Evans GW, Chen A: The potential role of effort. In Berglund B, Bergland U, Karlsson J, Lidnvall T (eds): Proceedings of the Fifth International Congress on Noise as a Public Health Problem, Vol. 3. Stockholm, Swedish Council for Building Research, 1988, pp 95–100.

247. Tannenbaum AS, Rozgonyi T: Authority and reward in organizations: An international research. Ann Arbor, The University of Michigan, 1986.

248. Task Force of the European Society of Cardiology and the North American Society of Pacing and Electrophysiology: Heart rate variability standards of measurement, physiological interpretation, and clinical use. Eur Heart J 17:354–381, 1996.

249. Taylor F: The Principles of Scientific Management (1911). New York, Norton, 1967.

250. Reference deleted.

251. Theorell T, Karasek R: Current issues relating to psychosocial job strain and cardiovascular disease research. J Occup Health Psychol 1:9–26, 1996.

252. Theorell T, Karasek R: The demand-control-support model and cardiovascular disease. Occup Med: 2000.

253. Theorell T, Perski A, Akerstedt T, et al: Changes in job strain in relation to changes in physiological states—A longitudinal study. Scand J Work Environ Health 14:189–196, 1988.

254. Theorell T, Perski A, Orth-Gomer K, et al: The effects of the strain of returning to work on the risk of death after a first myocardial infarction before age of 45. Int J Cardiol 30:61–67, 1991.
255. Theorell T, Tsutsumi A, Hallqvist J, et al (SHEEP Study Group): Decision latitude, job strain, and myocardial infarction. Am J Public Health 88:382–388, 1998.
256. Tokyo Declaration on work-related stress and health in three post-industrial settings: EU, Japan, and USA. Tokyo, Department of Preventive Medicine and Public Health, Tokyo Medical University, 1998.
257. Transport Workers Union: Local 250-A and San Francisco Municipal Railway's Plan to Reinvent MUNI, 1996.
258. Ullsperger P, Metz AM, Gille HG: The P300 component of the event-related potential and mental effort. Ergonomics 31:1127–1137, 1988.
259. Van Winsum W, Sergeant J, Geuze R: The functional significance of event-related desynchronization of alpha rhythm in attentional and activating tasks. Electroencephalogr Clin Neurophysiol 58:519–524, 1984.
260. Volpert W: The model of the hierarchical-sequential organization of action. In Hacker W, Volpert W, von Cranach M (eds): Cognitive and Motivational Aspects of Action. Amsterdam, North-Holland, 1982, pp 35–51.
261. Volpert W: The model of the hierarchical-sequential organization of action. In Hacker W, Volpert W, von Cranach M (eds): Cognitive and Motivational Aspects of Action. Amsterdam, North-Holland, 1982, pp 35–51.
262. Vrijkotte TGM, van Doornen LJP, de Geus EJC: Work stress and metabolic and hemostatic risk factors. (Submitted), 1999.
263. Reference deleted.
264. Walker EA, Katon WJ: Psychological factors affecting medical conditions and stress responses. In Stoudemire A (ed): Human Behavior. Philadelphia, Lippincott-Raven, 1998, pp 85–108.
265. Walton P, Callaway E, Halliday R, Naylor H: Stimulus intensity, contrast, and complexity have additive effects on P300 latency. Electroencephalogr Clin Neurophysiol 40 (Suppl):284–292, 1987.
266. Walton P, Gamble A: From Alienation to Surplus Value. London, Sheed and Ward, 1972.
267. Weber M: The Protestant Ethic and the Spirit of Capitalism. New York, Scribners Press, 1904.
268. Weber M: Economy and Society. Berkeley, University of California Press, 1978.
269. Welford AT: The measurement of sensory-motor performance: Survey and reappraisal of twelve years' progress. Ergonomics 3:189–230, 1960.
270. Wenckebach KF, Winterberg H: Die Unregelmassige Hertzatigkend. Leipzig, Engelman, 1927.
271. White R: Motivation reconsidered: The concept of competence. Psychol Rev 66:297–333, 1959.
272. WHO: Health effects of combined exposures in the work environment. Geneva, World Health Organization, 1981.
273. WHO: Health for All in the 21st Century. Geneva, World Health Organization, 1998.
274. Whyte WF: Human relations in the restaurant industry. New York, McGraw-Hill, 1948.
275. Wickens CD: Processing resources in attention. In Parasuraman R, Davies DR (eds): Varieties of Attention. London, Academic Press, 1984.
276. Wilkinson R: What health tells us about society. Bull Inst Develop Studies 29:77, 1998.
277. Wilkinson RG: National mortality rates—The impact of inequality. Am J Public Health 82:1082–1084, 1992.
278. Wilkinson RG: The epidemiologic transition—From material scarcity to social disadvantage. Daedalus 123:61–77, 1994.
279. Williams DR, Collins C: US socioeconomic and racial differences in health: Patterns and explanations. Annu Rev Sociol 21:349–386, 1995.
280. Wolf MM, et al: Sinus arrhythmia in acute MI. Med J Australia 2:52–53, 1978.
281. Wolff HG: Stress and Disease. Springfield, Charles C Thomas, 1953.
282. Zubin J, Kietzman ML: A cross-cultural approach to classification in schizophrenia and other mental disorders. In Hoch PH, Zubin J (eds): Pasychopathology of Schizophrenia. New York, Grune & Stratton, 1966, pp 482–514.

THE CENTRAL NERVOUS SYSTEM: BRIDGE BETWEEN THE EXTERNAL MILIEU AND THE CARDIOVASCULAR SYSTEM

THE ENVIRONMENT-BRAIN-HEART CONNECTION: ECONEUROCARDIOLOGY   *by Stewart Wolf, MD*

The concept of neurocardiology emerged in the medical literature for the first time in an editorial by this author in the February, 1967 issue of the Oklahoma State Medical Journal.[62] The editorial introduced the manuscripts of 12 investigators collaborating on a project supported by the National Heart Institute (NHI) of the National Institutes of Health. Six years later, this neurocardiology research program culminated in a report at an international colloquium in Lindau on Bodenzee, West Germany—The Artery And The Process of Arteriosclerosis: Measurement and Modification.[55]

"Eco" was added to the term neurocardiology to acknowledge the fact that the brain's activities are largely governed by life experience and environment, as proposed by John Locke in the early 16th century.[30] "Eco" derives from a Greek word meaning house, and ecology implies an interdependent relationship between the inner and outer aspects of a system, our ecosystem. Many aspects of our environment are capable of activating neuroregulatory mechanisms to develop, enhance, enrich, adapt, protect, or challenge our capacity for fulfillment on this planet. Most commonly the environmental forces at work are people. The emotionally significant events that take place in our relationships with parents, siblings, colleagues, mates, and children may set off almost any type of cardiovascular (CV) effect through their impact on the forebrain mechanisms.

Among the first to discover the importance of the forebrain in CV regulation was René Leriche, a pioneer in peripheral neurosurgery.[27,28] His demonstration that stimuli from higher neural centers are required to achieve fatal arrhythmia has been confirmed by several subsequent investigators.[1,9,29,33,34,51,61,65]

In 1985, Natelson published a comprehensive paper on neurocardiology.[37] Within the next 10 years, as if in response to a call, two books appeared under the title "Neurocardiology."[1,26] Despite the massive body of evidence published over the past 67 years that documents the importance of forebrain discharges in causing fatal cardiac arrhythmia, the findings have been neglected by the most recent and widely quoted cardiovascular textbooks.

It has taken a long time to dispel the many popular dogmas that have emerged in relation to the disorder generally labeled "heart attack." Evidence that established the role of the brain in CV control, including internal vascular changes involved in atherosclerosis[56] and the process of MI,[55] has been widely ignored. Early recognition of the importance of the nervous system to CV development and disease was slow coming to confirmation, but the data have been supplemented recently with direct evidence that higher neural forebrain mechanisms affect all aspects of cardiovascular function.[23] Although it has been well established that intracranial neural mechanisms may support or impair multiplex CV functions, there needs to be further inquiry into the molecular sequences whereby a life experience communication with intracranial axon cones enables the axons to trace long distances throughout the forebrain cortex. We owe the discovery of this extraordinary and indispensable communicative process to the work of Santiago Ramon y Cajal nearly a century ago.[44]

Failure to appreciate the most relevant regulatory forces governing cardiac function and dysfunction may have emerged from the unfortunate pedagogic error of medical schools to subdivide medical teaching of residents and fellows into clinical specialties. That narrow focus has been carried over into the leading CV specialty textbooks,[54] which fail altogether to deal with neuroregulatory mechanisms, except for a few autonomic reflexes.

Among the most important and frequently involved forebrain areas is the site on the ophthalmic branch of the fifth cranial nerve that connects to autonomic efferents producing the O_2-conserving dive reflex, which affects the sinoatrial node.[23] These regulatory efferents may be activated during the brain's interpretation of emotionally laden life experience, and thereby may influence all aspects of cardiac function and vulnerability. In 1962, recognizing the importance of higher neural mechanisms to most cardiovascular functions, the NHI established a special program in neurocardiology at the University of Oklahoma School of Medicine. The program supported a 10-year prospective study of 79 subjects who had experienced MI in the past, matched with an equal number of subjects who had been free of CV disorders.

Among the studies that emerged from that program was the first report on the relationship of reduced RR variability to sudden arrhythmic death.[45] The prospective findings were so novel that the paper was turned down for publication by two of the leading heart journals. The work was later presented at the cardiovascular conference in Lindau, West Germany in 1971.[45]

Thereafter, the data from the entire 10-year prospective study were re-examined, fully analyzed, and published.[61] The findings that emerged established a validity of reduced RR variability being predictive of subsequent sudden cardiac death. Not all of the fatal heart attacks were associated with a fresh MI, or even other evidence of occlusive disease of the coronary arteries. Some were fatal arrhythmias.

In the 1950s and 1960s a great deal was learned about the autonomic nervous system, but inattention to brain mechanisms that governed autonomic functions still prevailed. The voices that implicated the intermediate forebrain in cardiac disorders were not heard until the 1970s and 1980s, when reports linked forebrain influences to control of autonomic reflexes as well as more direct neural pathways to the heart. Such channels were found to derive from numerous forebrain sites, including the insular cortex, hypothalamus, medial frontal cortex, septum, thalamus, zona incerta, amygdala, and bed nucleus of the stria terminalis.[1]

These and other data led to an investigation of a possible involvement of forebrain functions with sudden arrhythmic death independent of MI or other cardiac injury. A search of the literature provided considerable support for this view, and a series of experiments with Paul Houk provided strong confirmation.[23]

The claim that environmental forces may arouse physiological and pathological manifestations does not usually refer to some change in the *physical* environment, but more likely to the *social* environment, especially the phenomenon that Horsley Gantt called **the effect of person**.[17] Our social interactions may powerfully affect the heart and influence its performance in many ways. It appears that the CV systems contain structures most susceptible to the influence of person. Vivid examples range from the facial blush in response to an embarrassing comment, to sudden death, including angina pectoris, hypertension, and MI. The mechanisms responsible for such effects have been brought to light by recent experiments exploring sites rostral to autonomic nerve origins in forebrain areas that elicit and control autonomic responses. The activities of these forebrain structures are, of course, activated by sensory signals that may originate from the environment in the form of a word or a threat from a person. They may be relayed by the afferent fibers of the ophthalmic branch of the trigeminal nerve, as in the diving reflex that is important in inducing fatal ventricular fibrillation. Other examples include cardiac stand-still during drowning; during intubation of the trachea under anesthesia; from trauma to the pleura or to the surface of the heart itself, as may happen during cardiac catheterization; or even from the fright that sometimes is associated with this latter procedure.

Anecdotes abound concerning the "infliction" of sudden death throughout history. For example, it was described among certain New England women in relation to the sociological treatment known as "shunning." Among the ancient Greeks, sudden death to the person being socially excluded was inflicted by ostracism, by simply writing the victim's name on an oyster shell and throwing it out to sea. Comparable techniques have been described in other civilizations, such as voodoo in Central America or pouri-pouri in the Pacific Islands. We cannot exclude the possibility that these techniques activated the victim's forebrain mechanisms to turn off the heart with a fatal arrhythmia. As Ben Natelson expresses it, "The brain adapting the heart to the circumstances of its surroundings is econeurocardiology."[37] Some of the most convincing data that support the "eco" aspect of econeurocardiology have emerged from human experiments in which cardiac arrhythmias, anginal pain, blood pressure elevations, and angina pectoris have been induced by the technique of stress interviews.[63]

THE FOREBRAIN: CENTRAL STRESS MECHANISMS
AND CARDIOVASCULAR RESPONSES   *by Karen Belkić, MD, PhD*

The concept of econeurocardiology renders plausible the various theoretical constructs of work stress as they relate to CVD. It also offers a framework in which the reader can integratively grasp how these stress mechanisms give rise to various cardiovascular target organ responses. The following text provides empirical grounding, focusing on animal studies in which CNS mediation of stress mechanisms, as it relates to cardiovascular responses, is specifically examined. Particular attention is paid to CNS triggering of cardiac electrical accidents. Detailed reviews of the anatomic connections between the brain and the heart and of experimental and clinical data on the role of the CNS in cardiac dysfunction can be found elsewhere.[37,38] These reviews point out that "links between emotional states, neural control, and cardiac function have been investigated since Cannon's classic studies in the 1920s and those from Selye in the 1930s." They not only explore "the role of the nervous system in the pathogenesis of lethal ventricular arrhythmias," but also "the role of stress in turning on the neural link that connects the environment to the heart."

Forebrain Mechanisms and Cardiac Electrical Accidents

The critical importance of stimuli from higher neural centers in fatal arrhythmia has been well appreciated since the 1930s.[27,28] Cardiac electrical accidents can occur "with or without associated myocardial infarction, [and] may often be attributable to undamped autonomic discharges in response to either afferent information from below, or to impulses resulting from integrative processes in the brain involved in adaptation of life experience, or both."[57]

THE DEFENSE RESPONSE AND VULNERABILITY TO VENTRICULAR FIBRILLATION

Skinner has developed an econeurocardiologic model in which environmental stressors are linked to vulnerability to ventricular fibrillation (VF) via brain mechanisms originating in the frontal cortex[49] (Fig. 1). The stressor event evokes electrochemical responses that can be transmitted via frontocortical-brainstem pathways. Particularly in the setting of myocardial ischemia, activation of these pathways can trigger VF. According to Skinner's experimental findings, three independent, CNS-mediated interventions prevent VF in psychologically-stressed pigs after acute coronary artery occlusion: (1) learned behavioral adaptation to the stressor, (2) cryogenic blockade of the frontocortical brainstem pathway, and (3) intracerebral injection of the beta-receptor blocking agent l-propranolol (but not intravenous injection of d, l-propranolol).[49] Based on the latter experimental findings, Skinner concludes that "beta-receptor antagonists prevent VF in the ischemic myocardial by their effect on the brain and not the heart."[48] Thus, *central* beta-adrenergic mechanisms are implicated in stress-related lowering of the VF threshold.[42]

The visual system, with its hierarchically primary demand on attention,[47] may be of particular importance in the activation of these processes. Cortical noradrenergic and beta-receptor functions are required for the detection of a change in visual input. These neurochemical changes appear to be involved in local, event-related, slow potential formation, which may mediate these processes.[49] The finding of heightened electrocortical event-related slow potential responses among professional

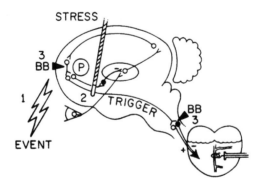

FIGURE 1. Theoretic model of the cerebral mechanism that mediates the deleterious effects of psychosocial stressors on cardiac vulnerability. An environmental stressor (EVENT) evokes a cerebral process in the frontal lobes (P) that determines whether activity occurs in the frontocortical-brainstem pathway (TRIGGER). The activity in this pathway results in dual autonomic outflow (+/−) and inhibits homeostatic reflexes. The projected autonomic activity, either alone or in combination with MI, triggers the initiation of VF. (From Skinner JE: Regulation of cardiac vulnerability by the cerebral defense system. J Am Coll Cardiol 5:88B–94B, 1985; with permission.)

drivers to cognitively-relevant visual signals has been broadly viewed in light of Skinner's model as a possible econeurocardiologic mechanism of cardiac vulnerability in this stressed occupational group.[2]

In contrast to the role of brain norepinephrine, elevated cerebral levels of serotonin *raise* the threshold for VF.[31] Other experimental findings of Lown and colleagues also illustrate the role of forebrain mechanisms in VF. In dogs, stimulation of the posterior hypothalamus in the face of experimentally-induced myocardial ischemia proves to be the critical factor in inducing VF.[32]

Alerting and the defense response are elicited with stimulation of the posterior hypothalamus.[22] Stimulation of the "defense area" of the hypothalamus in conscious rabbits gives rise to furious running such as would be expected in escape behavior. The cardiovascular-respiratory responses are consistent with a flight-or-fight pattern: tachycardia, hyperventilation, and augmented blood pressure (BP) with blood flow directed to the skeletal muscles at the expense of the viscera.

Other brain structures involved in the defense response are the amygdala and periaqueductal gray matter of the midbrain.[8] Neural traffic from the amygdala contributes to the risk of life-threatening ventricular tachyarrhythmias in the face of myocardial ischemia. Electrical stimulation of the midbrain reticular formation also lowers the threshold for VF.[35]

THE DIVE REFLEX AND CARDIAC ASYSTOLE

The ophthalmic branch of the fifth cranial nerve connects to autonomic efferents producing the oxygen-conserving dive reflex. Activation of this reflex can trigger sudden asystolic cardiac death. The dive reflex is a complex patterned reaction mediated by the reticular-activating system. Along with vasoconstriction and vagally-mediated bradycardia and cardiac conduction abnormalities, metabolic changes consistent with hypoventilation are found.[24,60,62] In addition to noxious agents and hypoxia, this reflex can be evoked by threatening symbolic stimuli. The dive reflex is basically a conservative reflex, but it may be inappropriately activated under circumstances of hopelessness, extreme fear, or exhaustion.

Besides the defense response, another CNS integration of CV and behavioral stress responses has been identified by McCabe and colleagues.[36] Quite reminiscent of the dive reflex, stimulation of the medial part of the lateral hypothalamus and the ventrolateral periaqueductal grey area of the midbrain in conscious rabbits elicits the **vigilance response**, with behavioral immobilization and a cardiovascular-respiratory pattern of vagally mediated bradycardia, bradypnea (to the point of inspiratory apnea), and elevated BP but with diminished blood flow to skeletal muscle *and* to the viscera.[8,36]

The insular cortex has been identified as a site that mediates stress-induced ventricular asystole. As described by Cechetto, this site receives an "organized representation of visceral information," as well as "highly processed association cortex information. The insular cortex is also highly interconnected with many subcortical limbic and autonomic regions. This combination of sensory input and limbic/autonomic connectivity would be necessary to permit the insular cortex to be a critical site for the integration of emotional and autonomic responses."[7] Prolonged phasic stimulation of the posterior insular cortex has been shown in rats to lead to progressive degrees of heart block, together with increased plasma norepinephrine and myocardial damage, and finally to asystolic death.[40]

The fight-or-flight defense response pattern may occur in rapid alternation with the vigilance response. This alternation may represent yet another centrally-mediated mechanism leading to cardiac electrical accidents.

PROFOUND CONFLICT: RAPID ALTERNATION OF FIGHT-OR-FLIGHT
AND PLAYING DEAD

It has been proposed that rapid alternation between these two mechanisms leads to forebrain-mediated cardiac electrical accidents. Buell and Eliot observed the behavioral backdrop typical of sudden cardiac death in animals as a combination of arousal and enforced helplessness, plus profound conflict.[5] They suggested that this combination may lead to a "breakdown of reciprocity between the flight-or-fight reaction and the playing-dead reaction."[5] Under overwhelming stress, both systems may activate simultaneously or in rapid alternation with each other, constituting the basis of the behavioral disorganization "typically exhibited by animals under extreme stress. The dog that startles, crouches, trembles, moves about aimlessly, barks, whines, salivates, urinates, defecates, pants, piloerects, and sometimes momentarily dozes. All these activities indicate simultaneous or rapidly alternating sympathetic and parasympathetic activation."[5]

The retrospective, content-analytical study by Engel of 170 victims of sudden cardiac death provides some anecdotal corroboration.[13] The following patterns were repeatedly observed among these victims: (1) the individual faces overwhelming excitement, (2) there is a personal dilemma or conflict about a course of action, (3) the situation is overwhelming, and the individual attempts to cope or he/she gives up completely, and (4) the events that occur cannot be ignored by the individual.

While these observations require neurophysiologic support, they are coherent with the dual regulation of increased vulnerability of the heart as elaborated by Skinner.[49] He proposes that combined high sympathetic and parasympathetic tone lead to a state of electrical instability. Wolf considers that autonomic control requires an autonomic nervous system inhibitory network; this can be disturbed in overwhelming, unavoidable, conflicting situations, resulting in a loss of regulatory inhibition.[57] These findings are conceptually reminiscent of Pavlov's formulation of conflict as the "difficult meeting of excitation and inhibition" in the brain.[43]

Stress-Mediated Forebrain Mechanisms and Control of Blood Pressure and Heartbeat Dynamics

BLOOD PRESSURE

Repeated elicitation of the defense response appears to play a critical role in the development of primary hypertension.[14] Henry states: "Chronic arousal of the defense response with catecholamine and renin release provides a physiological mechanism giving rise to sustained hypertension."[19] Loss of control/giving-up as a consequence of prolonged exposure to overwhelming stress is also implicated as an important mechanism of primary hypertension.[14] Experimental studies reveal that strong control over animals' behavior elicits hypertensive responses.[3,16] Signaled and unsignaled avoidance conditioning in dogs and monkeys is associated with an increase in BP, as well as heart rate. When exposure to this type of paradigm is sustained over several months, the animals become hypertensive.[46] In general, induction of hypertension in experimental animals requires several months of repeated exposure to stressful situations.[15,16] Henry also has found that long-term stressful life conditions in crowded cages leads to permanent hypertension among rats.[21]

Stimulation of the lateral hypothalamus in rabbits evokes a defeat-type pattern with motoric immobilization, *generalized* vasoconstriction, and vagally mediated bradycardia.[8,36] Short-lived but repeated stimulation of the lateral hypothalamus for several days to weeks in rats is found to lead to a progressive, sustained rise in arterial BP.[18]

Microstimulation of the rostral portion of the posterior insular cortex evokes arterial pressor responses in rats.[64] Szilagyi and colleagues have demonstrated, in rats with experimental hypertension, that synaptic cryoblockade of the ventromedial region of the frontal cortex leads to a significant fall in arterial BP.[53] This frontal cortical site projects via the anteroventral hypothalamus to brainstem cardioregulatory loci. Other forebrain loci that have been identified as important in blood pressure regulation include the amygdala, the septal nuclei, and the cingulate cortex. Oparil and colleagues state: "Since these areas are involved in learning, emotional responses (especially the defense reaction), and the integration of information from higher centers, they are likely to be most important in the pathogenesis of hypertension that is related to environmental stress."[39] These authors provide a detailed review of neuroanatomic and neurochemical pathways as they relate to the development of hypertension.

HEARTBEAT DYNAMICS

Heart rate variability (HRV) has been noted to provide one important mechanistic link between exposure to mental stress and risk of cardiac events. Using a deterministic measure of HRV that tracks non-stationarities,[52] injection of intracerebral l-propranolol in pigs has been found to increase HRV.[50] This landmark finding illustrates the role of central noradrenergic mechanisms in control of HRV.

Econeurocardiology and Clinical Outcomes

The econeurocardiologic model of Skinner[49] can be expanded to the realm of human psychosocial experience, for which symbolic stimuli often play a particularly important role:

Bodily responses triggered by a thought or by a perception of one's surroundings are attributable, of course, to symbolic as contrasted with tangible stimuli. The bodily changes observed constitute a part of the behavior of a person, behavior that is governed by the significance of the situation to the implicated individual. There is, indeed, a vast repertoire of behaviors that adapt the individual to life experiences of all sorts. Each involves discrete patterned responses that are activated and coordinated by the nervous system, and may involve voluntary as well as involuntary behavior.[59]

The impact of these mechanisms on clinical CV events has been appreciated since early times. One particularly important sociological example has been called the "Roseto effect," in which a consistently lower mortality rate from myocardial infarction was observed over 30 years in a homogeneous Italian-American community, compared to adjacent towns with greater acculturation and lower social cohesion. Further followup revealed that with erosion of social networks in Roseto, a dramatic rise in deaths from MI occurred, most notably among the young of both genders and older women.[10,57] These findings are highly consistent with the burgeoning literature on social isolation as a potential risk factor for clinical CV events.[4,41]

HYPERFUNCTIONAL OVERDRIVE: ACQUIRED CARDIOVASCULAR DISORDERS

In 1974, R.S. Eliot introduced the concept of "acquired cardiovascular disorders." These include: acute MI, angina pectoris, arterial hypertension, and sudden cardiac death. The common feature of these disorders may be a stress-related component mediated by the CNS, resulting from "hyperfunctional overdrive," i.e., overstimulation by the catecholamine system (see Chapter 5). Eliot broadly outlined the environmental backdrop for CNS-mediated overactivity of the sympathetic nervous system, noting "the social inpropriety" of the flight-or-fight reaction in modern day life, such that most stressors are chronically present and cannot be resolved in a physical way.[12] The consequence is a "chronic alarm reaction" in which there is a "constant state of visceral-vascular readiness" whereby the heart and blood vessels are activated irrespective of the actual metabolic needs of the organism.

The acquired CV disorder formulation could be expanded to include loss of control—a defeat or "giving-up" dimension—which also is associated with untoward CV outcomes. Henry presents a model in which the deleterious effects of the latter are highlighted.[20] In working life, a particularly cardionoxious combination is arousal plus low control or defeat, i.e., job strain, which would imply the activation of both branches of Henry's model.[25]

REFERENCES

1. Armour JA, Ardell JL: Neurocardiology. New York, Oxford University Press, 1994.
2. Belkic K, Savic C, Theorell T, et al: Mechanisms of cardiac risk among professional drivers. Scand J Work Environ Health 20:73–86, 1994.
3. Benson H, Gutmann MC: The relation of environmental factors to systemic arterial hypertension. In Eliot RS (ed): Stress and the Heart. Mt. Kisco, Futura Publishing Co., 1974, pp 13–31.
4. Berkman LF, Leo-Summers L, Horowitz RI: Emotional support and survival after myocardial infarction. Ann Intern Med 117:1003–1009, 1992.
5. Buell JC, Eliot RS: Psychosocial and behavioral influences in the pathogenesis of acquired cardiovascular disease. Am Heart J 100:723–740, 1980.
6. Carpeggiani C, Landisman C, Montaron MF, Skinner JE: Cryoblockade in limbic brain (amygdala) prevents or delays ventricular fibrillation after coronary artery occlusion in psychologically distressed pigs. Circul Res 70:600–606, 1992.
7. Cechetto DF: Identification of a cortical site for stress-induced cardiovascular dysfunction. Integ Physiol Behav 29:362–373, 1994.
8. Duan Y-F, Winters RW, McCabe PM, et al: Modulation of neuronal firing in the medullary solitary complex by electrical stimulation of the hypothalamic defense and vigilance areas in rabbits. Brain Research 643:218–226, 1994.
9. Ebert PA, Allgood RJ, Sabiston DC: Effect of cardiac denervation on arrhythmia following coronary artery occlusion. Surgery Forum 18:114, 1967.
10. Egolf B, Lasker J, Wolf S, Potvin L: The Roseto Effect: A 50-year comparison of mortality rates. Am J Public Health 82:1089–1092, 1992.
11. Eliot RS: Stress and the Heart. Mt. Kisco, NY, Futura Publishing Co., 1974.
12. Eliot RS: Stress and the Major Cardiovascular Disorders. Mt. Kisco, Futura Publishing Co., 1979.
13. Engel GL: Sudden and rapid death during psychological stress. Ann Intern Med 74:771–782, 1971.
14. Folkow B: Autonomic nervous system in hypertension. In Swales JD (ed): Textbook of Hypertension. London, Blackwell Scientific Publications, 1994, pp 427–438.
15. Forsyth RP: Blood pressure responses to long-term avoidance schedules in the unrestrained rhesus monkey. Psychosom Med 31:300–309, 1969.
16. Friedman R, Dahl L: The effects of chronic conflict on the blood pressure of rats with a genetic susceptibility to experimental hypertension. Psychosom Med 37:402–416, 1975.
17. Gantt WH: Effect of person. Conditional Reflex 1:18–34, 1966.
18. Gilmore JP: Physiology of Stress. Stress and the Heart. Mt. Kisco, Futura Publishing Co., 1974.
19. Henry JP: Psychosocial stress and hypertension. The relevance of animal studies. In Swales JD (ed): Textbook of Hypertension. London, Blackwell Scientific Publications, 1994, pp 633–639.
20. Henry JP: Biological basis of the stress response. Integ Physiol Behav 27:66–83, 1992.
21. Henry JP, Meehan JP, Sephens PM: The use of psychosocial stimuli to induce prolonged systolic hypertension in mice. Psychosom Med 29:408–432, 1967.
22. Hilton SM: Hypothalamic regulation of the cardiovascular system. Br Med Bulletin 22:243–248, 1966.
23. Houk P, Smith V, Wolf S: Brain mechanisms in fatal cardiac arrhythmia. Integrative Physiol Behav Sci 31:(In press), 1999.
24. Hughes T, Carter J, Wolf S: Disorders of cardiac conduction accompany the dive reflec in man. Pavlov J Biol Sci 16:25–33, 1981.
25. Karasek RA: Job demands, decision latitude and mental strain: Implications for job redesign. Adm Sci Q 24:285–308, 1979.
26. Kulbertus H, Frank G: Neurocardiology. Mt. Kisco, NY, Futura Publishing Co., 1988.
27. Leriche RL, Fontaine R, Kunlin J: Contribution a l'etude des vaso-moteurs coronariens. Compt Rend Soc de Biol 110:299, 1932.
28. Leriche RL, Herman L, Fontaine R: Ligature de la coronaire gouche et fonction ches l'animal intact. Compt Rend Soc de Biol 107:545–546, 1931.

29. Leroy GV, Snider SS: The sudden death of patients with few symptoms of heart disease. J Am Med Assoc 117:2019, 1941.
30. Locke J: An essay concerning human understanding. In Nidditch PH (ed): The Claredon Edition of the Works of John Locke. London, Oxford University Press, 1979.
31. Lown B: Sudden cardiac death: Biobehavioral perspective. Circulation 76 Suppl I:I-186–I-195, 1987.
32. Lown B, Verrier RL: Neural activity and ventricular fibrillation. N Engl J Med 294:1165–1170, 1976.
33. Malliani A, Lombardi F: Neural reflexes associated with myocardial ischemia. In Schwartz PJ, Brown AM, Malliani A, Zanchetti A (eds): Neural Mechanisms in Cardiac Arrhythmias. New York, Raven Press, 1978, p 209.
34. Manning GW, McEachern CG, Hall GE: Reflex coronary arery spasm following sudden occlusion of coronary branches. Arch Intern Med 64:661–674, 1939.
35. Matta R, Lawler JE, Lown B: Ventricular electrical instability in the conscious dog. Am J Cardiol 38:594–598, 1976.
36. McCabe PM, Duan Y-F, Winters RW, et al: Comparison of peripheral blood flow patterns associated with the defense reaction and the vigilance reaction in rabbits. Physiol Behav 56:1101–1106, 1994.
37. Natelson BH: Neurocardiology: An interdisciplinary area for the 80s. Arch Neurol 42:178–184, 1985.
38. Natelson BH, Chang Q: Sudden death: A neurocardiologic phenomenon. Neurol Clin 11:293–308, 1993.
39. Oparil S, Chen YF, Berecek KH, et al: The role of the central nervous system in hypertension. In Laragh JH, Brenner BM (eds): Hypertension: Pathophysiology, Diagnosis, and Management. New York, Raven Press, Ltd., 1995, pp 713–740.
40. Oppenheimer SM, Wilson JX, Guiraudon C, et al: Insular cortex stimulation produces lethal cardiac arrhythmias. Brain Res 550:115–121, 1991.
41. Orth-Gomer K, Unden AL, Edwards ME: Social isolation and mortality in ischemic heart disease: A 10-year follow-up study of 150 middle-aged men. Acta Med Scand 224:205–215, 1988.
42. Parker GW, Michael LH, Hartley CH, et al: Central beta-adrenergic mechanisms may modulate ischemic ventricular fibrillation in pigs. Circul Res 66:259–270, 1990.
43. Pavlov I: Conditional Reflexes: An Investigation of the Physiological Activity of the Cerebral Cortex. (G.V. Anrep, Trans.) New York, Oxford, 1927.
44. Ramon y Cajal S: Degeneration & Regeneration of the Nervous System. (R.M. May, Trans.) London, Oxford University Press, 1928.
45. Schneider RA, Costiloe JP, Wolf S: Arterial pressures recorded in hospital and during ordinary daily activities: Contrasting data in subjects with and without ischemic heart disease. J Chron Dis 23:647, 1971.
46. Schneiderman N: Animal models relating behavioral stress and cardiovascular pathology. In Dembroski TM, et al (eds): Coronary-Prone Behavior. New York, Springer-Verlag, 1978, pp 155–181.
47. Singleton WT: Introduction a L'ergonomie (Introduction to ergonomics). Geneva, Organization Mondial de la Sante, 1974.
48. Skinner JE: Neurocardiology shows that the central, not peripheral, action of propranolol reduces mortality following acute coronary occlusion in the conscious pig. Integ Physiol Behav 26:85–97, 1991.
49. Skinner JE: Regulation of cardiac vulnerability by the cerebral defense system. J Am Coll Cardiol 5:88B–94B, 1985.
50. Skinner JE: The role of the central nervous system in sudden cardiac death: Heartbeat dynamics in conscious pigs during coronary occlusion, psychologic stress and intracerebral propranolol. Integ Physiol Behav 29:355–361, 1994.
51. Skinner JE, Lie JT, Entman ML: Modification of ventricular fibrillation latency following coronary artery occlusion in the conscious pig: The effects of psychological distress and beta-adrenergic blockage. Circulation 51:656–667, 1975.
52. Skinner JE, Molnar M, Vybiral T, Mitra M: Application of chaos theory to biology and medicine. Integ Physiol Behav 27:39–53, 1992.
53. Szilagyi JE, Taylor AA, Skinner JE: Cryoblockade of the ventromedial frontal cortex reverses hypertension in the rat. Hypertension 9:576–581, 1987.
54. Willerson JT, Cohn JN: Cardiovascular Medicine. New York, Churchill Livingstone, 1995.
55. Wolf S: The Artery and the Process of Arterosclerosis: Measurement and Modification. New York, Plenum Press, 1972.
56. Wolf S: The Artery and the Process of Arteriosclerosis: Pathogenesis. New York, Plenum Press, 1971.
57. Wolf S: Psychosocial forces in myocardial infarction and sudden death. Circulation 40:IV-74–IV-83, 1969.
58. Reference deleted.
59. Wolf S: Discrete, patterned, and purposeful adaptive physiological adjustments integrated by forebrain influences. Integ Physiol Behav Sci 30:190–200, 1995.
60. Wolf S: Sudden death and the oxygen-conserving reflex. Am Heart J 71:840–841, 1966.
61. Wolf S: Oscillatory functions affecting outcome of coronary heart disease: The hazard of too much or too little stability. Integ Physiol Behav Sci 30:118–126, 1995.
62. Wolf S: Neurocardiology (Editorial). Oklahoma State Med J 60:61, 1967.
63. Wolf S: Social Environment and Health. Seattle, University of Washington Press, 1981.
64. Yasui Y, Breder CD, Saper CB, Cechetto DF: Autonomic responses and efferent pathways from the insular cortex in the rat. J Comp Neurol 303;355–374, 1991.
65. Zipes DP: Influence of myocardial ischemia and infarction on autonomic innervation of the heart. Circulation 82:1095–1105, 1990.

EVIDENCE FOR MEDIATING ECONEUROCARDIOLOGIC MECHANISMS

CARDIAC ELECTRICAL STABILITY AND ENVIRONMENTAL STRESS   *by Karen Belkić, MD, PhD*

Sudden arrhythmic death is the most common mode of death among adults under the age of 65 in industrialized countries, accounting in the U.S. alone for approximately half of all CV mortality, or an estimated 250,000 to 350,000 deaths annually.[31,62,155,221,245,261] Most of the arrhythmias leading to these deaths are ventricular tachyarrhythmias.[56,89,261] A substantial number, in some series up to 50%, of these victims have had no previous history of known heart disease; in other words, the first cardiac episode proves to be the last.[305] Bernard Lown has stated: "[Sudden cardiac death] is not the expression of inexorable and irreversible pathomorphologic alterations. It represents instead an electrical accident that can be reversed and even prevented."[221] Thus, understanding the mechanisms underlying sudden cardiac death could be of critical public health importance, particularly for primary prevention, which remains the most elusive goal.

The relation between stress and sudden cardiac death (SCD) has long been appreciated. As stated by Eliot and Buell, "History is replete with anecdotes of persons who died suddenly in the throes of intense emotion. Now scientific study is beginning to shed light on the pathways and mechanisms responsible for these observations."[87] The role of the forebrain in life-threatening arrhythmias is discussed in Chapter 4. Here, the focus is on how these processes play out on the cardiac electrical substrate. Acute and chronic stress-related factors can contribute to destabilization of the electrical substrate of the cardiac ventricle, leading to life-threatening ventricular tachyarrhythmias by a number of mechanisms.

Major Stress-Mediated Mechanisms of Cardiac Electrical Destabilization

SYMPATHETIC OVERDRIVE

Catecholamine excess is arrhythmogenic. Based primarily on laboratory studies of isolated cardiac tissues, it can be concluded that catecholamines directly evoke tachyarrhythmias by three mechanisms: (1) increased automatic activity (increased slope of phase 4 depolarization and in slow inward calcium current in partially depolarized cells), (2) augmented early and late triggering (facilitation of calcium influx), and (3) re-entry (lowered phase 4 potential slows conduction, increases internal resistance, and diminishes cell-to-cell conduction, which promotes asynchronous repolarization.[295,344,402,410] These arrhythmogenic effects have been attributed primarily to beta, but also to alpha-1 adrenergic mechanisms.[138,221,330,340,356] Furthermore, catecholamine damage to myocardial tissue can provide a morphologic substrate for lethal arrhythmogenesis.[87,243,400]

OTHER AUTONOMIC IMBALANCES

Unopposed sympathetic outflow is not the only stress-related mechanism by which autonomic imbalance destabilizes the heart. The balance of sympathetic outflow between the right and left stellate ganglion, as well as vagal/sympathetic ratio and its temporal relation to the cardiac cycle, are also autonomic determinants of cardiac electrical stability. Vagal outflow usually stabilizes the electrical substrate of the heart by increasing the resting potential of cardiac fibers.[221,366] Low parasympathetic relative to sympathetic tone as reflected by heart rate variability (HRV) has been found on Holter recordings to precede spontaneous episodes of ventricular tachycardia.[155] This finding provides pathophysiologic corroboration for the clinical-epidemiologic association reported between altered HRV and sudden arrhythmic death.[155,268]

After transmural myocardial infarction (MI), sympathetic as well as vagal efferent innervation can be compromised in noninfarcted portions of the myocardium apical to the infarct, with reduction in norepinephrine and acetylcholine concentrations. As a consequence, this denervated tissue demonstrates supersensitivity with exposure to adrenergic agents. These changes may promote cardiac electrical instability.[411]

The temporal relations between vagal and sympathetic outflow also must be considered. Levy has demonstrated in experimental studies that varying temporal sequences of vagal and sympathetic stimulation can have disparate effects on autonomic interactions.[213] Furthermore, abrupt withdrawal of sympathetic vasoconstrictor tone and sudden vagal outflow can lead to hemodynamic collapse as well as asystole, implicated in some animal models of sudden cardiac death,[60,61,123] as well as clinical syndromes.[193,322] The dive reflex falls into this category.

While stimulation of either stellate (sympathetic) ganglion lowers the threshold for ventricular fibrillation, the left stellate, which increases the temporal dispersion of repolarization and thereby prolongs the corrected QT interval, is twice as effective.[145,330,386] Dynamic prolongation of the QT interval during daily activity in post-MI patients is a potential marker of risk for life-threatening ventricular arrhythmias.[153] Exposure to sensory and/or emotional stressors, as well as physical exercise, can increase vulnerability to developing life-threatening ventricular tachyarrhythmias among patients with the idiopathic long QT syndrome.[123,389]

LEFT VENTRICULAR HYPERTROPHY

Cardiac electrical stability is also jeopardized by left ventricular hypertrophy (LVH), which has a particularly close association to work-related stress. Mechanisms by which LVH may be arrhythmogenic include: (1) increased automatic activity from stretching of the myocardial fiber sheaths, (2) induction of triggered activity from disturbed calcium homeostasis, and/or (3) re-entry occurring in electrically silent areas that arise from the hypertrophied myocytes and from areas of interstitial fibrosis.[162,242,248,357] Hypertensive patients with LVH have significantly greater prevalence, overall number, and severity of ventricular as well as supraventricular arrhythmias compared to those without LVH.[206,266]

MYOCARDIAL ISCHEMIA

Acute myocardial is perhaps the best recognized and most well-investigated cause of lethal tachyarrhythmias. Experimental studies reveal that the immediate effects of acute myocardial ischemia produced by abrupt coronary artery (CA) occlusion include acidosis and depletion of high-energy phosphates, leading to a loss of resting membrane potential with altered refractoriness and excitability. Conduction becomes slowed and inhomogeneous. Re-entry mechanisms appear to predominate, although automatic and triggered activity also can occur.[18,37,123,173,245] Ischemic myocardium also triggers reflex sympathetic outflow with attendant catecholamine-related arrhythmogenesis, by the above-described mechanisms.[198,378] During this early phase, lasting approximately 30 minutes, irreversible morphologic changes have still not occurred—yet mortality is high in experimental investigations.[245] This phase seems to be the correlate of very rapidly occurring death due, in the clinical setting, to primary arrhythmic events.[173,245]

After about 90 minutes of coronary occlusion, lethal arrhythmias appear to arise in the interface between viable and infarcted tissue. The clinical correlate of this phase is arrhythmias that develop several hours after the onset of symptoms of acute MI. Life-threatening ventricular tachyarrhythmias also have been recorded in association with episodes of coronary artery spasm.[77,156,236,292] Animal studies reveal that lethal ventricular arrhythmias may occur during reperfusion after a short episode of CA occlusion,[114,174] especially when the occlusion was only partial, suggesting that the risk of ventricular fibrillation after CA spasm may be increased among patients with minimal CA disease.[335]

The Critical Role of Higher Nervous Activity in Cardiac Electrical Stability

Mehta and colleagues point out that "despite a substantial understanding of the biochemical aspects of acute myocardial ischemia, our knowledge of which patients with acute myocardial ischemia will develop sustained ventricular tachyarrhythmias remains unclear."[245] Superimposed exposure to acute stressors in the face of ischemic myocardium can represent the critical trigger of lethal cardiac electrical instability. Animal studies reveal that a number of stressful paradigms, such as threat of electric shock, food access denial, altered or unfamiliar laboratory environment, and avoidance task performance, significantly lower the threshold for ventricular fibrillation under conditions of experimental myocardial ischemia. It is noted that without exposure to such stressors, lethal arrhythmias rarely occurred in these animals, despite ongoing ischemia.[44,179,221,222,348] Thus, myocardial ischemia alone may not be sufficient to trigger life-threatening arrhythmias; rather, autonomic outflow may be needed in addition.[347] Stimulation of the posterior hypothalamus, which potentiates sympathetic outflow, lowers the ventricular fibrillation threshold in dogs with normal coronary arteries and, with experimentally-induced myocardial ischemia, proves to be the critical factor in the electrical stability of the heart.[223] Skinner demonstrated the role of higher cortical centers in cardiac electrical stability, using the pig model.[347] With blockade of either the frontocortical-brainstem pathways or the amygdaloid nuclei, psychologically-stressed pigs with acute myocardial ischemia were prevented from developing ventricular fibrillation.

Chemical Exposures and Cardiac Electrical Stability

Life-threatening cardiac arrhythmias and SCD can occur after a single, excessive exposure to carbon monoxide (CO) or to other substances that produce myocardial ischemia, although low levels of CO exposure (3–5% carboxyhemoglobin) do not appear to be proarrhythmic.[45,63,306,307] A number of organic solvents, especially those that are halogenated, have been shown to sensitize the myocardium to catecholamine and thereby compromise the heart's electrical stability. Fatal outcomes after heavy exposure to these substances have been reported in the industrial setting.[164,197,210] Acute re-exposure to nitrate esters, notably ethylene glycol dinitrate, among workers in the explosives industry has been associated with sudden cardiac death. There are numerous reports of these deaths occurring upon return to work after a brief period of absence from dynamite manufacturing work: "Monday Morning Sudden Cardiac Death."[197,306,307,382,388,391]

Monday Morning Sudden Cardiac Death

The over-representation of SCD and other acute cardiac events in the early morning hours of Mondays may not be limited to workers in the explosives industry. There is substantial data demonstrating a circadian variation in SCD and MI, with a peak in the morning hours after waking.[119,256,257,397,398] A number of the preconditions for plaque rupture and thrombus formation are present at that time of day. In the morning hours after waking, systolic blood pressure increases by about 20–30 mmHg, heart rate and vascular tone rise, platelets are hyper-reactive, and fibrinolytic activity is at its low.[375] Sympathetic activation occurs upon assuming the upright position, and in the early morning cortisol is at its peak. This can result in a glucocorticoid-related increase in coronary-artery sensitivity to catecholamine-mediated vasoconstriction.[123,375,400] Beta-adrenergic blockade is found to attenuate this early morning peak in SCD.[398,400] Willich and colleagues point out that besides assuming the upright posture, other morning activities may trigger an increase in sympathetic outflow.[400]

A weekly variation in the occurrence of acute MI with a peak on Mondays has been reported among patients who had been working, but not in those who were not employed at the time of MI.[399] In that series a similar trend was not observed, however, for SCD. In contrast, among a cohort study of 3983 men without manifest IHD, an excess proportion of sudden cardiac deaths, but not MI or cancer deaths, was found on Mondays.[296]

Epidemiologic studies of unmonitored, out-of-hospital SCD are fraught with methodologic difficulties; death certificates lack both sensitivity and specificity; and major definitional dilemmas still exist.[56,92,305,376] Sudden death at work has been underestimated by death certificates.[305] An investigation of coroners' reports reveals an annual, age-adjusted rate of sudden death at work twice that of fatal work injuries.[305] Systematic examination of the incidence of life-threatening ventricular tachyarrhythmias among 683 patients with third-generation automatic implantable cardioverter defibrillators (AICD) reveals a highly significant septadian distribution of these arrhythmias, with the largest percentage (21%) of AICD activations occurring on Mondays, twice greater than the number of episodes during the weekend.[282] Employment data was not available on these patients.

These epidemiologic findings along with the biological data render plausible the conclusions that "the stress of work after a weekend of respite may have been the precipitant of a lethal arrhythmia"[220] and that "an increase in physical and mental burden from leisurely weekend activities to stressful work on Monday in the majority of working patients" is causally related to the occurrence of acute MI.[400]

MECHANISMS LEADING TO HYPERTENSION AND CV MORBIDITY   *by Joseph Schwartz, PhD, Karen Belkić, MD, PhD, Peter Schnall, MD, and Thomas Pickering, MD, DPhil*

The relationship between elevations in blood pressure (BP) and cardiovascular risk is "strong, continuous, graded, consistent, independent, predictive, and etiologically significant for those with and without CHD."[7] From the age of 20 on, in the U.S. and other industrialized settings, BP increases progressively with age for the population as a whole, so that by age 60 approximately 50% of the population has hypertension, according to the standard definition of BP > 140/90 mmHg.[392] It is now clear that an increase in BP, even for those at a far lower level of BP than the current definition of hypertension, is associated with an increase in CHD risk.[7] With heart disease and stroke representing the first and third leading causes of death in the U.S., respectively, the public health implications of the hypertension epidemic are clear.[263]

Essential hypertension is a chronic disease process defined by the presence of persistently elevated (not just acutely elevated) BP, without secondary causes. Epidemiologic evidence reveals that essential hypertension is a disease of industrialized society, as there is a minimal hypertension disease burden among hunter-gatherers, nonmarket agricultural communities, and other nonindustrialized societies.[329,387] Within industrial society, hypertension is socially patterned by class, race, and gender.[137,291,392]

Current evidence suggests that the "unidentified" cause(s) of essential hypertension most likely include one or more ubiquitous exposures. Thus, diet, lifestyle, work, and community should be examined. An adequate explanatory risk factor would also have to be consistent with the above-mentioned social patterning of the disease. Migration studies strongly suggest that genetic factors are not the primary determinants of hypertension. This is dramatically demonstrated by the fact that African-Americans have among the highest rates of hypertension in the world,[7] whereas in rural West Africa (from whence African-Americans underwent forced migration to the U.S.) the prevalence of hypertension is among the lowest in the world.[59]

The contemporary work environment is a ubiquitous environmental exposure. It is the locus in which adults now spend the majority of their waking time. The work environment is frequently the source of exposures to psychosocial, physical, and other cardionoxious factors.

We know that BP is higher during working hours, compared to leisure time, within a 24-hour period.[328] Furthermore, mean 24-hour BPs are lower on nonwork days compared to work days.[286] These observations have been made possible by the development of ambulatory blood pressure (AmBP) devices, and their use in working populations. In comparison to casual clinic BP, AmBP is a better reflection of "true blood pressure" and has been demonstrated to be superior to the former in predicting target organ damage (such as left ventricular hypertrophy) and clinical prognosis.[8,277,278,383] Thus, studies using AmBP provide indispensable insights into the link between environmental/situational factors and hypertension.

Whether, how, and when repeated acute rises in BP transform into the chronic process of essential hypertension are only partially understood. Clearly, longitudinal studies that follow this process over time are critical to our understanding of the mechanisms involved. Our goal is to present the current biological models and existing empirical evidence, to identify where the argument of biological plausibility is best substantiated.

Workplace Stressors and Hypertension

Occupations at High Risk

A number of the occupational groups that are at high risk for developing ischemic heart disease (IHD) also show an elevated risk for hypertension and/or elevated resting BP. These include professional drivers,[16,24,25,297,408] air traffic controllers,[57] and sea pilots.[90] These occupations can be characterized as predominantly threat-avoidant vigilant jobs, with a high total burden of occupational stressors. Cumulative exposure to this occupational stress burden emerges as a significant, independent predictor of hypertension among urban transit operators.[298] Among San Francisco urban transit operators aged 45–54 with over 20 years on the job, 52.2% had hypertension. In comparison, the prevalence of hypertension was 42.9% among those of the same age strata who had been on the job less than 10 years, and 48.8% among those with 10–20 years on the job. Prior to employment as an urban transport operator, the prevalence of hypertension among a group of the same age was 36.7%.

Elevations in AmBP have been found during working hours among urban transport operators, compared to workers whose overall occupational stress burden is much lower.[379] Acute rises in AmBP have been observed during emergency situations among healthy, middle-aged train drivers whose BP increased by +12.7/+9.4 mmHg compared to resting values.[194]

Chronic Exposure to Job Strain and Effort-Reward Imbalance

Of the psychosocial work stress models relevant to cardiovascular disease (CVD), the Job Strain Model has been one of the most intensively investigated in relation to hypertension. Strong empirical evidence links exposure to job strain with elevations in AmBP, greatest at work but also evident at home and during sleep. Besides the consistent body of cross-sectional data in men and women and the demonstration of a dose-response relationship, recent longitudinal studies reveal a significant cumulative effect, as well.[201,325] In the Cornell Work Site Blood Pressure Study, the adjusted worktime AmBP of men who were exposed to job strain at baseline as well as 3 years later was greater by 11.1/9.1 mmHg, compared to those without exposure at either time.[325] Exposure to high effort together with low rewards at work also has been demonstrated to predict hypertensive status prevalence in combination with hyperlipidemia.[341,343]

Physical and Chemical Exposures

Empirical evidence links exposures to certain physical and chemical agents with hypertension. With regard to noise, the literature is abundant, but not entirely consistent. However, several fairly recent studies were positive,[76,93,251,365] and three of these took into account length of exposure.[76,251,365] In the study of Talbott, et al., cumulative occupational noise exposure was a significant independent predictor of systolic BP in the two plants studied, while it predicted diastolic BP in only one of the plants.[365] The authors attribute this latter finding to a possible threshold effect. Among male industrial workers aged 25–44 with normal BP, Green and colleagues found a +3.2/+2.3 mmHg effect on work AmBP among those exposed to > 85 dB noise (p < 0.001), after controlling for potential confounders.[126] No significant effect was seen among those over 44 years of age. However, in another study from the same center in Israel, work AmBP was not significantly associated with noise intensity among male or female blue-collar workers.[196] Some evidence suggests that exposure to lead or to arsenic may be associated with an increased risk of hypertension.[52,143]

LONG WORK HOURS AND SHIFTWORK

Studies by Hayashi, et al.[136] and by Iwasaki, et al.[159] have shown that long working hours are associated with elevations in AmBP as well as casual BP. Shift workers appear to reverse the usual circadian BP pattern, showing peak levels at night while working. Chau and colleagues found that while the mean BP during the high pressure span was the same for three shift schedules, the duration of the high pressure span was longest during the night shift, and shortest during the afternoon shift.[50] There is also evidence that shift workers' BP during sleep fails to drop to the levels seen among day workers. In a study of approximately 100 nonhypertensive nurses, Yamasaki, et al. showed that those who worked evening/night shifts had higher BP during sleep than those who worked day shift.[404] As a result, shift workers exhibited less "nocturnal dipping," the lack of which has been associated with increased left ventricular mass according to Verdecchia, et al.,[384] although not according to Bhatt, et al.[30] A recent longitudinal study by Morikawa and colleagues indicates that among young (< 30 y.o.), initially normotensive, blue-collar working men in a single factory, the relative risk of developing hypertension during the 5-year followup was 3.6 for those who rotated shifts compared to those who worked day shift only, after adjusting for age, BMI, alcohol intake, and baseline systolic BP.[255] This effect was not seen among older workers, however.

Human Blood Pressure Responses to Simulated Work Stressors

ECOLOGICAL RELEVANCE

A large body of research examines human CV responses to various stressful paradigms. While acute elevations of BP and heart rate are achieved, these paradigms often bear little or no resemblance to real aspects of working life. Besides the artificiality of the laboratory environment itself, the tasks have not usually been chosen for their similarity to the cognitive exigencies of the subjects' jobs. Very few studies have, by design, examined between-subject responses to laboratory stressors that are similar to the subjects' workplace exposure. It is therefore not surprising that many of these studies have failed to find that BP reactions to laboratory stressors reflect real-life BPs during a workday.[121,287,352] Pickering concludes that "viewed as a whole, these studies suggest that if there is an association between reactivity measured in the laboratory and the BP variability or reactivity of daily life, it is rather weak, or is obscured by the problems of measurement error."[287]

Pickering notes, however, that when the laboratory stressors closely resemble task performance during real life, a significant correlation in BP responses has been found. He cites a study by Matthews, et al., in which BP changes during a laboratory speaking task were compared to a similar task in the classroom.[238] Concordantly, Steptoe and Vögele emphasize the importance of "ecological validity" of laboratory mental stress tests, which should be designed "to model processes that will be important to CV health only if they are repeated or sustained in everyday life over many years."[352]

BP response during an interview in which stressful workplace events are discussed can be informative, precisely because of the personal relevance of the subject. For example, among 22 young, healthy, mainly blue-collar, male workers, a short semi-structured laboratory interview about intensely stressful events related to work (e.g., work accidents, interpersonal conflicts) produced a greater pressor response (+12.4/+15.1 mmHg) than any of the standardized mental stress tests, (mental arithmetic, quiz, auditory and visual choice-reaction time tasks).[19]

MENTAL STRESS

A body of laboratory-based cardiovascular research provides insight into some of the more generic aspects of workplace mental stress, most notably job strain. For example, external pacing, an important component of low control during performance of mental arithmetic is associated with increased systolic and diastolic BP responses.[34,120] Peters and colleagues found that both increasing effort in a mental task and lowered control provoked elevations in BP and plasma norepinephrine.[281] Uncontrollability also was associated with elevations in salivary cortisol. Furthermore, an effort-control interaction effect was observed with respect to diastolic BP response. Steptoe and colleagues found that BP reactions to an externally paced (low control) task were greater in teachers with high as compared to low job strain.[351] In contrast, BP responses to a self-paced (high control) task did not differ significantly between these two groups.

The ameliorating effects of social support also have been demonstrated in the laboratory setting. During performance of a speech task, BP reactivity was attenuated when an audience observer behaved in a supportive manner (nodding and smiling) as compared to acting neutrally.[54]

PHYSICAL STRESS

One ecologically valid, laboratory-based model of a work-related physical stressor is the **glare pressor test** (GPT), in which a standardized stimulus mimics the commonly occurring circumstance of facing an oncoming headlight during night driving. Studies using the GPT were designed to compare exposed groups (professional drivers) to those with no driving experience whatsoever. Compared to matched working nondriver referents, young normotensive professional drivers showed diastolic hyperreactivity to the GPT, together with digital vasoconstriction and signs of central arousal (EEG desynchronization).[23] It has been postulated that BP reactivity to the GPT represents an early phase of sensitization (a conditioned defense response) to threatening stimuli in the driving environment which, with continued exposure, may lead to sustained hypertension.[26] Longitudinal study is needed to further test this hypothesis.

Some laboratory paradigms of **noise exposure** have provoked significant elevations in BP, while others have not. Among 18 healthy males, 95 dB of industrial noise induced significant elevation in diastolic BP, which persisted during the 20-minute exposure period. Total peripheral resistance (TPR) increased significantly, while stroke volume and cardiac output fell.[5] Sawada also found an increase in TPR, together with a reproducible, persistent elevation in BP, when a similar group of subjects was exposed to 100 dB of pink noise.[319] A significant elevation in systolic BP associated with noise exposure during performance of mental arithmetic has been reported by Linden,[218] but not by Tafalla and Evans.[359]

The **cold pressor test** (immersion of the hand into cold water for 1–3 minutes) induces significant increases in systolic and diastolic BP and marked elevations in norepinephrine and epinephrine levels.[14,19,27,146,262,304] Several studies applying the cold pressor test found no relation between reactivity and future level of BP.[287] The study of Menkes, et al., however, revealed that even after statistically controlling for other risk factors, including family history of hypertension, hyperreactivity to the cold pressor test was a significant predictor of hypertension among 1000 medical students followed for 20–36 years.[247]

Isometric handgrip is also an extremely potent pressor stimulus. Both systolic and diastolic BP rise out of phase with heart rate, and the baroreceptor set point is changed such that a disproportionate pressure load is placed on the heart. Neurogenic mechanisms along with local factors such as afferent reflex stimulation and mechanical hindrance to blood flow, contribute strongly to these cardiovascular changes.[13,338] In normal subjects, isometric handgrip to one-third maximal capacity for 3 minutes evoked the greatest diastolic BP rise of a series of ten powerful cardiovascular stressors.[19] It also was associated with a significant rise in norepinephrine and epinephrine.[14] Among borderline hypertensive men, mean peak BP during isometric handgrip was 181.8/114.9 mmHg.[66] At 1-year followup BP reactivity while performing isometric handgrip and mental arithmetic was significantly correlated with the risk of developing established hypertension, but this association became nonsignificant after controlling for basal diastolic BP and mean ambulatory systolic BP during the day.

Among 33 post-MI patients, **carrying graded loads** of 20–50 lbs. while walking on a treadmill was associated with diastolic BP levels > 120 mmHg.[337] Hietanan reported that static exercise training (e.g., weight lifting, hammer throwing) was associated with increased ventricular wall thickness, and noted that increased afterload is the physiologic adaptation to static exercise (as opposed to increased pre-load for dynamic exercise).[144]

Thus, a number of physical stressors can provoke substantial acute rises in BP. However, the relationship between acute BP changes to these stimuli in the laboratory and tonic BP elevations brought about by chronic occupational exposure needs exploration.

Biological Mechanisms: I. The Defense Response

THE ACUTE REACTION: PREPARATION FOR "FIGHT OR FLIGHT"

The defense response comes into play when the organism is called upon to actively cope with a threat or challenge. The cardiovascular system is geared up for the anticipated physical activity (fighting or fleeing): cardiac output increases, with blood flow directed to the heart, brain, and skeletal muscle at the expense of the viscera. Skeletal muscle vasodilatation ensues, as a result of CNS inhibition of vasoconstrictor activity to skeletal muscle fibers and circulating epinephrine binding to beta-2 receptors in muscle resistance vessels. Higher CNS centers inhibit baroreceptor vagal activity, such that heart rate is simultaneously elevated. Efferent renal sympathetic nerves increase their firing, leading to diminished renal blood flow; the renin-angiotensin system activates; the glomerular filtration rate falls; sodium retention is enhanced; and blood volume increases. The net hemodynamic result of activating the defense response is a rise in BP, with a hyperkinetic heart and with total peripheral resistance (TPR) usually within normal levels, although TPR is high relative to cardiac output.[78,97,166,287] The defense reaction to an acute threat is a rapid-acting, and arguably the best understood, biological mechanism for regulating BP and heart rate. The release of catecholamines triggered by the sympathetic nervous system produces nearly instantaneous increases in BP and heart rate, increasing the supply of oxygen and energy to the musculoskeletal system so as to facilitate active physical responses to environmental challenges.

RELATION OF THE DEFENSE RESPONSE TO SUSTAINED HYPERTENSION

The defense reaction is phylogenetically a very old response and is adaptive when the challenges faced by the organism are primarily direct, calling for a physical response. Levi notes that this reaction was "of practical value to Stone Age people confronted by a pack of wolves . . . (but that) we still prepare for bodily activity and muscular exertion when we encounter changes in our environment and the demands for adjustment that they imply. Our environment—most of all, our work environment—however, has undergone drastic changes over the millennia. The demands placed on our adaptability have altered in character, while our genes have hardly changed."[212]

Gilmore in paraphrasing Charvat, Dell, Folkow, and Folkow[48] graphically illustrates this point as follows:

> When a gazelle hears a predator approaching cardiovascular and humoral changes develop immediately, while the somatomotor or muscular response is perhaps only an alerting reaction. Later, as the predator comes closer, the gazelle explodes into an all-out flight response, with his cardiovascular system being already prepared.
>
> In contrast, civilized man is faced with stress-producing situations (which) seldom relate to physical danger, such that the defense response is no longer well coordinated, the autonomic-humoral component being dissociated from the somatotropic or muscular response. Since the cardiovascular or metabolic resources intended to support heavy or violent physical exertion will not be utilized in the natural way, the hormonally produced changes of the blood, and thus, the chemical environment of the blood vessels and the heart will be more long-lasting than when violent muscular activity occurs. In addition, since the neurogenically induced cardiovascular changes are not modified by the additional vasodilatation due to muscular activity itself, the pressure load on the heart and blood vessels will be greater than if muscular activity occurred.[122]

The idea that intermittent elevations of BP, occurring in response to repeated exposure to environmental stressors and elicitation of the defense response, could result in sustained hypertension was first proposed by Folkow.[94,98] Folkow notes that when physical activity is suppressed, the magnitude of the pressor response to sympathetic activation becomes greater because there is no exercise-induced muscle vasodilatation. This is seen as a "forced dissociation of normal response patterns,"[97] which Eliot has described as a "constant state of visceral-vascular readiness,"[86] whereby the heart and blood vessels are activated irrespective of the actual metabolic needs of the organism. Thus, while the defense reaction, including the acute elevation in BP, is adaptive in the short run under certain circumstances, it may be maladaptive in the long run.

Still unknown are the precise dynamics by which repeated evocation of the defense reaction without physical fight-or-flight behavior translates into sustained hypertension. Elevations in BP do not necessarily lead to hypertension. As shown by Julius, et al., mechanical compression of the thighs in dogs can produce an acute increase of BP for as long as the compression is applied, but without causing any upward drift of the resting pressure.[169] Chronic instrumental CV conditioning in nonhuman primates provokes repeated elevations in BP, but does not consistently evolve into sustained hypertension after the conditioning paradigm is discontinued.[377] Henry and colleagues have found that long-term social disruption leads to hypertension in some but not all initially normotensive rats.[141] While heart and adrenal weights, adrenal catecholamine synthetic enzymes, and pathohistologic changes in the heart, aorta, and kidney in several rat strains generally paralleled the BP changes, the Wistar-Kyoto hyperactive strain showed stress-induced increases in heart and adrenal weights, but no BP changes. Thus, many questions are unanswered. The length and intensity of exposure to the stressor, and its nature, clearly are issues of importance.

The Role of Adrenergic Activity in the Early Stages of Hypertension

BP changes occur over various time frames, and the factors that cause acute changes may not be the same as those that contribute to chronic changes. The fluctuations that occur throughout the day in response to environmental circumstances have been collectively called the "phasic" component of BP; the "tonic" (long-term resting level) component changes only gradually over time.[285] Essential hypertension is defined as an elevation of the tonic component.

There is evidence of a subtle increase in the level of sympathetic nervous system (SNS) activity in many patients during the early stages of hypertension, and this increase is primarily tonic rather than phasic. For example, several (but not all) studies have demonstrated that subjects with mild hypertension have increased resting catecholamine excretion, heart rate, and cardiac output,[124,165,283] as well as enhanced catecholamine responses to stressors.[123] Oparil and colleagues review a number of lines of evidence implicating SNS activity in essential hypertension. They state that "SNS activity is elevated in nearly every form of human and experimental hypertension, and reduction of this activity decreases arterial pressure" and note that "chemical or surgical lesions of the SNS lower arterial pressure in most hypertensive individuals."[270] Concordant conclusions are drawn by Mancia, particularly focusing on direct measurement of sympathetic nerve traffic to skeletal muscle circulation, which is found to increase with progressively more severe degrees of essential (but not secondary) hypertension.[231]

Pharmacologic studies, predominantly conducted by Majewski and Rand, have identified one potential mechanism by which adrenaline (epinephrine) might mediate stress-linked hypertension.[228] Both in vitro and in vivo studies have shown that infusion of epinephrine in low doses (equivalent to the levels seen during naturally occurring stress) can enhance norepinephrine release from sympathetic nerve terminals.[227] Although sustained experimental neurogenic hypertension has been quite hard to produce in practice, Majewski, et al. achieved it in rats using a slow-release depot implantation of epinephrine.[229] After the 8th week, when excess epinephrine could no longer be detected in the plasma, BP (but not heart rate) was still elevated.

Similarly, Blankenstijn, et al. showed that the arterial pressure of humans infused with epinephrine was at first reduced, but by the end of the infusion (6 hrs) was above the baseline value, and remained elevated throughout the night.[32] The pressor effect of epinephrine was most marked during periods of increased sympathetic activity—for example, when the subjects were active—and not when they were at rest. Infusion of norepinephrine produced an initial elevation of pressure, but no sustained effects.

Structural Changes in Resistance Vessels

Through repeated elicitation of the defense reaction—i.e., repeated pressor episodes—structural changes may gradually occur in the cardiovascular system, and these can result in a higher basal BP. Adrenergic neurotransmitters and other substances (e.g., angiotensin and insulin) that rise in association with the defense response act as "growth promoters" on vascular smooth muscle.[172] Prolonged exposure of resistance vessels to these substances can result in vascular structural changes (hypertrophy) and increased smooth muscle contractility. This is precisely what occurs during repeated exposure to mental stress, due to the lack of skeletal muscle vasodilatation. Furthermore, mechanical factors related to increased wall pressure, tension, or stress promote increased vessel wall thickness.[355]

According to Folkow and colleagues, activation of smooth muscle during repeated exposure to acute stress, even if only intermittent, can stimulate an increase in smooth muscle cell size (hypertrophy), thereby increasing the wall thickness of the resistance vessels and shrinking their internal radius.[98,98a] The net result is an increase in peripheral resistance. These hypertrophied vessels are rendered hyper-responsive to vasoconstrictive stimuli. This could explain why stress responses of hypertensive individuals are predominantly characterized by vasoconstriction with elevation of TPR, while the response of normotensive individuals is usually an increase in cardiac output.[38,123] Egan and colleagues have demonstrated increased forearm vascular resistance responses to norepinephrine and angiotensin II in patients with mild hypertension, compared to weight-matched normotensive controls.[83] The net outcome is a chronically increased TPR, usually with a down-regulation of beta-adrenergic receptors in the heart, leading to a normal cardiac output, as seen in established hypertension.[97,167,172]

RENAL MECHANISMS AND LONGER-TERM CHANGES IN ARTERIAL BP

Besides structural changes in resistance vessels, longer-term changes in arterial BP appear to be strongly influenced by renal mechanisms. Guyton provides a possible explanation of how neurogenic mechanisms could contribute to chronic hypertension by their effects on the kidney.[129] With SNS activation, the renal vasculature becomes severely constricted, compromising renal blood flow. For example, chronic infusion of norepinephrine can permanently damage the renal arteries. Severe essential hypertension is characterized by approximately half the normal renal blood flow and a two- to fourfold increase in renal vascular resistance. In order to maintain an adequate glomerular filtration rate, the arterial pressure must be maintained at a high level. Furthermore, there is evidence that environmental stress can cause sodium retention, mediated via renal sympathetic nerve activity in animals[4,190] and in humans.[216] Hollenberg, et al. showed that the effects on renal blood flow of a behavioral challenge lasted much longer than the effects on BP.[152] This, in turn, can lead to sodium retention and a gradual increase in tonic BP.

Increased salt intake may exacerbate this process. Poulter and Sever present a model by which neurogenic pressor mechanisms (repeated elicitation of the defense response) combined with increased dietary sodium may together account for the elevated BP among persons migrating from environments with a low to those with a higher prevalence of hypertension.[291] However, Waldron and colleagues reported that the higher BPs that developed in the latter settings (e.g., those affected by the market economy, economic competition, breakdown of family ties) appeared to be independent of salt intake.[387]

FURTHER INSIGHTS FROM PSYCHOSOCIAL STRESS MODELS IN ANIMALS

Henry notes that in the early stages of psychosocial stimulation (continuing conflict resulting in social instability) in mice, adrenal catecholamine synthetic enzymes approximately double, and plasma renin is very high.[139] After about 3 weeks, however, although systolic BP is elevated, plasma renin levels have fallen. Subsequently, the renal and hindquarter vessels show greatly enhanced sensitivity to angiotensin. Induction of hypertension in experimental animals requires several months of repeated exposure to stressful situations.[101,142] These experimental results provide a biological rationale for the finding that an induction period appears to exist before exposure to job strain gives rise to an increased risk of established hypertension.

WORK STRESSORS, DEFENSE RESPONSES, AND HYPERTENSION: IS THERE A LINK?

The threats and challenges of working life are clearly capable of provoking arousal, as characterized by the defense response. Because these threats and challenges are often of a chronic nature, and are rarely, if ever, resolved by a physical fight-or-flight reaction, a prolonged state of "visceral-vascular readiness" is likely to emerge. Elevations in catecholamine excretion, typical of the defense response, have been associated with exposure to numerous acute and chronic work stressors. Furthermore, elevations in BP and catecholamine excretion during stressful work appear to be related. Among women who perceived work as the greatest source of stress, systolic BP at work was significantly higher compared to women who cited home as the greater stressor. In the former group, the percent changes in BP and catecholamine excretion during waking hours (relative to sleep) were significantly correlated. In contrast, among the women who cited home as more stressful, these waking BP changes were not correlated with changes in urinary catecholamines.[161]

Studies among professional drivers have demonstrated that laboratory stressors that are reminiscent of the threats and challenges of the work environment elicit signs of electrocortical arousal characteristic of the defense response, especially in hypertensive transport operators.[88] Other studies in which ecologically valid work stressors have been simulated in the laboratory indicate that these are capable of eliciting significant acute BP elevations.

However Schwartz, Pickering, and Landsbergis note that for work stress to contribute to a tonic elevation in BP, "the blood pressure of the exposed individuals would have to be elevated not only in the presence of a stressor but also during rest."[329] Thus, the focus should be on "exposure to chronic low- or moderate-grade stress rather than on discrete events that are widely acknowledged to produce brief spikes in the blood pressure profile."[329] The large, consistent body of data on AmBP and exposure to job strain indicates that these elevations are indeed persistent. They occur not only at work, but also at home and, in some studies, during sleep. Finally, and probably most compelling, are the data indicating that there may be a cumulative effect of chronic exposure to job strain on AmBP.

Biological Mechanisms: II. The Defeat Reaction and Glucocorticoids

Although most attention has been paid to the SNS as the prime mediator of stress-induced increases in BP, evidence also suggests that activation of the hypothalamic-pituitary-adrenocortical (HPA) axis may be involved. During exposure to some acute stressors, particularly those that are psychologically threatening (e.g., public speaking), cortisol is released over a period of about 15–20 minutes. This release is much more gradual, but also persists much longer after termination of the stress condition, than that of epinephrine and norepinephrine.[180]

Animal studies reveal that when repeatedly faced with noxious events that cannot be controlled, motivation becomes undermined, resulting in passive behavior and giving-up. In animals this pattern has been labeled the "defeat reaction,"[142] while in humans it is perhaps most closely linked to the construct of learned helplessness.[331] According to Folkow, defeat reactions, if prolonged, "may exert more harmful effects than strong and prolonged defense reactions."[97] Defeat reactions tend to activate the HPA axis to release glucocorticoids. Glucocorticoids have a likely pressor role, both singly and as potentiators of reactivity to adrenergic and angiotensin II stimulation.[258,270,318,394] They also have a weak mineralocorticoid effect, leading to renal sodium reabsorption at higher doses.[395] Thus, it is possible that glucocorticoids play a major role in mediating the effects of chronic stress.

Experimental studies have shown that strong control over an animal's behavior provokes hypertensive responses.[28] An integrated CNS-behavioral stress response pattern, distinct from the defense response and characterized by passive behavior (motoric immobilization, lying still, "playing dead"), generalized vasoconstriction, and vagally mediated bradycardia has been identified.[81,239] This "defeat-type" reaction pattern is typical of the "dive reflex,"[403] and can be activated under conditions of hopelessness, extreme fear, or exhaustion. A similar pattern also has been evoked by stimulation of the lateral hypothalamus in rabbits.[81] Finally, short-lived, repeated stimulation of the lateral hypothalamus for several days to weeks in rats leads to a progressive, sustained rise in arterial BP.[122,140] The role of the HPA axis in these processes needs to be further investigated.

CHRONIC DEFEAT REACTIONS AND HYPERTENSION

While pointing out the pitfalls of extrapolating from animal or human laboratory studies to real life, Lennerlöf hypothesized that "jobs that are characterized by little control, influence, learning and development entail risks of helplessness learning."[207] Some empirical support for this hypothesis comes from the Cornell Work Site Blood Pressure Study (WSBPS), in which Landsbergis and colleagues examined questionnaire responses of participants whose jobs were characterized as passive, i.e., low control, but also low demand.[202] These workers' responses to Seligman's Attributional Style Questionnaire indicated high levels of learned helplessness. Kohn and Schooler reported similar findings concerning the relationship between job characteristics and personality, both cross-sectionally and longitudinally.[191] However, contrary to expectation, the WSBPS participants in passive jobs did not show any elevation in BP compared to those in jobs with low demand and high control or high demand and high control.[327]

Empirical data links both acute (e.g., traffic peaks during bus driving) and chronic (e.g., heavy psychosocial job burden) exposure to work stressors with elevations in cortisol.[10,133] There is also some evidence that low job control is associated with elevated BP. For example, having undergone a forced job change was found to be a significant predictor, cross-sectionally, of hypertension among middle managers.[280] In a study by Härenstam and Theorell, low skill discretion predicted systolic AmBP among prison guards.[132] The meta-analysis of Pieper, et al. reported a significant association between low job decision-latitude and casual systolic BP.[288] However, there are also a number of studies in which low control, as a main effect, failed to show any association with BP. These include the AmBP studies of Light, et al.[217] and Schnall, et al.[327] as well as several casual BP studies, including the prospective investigation of Siegrist.[343] The outcome measure in the latter study was the co-occurrence of hypertension and hyperlipidemia (see Chapter 2 for further details). No single study has yet investigated each of the links in the hypothesized defeat reaction model as it applies to work stress and BP: low control → defeat reaction/learned helplessness → increased HPA axis activation → increased BP.

Biological Mechanisms: III. The Effort-Distress Model

Folkow states, "the ancient 'defense' and 'defeat' reactions, intended for quite different situations, are often activated by the artificial stimuli and symbolic threats inherent in today's hectic and competitive life . . . when intensely engaged over longer periods they can, indeed, profoundly disturb inner organ systems and metabolic events."[99] He notes that in stressful situations there often are shifts between the defense and defeat reactions.[97] Activation of both the sympathoadrenal medullary and the HPA cortical axes can be seen in such situations.[142] Frankenhaeuser observed that the activation of these two axes could be evoked in human laboratory studies by paradigms that demanded effort while providing little or no opportunity for control over the task performance, a condition she hypothesized would engender distress.[104] This led to the Effort-Distress Model, which was described as follows:

Effort with distress is probably the state most typical of our daily hassles. It is accompanied by an increase in both catecholamine and cortisol secretion. Most of our studies concern this category. For instance, mental work carried out under conditions of either stimulus underload or overload will typically evoke feelings of effort, as well as distress and, consequently, both the catecholamine and the cortisol level will rise. . . . The key question is how to achieve the state of effort without distress. Our data point to personal control as an important modulating factor in this regard. A lack of control is almost invariably associated with feelings of distress, whereas being in control may prevent a person from experiencing distress. Hence, personal control tends to act as a buffer, reducing the negative arousal effects, and thereby changing the balance between sympathetic-adrenal and pituitary-adrenal activity.[104]

One of the experimental paradigms applied in this context was performance of a monotonous vigilance task, as compared to a self-paced, reaction-time task. Both conditions required similar effort, but the former was associated with distress, while the latter was primarily enjoyable. During the vigilance task, both epinephrine and cortisol increased, whereas during the reaction-time task only epinephrine rose.[224] In a more recent study, Peters and colleagues applied a similar paradigm and registered BP as well as hormonal responses.[281] They found that when the effort involved in laboratory task performance increases and control is simultaneously diminished, not only do both catecholamines and cortisol rise together with BP, but an effort-control interaction effect is observed with respect to diastolic BP responses.

The Effort-Distress Model has not been tested as a predictor of sustained hypertension.[289a] It mainly has been applied in the human laboratory setting. However, neuroendocrine changes consistent with activation of both the sympathetic-adrenomedullary and the HPA axes have been demonstrated among metallurgists when performing paced assembly work with no control over the work pace.[374] These working conditions are clearly typical of job strain. The distress condition of the Effort-Distress Model is conceptually very similar to the high-strain condition of the Job Strain Model, though they are typically used to characterize laboratory versus actual workplace situations, respectively. While there is strong empirical evidence that chronic exposure to job strain is associated with the development of sustained hypertension, more investigation is needed to ascertain whether a combined catecholamine-glucocorticoid effect represents a major mechanism by which this process occurs.

Work Stress and Left Ventricular Hypertrophy

Schwartz, Pickering, and Landsbergis suggested that occupational stress may be of special etiologic importance in the progression from hypertension to IHD.[329] One of the mediating mechanisms may be increases in left ventricular mass (LVM), which is a major risk factor, independent of BP, for MI, cardiac electrical instability, and sudden cardiac death.[73,113,214,249,320]

Devereux and Roman contend that increased LVM occurs as a direct effect of chronic elevations in BP, due to increases in stroke volume together with impairment of myocardial contractile performance.[75] In contrast, Mancia argues that SNS activation is also crucial,[231] citing data indicating that increased LVM can be induced by sub-pressor doses of adrenergic agents,[272] and that lowering BP in spontaneously hypertensive rats prevents increased LVM only if not accompanied by high reflex sympathetic outflow to the heart.[333] Occupational stress can provoke both the hemodynamic and the adrenergic changes that promote increased LVM.

Ambulatory BP has been found to be more predictive of LVM or wall thickness than casual BP.[74,80,294,300,384] LVM is more highly correlated with average BP at work than at other periods, but a strong relation also has been observed between LVM and home BP measured on workdays.[15,74] Devereux and Roman interpret these findings as an indication of a "special impact on the heart of blood pressure responses to regularly recurring stress at work, with possible 'spillover' effect of home blood pressures on working days."[75] In addition, Schnall and colleagues found that exposure to job strain is associated with increased LVM index.[323] Synthesizing these results, we hypothesize that long-term exposure to job strain leads to a sustained elevation of BP that then causes structural changes in the left ventricle. Considering the strong, independent relation between increased LVM and cardiovascular morbidity, this pathophysiologic process may account for a substantial part of the reported association between job strain and CHD morbidity.[324]

MYOCARDIAL OXYGEN SUPPLY AND DEMAND: ENVIRONMENTAL TRIGGERS OF IMBALANCE
by Karen Belkić, MD, PhD

Whether or not accompanied by symptoms, myocardial ischemia has major prognostic importance. It is the consequence of an imbalance between the oxygen demand made by the myocardium and the available O_2 supply. Determinants of myocardial O_2 demand include: heart rate, blood pressure, myocardial contractility, size of the left ventricle (LV), and the duration of systole. Supply of O_2 to the myocardium is determined by coronary artery blood flow, the intraluminal size of the coronary arteries, the O_2 content of hemoglobin, the duration of diastole (during which approximately 85% of the coronary blood flow occurs), and coronary perfusion pressure (the difference between arterial pressure at the aortic root level and LV filling pressure).[49] Many of these determinants of myocardial O_2 supply and demand are affected by stress mechanisms and/or by chemical and other physical factors in the work environment. Exposure to these stressors has induced signs of myocardial ischemia among persons with various stable ischemic syndromes, and, in some instances, among apparently healthy workers.

Laboratory Studies of Mental Stress and Myocardial Ischemia
Laboratory studies have demonstrated that mental stress can trigger myocardial ischemia in 40–70% of patients with various stable ischemic syndromes. This is specifically associated with an adverse prognosis.[160,195] Among patients with single- or multiple-vessel coronary artery disease (CAD) LV ejection fraction assessed by radionuclide ventriculography as an indicator of myocardial ischemia was found to fall equally or more often in response to personally relevant mental stress as compared to exercise; this mental-stress induced ischemia was usually asymptomatic.[157,315] Patients with CAD who showed LV wall motion abnormalities during laboratory mental stress testing had a significantly increased likelihood of exhibiting myocardial ischemia during daily activities as assessed using ambulatory monitoring.[33,125] Laboratory mental stress–induced myocardial ischemia also is associated with a longer duration and increased frequency of ischemia during daily activity.[9]

Mental stress–induced myocardial ischemia invariably occurs at a lower double product than that evoked by exercise, while diastolic pressor responses to mental stress are larger.[157,195,316,321] Controlling for the change in double product, beta-endorphin secretion is greater in mental stress compared to exercise, which may explain the predominance of silent, as opposed to symptomatic, myocardial ischemia induced by mental stress.[252,339] It has been suggested that not only increased oxygen demand, but also decreased O_2 supply may contribute to myocardial ischemia during mental stress.[9]

Mechanisms of Decreased Myocardial O_2 Supply

CORONARY ARTERY SPASM

A major determinant of oxygen supply to the myocardium is the caliber of the coronary vessels. The luminal caliber of the coronary arteries can be compromised not only by stress-mediated processes and other environmental factors leading to atherosclerosis, but also by coronary arterial vasospasm. Coronary artery spasm is a dynamic mechanism that compromises blood flow in variant angina pectoris, as well as in ischemic heart disease in general.[405] Furthermore, vasospasm of epicardial coronary arteries can occur in response to increased adrenergic and vagal activity, thromboxane A2, and endothelin-1.[393] A number of substances that rise with the stress response, e.g., adrenergic neurotransmitters, angiotensin, and insulin, exert a trophic influence on vascular smooth muscle. These vessels with hypertrophied smooth muscle show an increased responsivity to vasoconstrictor substances.[97,167,172] In addition, endothelial damage, which can be mediated by stress-induced turbulent blood flow,[275] can render arteries vasoconstrictive, even in response to normally vasodilating substances such as acetylcholine.[115,188,276] Angiographic studies among patients with CAD reveal that mental stress can evoke vasoconstriction in atherosclerotic coronary vessels, especially at points of stenosis.[35,407] Experimental animal data links exposure to stressors such as social disruption to a paradoxical propensity for coronary arterial vasoconstriction in response to intracoronary acetylcholine.[396]

Stress mechanisms also are implicated among patients with Prinzmetal angina, for whom changes in autonomic outflow (withdrawal of vagal tone as indicated by diminished high frequency component of heart rate variability) were found to consistently precede episodes of ST segment elevation. This finding was irrespective of the presence or absence of coronary artery stenoses.[203]

Clinicians have long recognized that the vasospastic component of angina pectoris tends to be expressed more in the winter months. Exposure to extreme cold is unpleasant and evokes vasoconstriction by direct action upon the blood vessels and by a reflex increase in sympathetic activity. In coronary patients, as well as in normal subjects, the cold pressor test (immersion of the hand in cold water for 1–3 minutes) induces significant increases in systolic and diastolic blood pressure and marked elevations in norepinephrine and epinephrine levels.[14,20,27,146,262,304] Angiographic studies reveal that the cold pressor test can provoke coronary vasospasm in patients with Prinzmetal angina or with coronary atherosclerosis.[154,177,260,299,406] Female factory workers showed a significantly increased risk of ST segment depression during work in inverse relation to occupational temperature levels (OR 0.77, CI 0.62–0.95), after adjusting for age, type of work, smoking, and relative weight.[126]

Rebound coronary artery vasospasm also can result from withdrawal from exposure to nitrates among workers in the explosives industry. Nitroglycerin appears to reverse this effect.[306,391]

CARBON MONOXIDE EXPOSURE

Exposure to carbon monoxide (CO) impairs oxygen supply to the myocardium due to the high binding affinity of CO to hemoglobin and a leftward shift in the O_2 dissociation curve.[128] Among patients with CAD, exposure to low levels of CO (carboxyhemoglobin levels of 1.5–4%) is associated with a diminished exercise time to onset of ischemic ST changes and to angina pectoris.[1,189,306] (By way of reference, carboxyhemoglobin levels found in smokers range from 2–15%.[151])

REDUCTION IN CORONARY BLOOD FLOW VELOCITY

Another mechanism by which mental stress may act to compromise oxygen delivery to the myocardium is by diminishing coronary blood flow velocity. Acute mental stress can increase blood viscosity and decrease circulating plasma volume.[195] Among patients with syndrome X, performing mental arithmetic gave rise to a significant fall in coronary blood flow together with a significant increase in arterial norepinephrine; 13 of these 29 patients developed typical angina-like chest pain. There were, however, no significant changes in the diameter of the left anterior descending coronary artery during this mental stress.[51] Increased coronary microvascular resistance has been proposed as the mediating mechanism of myocardial ischemia in Syndrome X.[51,175]

LEFT VENTRICULAR HYPERTROPHY

LVH, which is closely related to workplace BP, can compromise myocardial oxygen supply. This is due to high end-diastolic pressure which compresses the intramyocardial vessels, as well as to a low capillary density of the large myocardial mass, with a lowered coronary flow reserve.[75,188,271,284]

Mechanisms of Increased Myocardial O_2 Demand

LEFT VENTRICULAR HYPERTROPHY AND ESSENTIAL HYPERTENSION

LVH also is associated with an augmented myocardial oxygen demand, due to increased pressure load and the burden of a large myocardial mass.[75] Myocardial oxygen demand is chronically increased in essential hypertension with or without LVH; this is related to elevated total peripheral resistance, which places an increased afterload on the heart. Based on these considerations, it is not surprising that patients with essential hypertension often have angina pectoris even in the absence of CAD.[188]

ELEVATED BLOOD PRESSURE AND/OR HEART RATE

Superimposed acute stressors create an inotropic and chronotropic demand for yet more oxygen to the myocardium. In patients free of manifest CAD but with stable essential hypertension with or without LVH, transient episodes of myocardial ischemia are found to be related to peaks in ambulatory BP.[12,266] In some,[266,293] but not all[12] reports, these episodes were significantly more frequent in hypertensive patients with LVH. Deedwania and colleagues found, by simultaneously recording ambulatory BP and ECG, that most episodes of silent myocardial ischemia in patients with CAD are preceded by an elevated systolic BP, as well as heart rate.[68,69]

Isometric stress elicits a powerful diastolic pressor response. In CAD patients, this response can lead to myocardial ischemia, which is attributed to augmented oxygen demand from LV afterload. Isometric maneuvers such as handgrip are less consistent triggers of myocardial ischemia than dynamic exercise; the latter leads to a greater increase in double product.[46,144,178] Upper extremity activity may entail a greater isometric component than lower extremity activity.[135]

Acute heat exposure, particularly with physical exertion, gives rise to a tachycardic response.[71,336] There are some reports of ST depression associated with heat-elicited tachycardia among workers in a precision casting factory,[358] as well as among normal subjects and CAD patients exposed to the intense heat of a sauna.[363] Other studies in milder conditions ($\leq 30°C$) failed to elicit any signs of myocardial ischemia in CAD patients.[2,336]

Elevations in the double product and in diastolic BP have been reported in response to short-term exposure to noise levels in the range of 85–95 dB,[6,385] although there are conflicting reports concerning chronic noise exposure and BP effects.[147,197,241,364] There is suggestion of a possible association between occupational noise exposure and risk of myocardial ischemia: noise-exposed male factory workers showed a borderline significant increase in odds ratio for ST depression during work (OR 1.07 CI 0.99–1.12), after adjusting for age, type of work, smoking, and relative weight.[126]

Empirical Data

Reported mental stress during general daily activities has been found to be associated with ischemic electrocardiographic changes in patients with coronary heart disease.[17,110,117] Gabbay and colleagues found that among 63 patients with CAD, "mental activities (appeared) to be as potent as physical activities in triggering daily life ischemia."[117] None of these studies, however, specifically examined stressful work activities.

There has been considerable attention paid to the circadian pattern of myocardial ischemia. Transient electrocardiographic signs of myocardial ischemia show a nadir during sleep and a peak in the morning hours after waking. This peak corresponds to the time of maximum heart rate and systolic BP, as well as high levels of catecholamine and cortisol which increase the sensitivity of coronary arteries to catecholamine-mediated vasoconstriction.[21,123,375,400] The relation of this circadian distribution of myocardial ischemia to shiftwork and other occupational factors remains to be determined.

Driving is known to be a highly stressful activity, and professional drivers are at inordinately high risk of developing ischemic heart disease (IHD).[22,380,401] While there are no published Holter monitoring studies among professional drivers with cardiovascular disease, recordings during driving have been reported among amateur drivers with IHD. In one study, a 20-minute drive in heavy London traffic elicited STT changes in 13 of 24 stable IHD patients.[362] Another also reported ischemic electrocardiographic changes among a series of IHD patients during driving.[204] A third study, however, did not find any driving-related ST changes in five patients with angina pectoris, but two of the five developed chest pain while driving.[219] More recent data reveals that among 22 IHD patients, driving into a speed trap was associated with a significant chronotropic effect, with some cases of silent, as well as symptomatic myocardial ischemia.[58]

There are a few reports of ambulatory monitoring during work made among subjects without apparent IHD. Green and colleagues made 1-hour Holter recordings during work among 2508 factory workers without a history of IHD to examine the relation between ST-segment depression and exposure to the physical factors of noise and cold.[126] Arstall and colleagues reported that among male police officers 45 years or older with 2+ cardiac risk factors but without known IHD, there was a 3.4% prevalence of ST-segment depression during 24-hour ambulatory monitoring, which included shiftwork; followup thallium perfusion scans were negative.[11] Of 18 precision casting factory workers examined by Taccola, et al., five exhibited tachycardia and STT changes during physical exertion and radiant heat exposure.[358] Asmar and colleagues found self-rated work stress levels were significantly higher among asymptomatic hypertensive patients who had ST-segment depression during ambulatory monitoring, compared to those without signs of myocardial ischemia.[12]

There is a general paucity of systematic study on myocardial ischemia in relation to work activity. In particular, comprehensive and integrative examination of the psychosocial, ergonomic, and physical-chemical work environment, as it affects the occurrence of myocardial ischemia, is lacking. Especially surprising is the lack of published data on this topic among series of patients who have returned to work after acute cardiac events. Kavanagh and Matosevic have provided descriptive reports on several post-myocardial infarction patients in whom laboratory exercise testing was normal, but who developed significant ST-segment depression during specific physically and mentally stressful work activities.[176] These authors consider that the work-site ambulatory data was essential for making recommendations concerning their patients' occupational activity.

Krantz and colleagues have stated: "Research on [myocardial] ischemia has provided a pathophysiologic model for understanding mechanisms by which mental stress may trigger clinical events."[195] Clearly, such a model needs to be focused on the work environment.

ATHEROGENESIS, COAGULATION, AND STRESS
MECHANISMS   *by Andrew Steptoe, DPhil, and Michael Marmot, PhD*

Atherogenesis is the process through which atherosclerosis is initiated and develops over the lifespan. Understanding of the early stages of atherogenesis has increased substantially over the past decade, with the recognition of the central importance of inflammatory responses and injury to the endothelial surface of the arterial vessel wall.[310] Endothelial damage, particularly at branching points of the arterial tree, results in plaque formation, involving the trapping of lipoprotein and adhesion of monocytes and T lymphocytes. Continued cell influx and proliferation leads to more advanced lesions and fibrous plaque formation. Pro-inflammatory cytokines (soluble proteins that regulate cellular behavior) such as interleukin 1, interleukin 6, and tumor necrosis factor-α are critically involved in atherogenesis.[29] They impair endothelial function and stimulate macrophage accumulation and migration of smooth muscle cells into lesions. These cytokines also are associated with insulin resistance and the cardiovascular metabolic syndrome[246] (see page 146).

Endothelial damage is most likely to occur at branching points on the arterial tree where there is turbulent blood flow. Hypertension has a major influence on shear stress at these sites, and also has direct pro-inflammatory effects, such as increasing the formation of free radicals.[200] Therefore, the influence of work stress on atherogenesis may be mediated in part by hypertension. Angiotensin II, an important component of the renin-angiotensin system, also may increase during stress, contributing to atherosclerosis by stimulating vascular smooth muscle cell growth.[53]

Direct evidence for the effects of stress on endothelial dysfunction is available in animal studies, since social stress in cynomolgus monkeys causes endothelial injury in atherosclerotic arteries.[346] This response is inhibited by beta-adrenergic blockade, implicating sympathetic nervous system (SNS) activation. Behavioral stress also has been shown in animal studies to stimulate the production of pro-inflammatory cytokines.[409] The function of the endothelium is dependent on nitric oxide (NO), which inhibits adhesion of platelets and white cells to vessel walls, and on the growth of vascular smooth muscle cells. NO has been found to be involved in the vasodilatory response to mental stress.[43] Hypertensive patients show blunted forearm vasodilation to mental stress, and this effect is mediated by impaired NO production.[42] Although no studies linking NO and cytokines with work stress have been described yet, these factors are potentially of great importance.

The role of inflammation in atherogenesis also has raised the possibility that infections contribute to coronary heart disease (CHD). Markers of systemic inflammation such as plasma C-reactive protein concentration are associated with future myocardial infarction and stroke.[302] Associations between CHD risk and persistent infection with *Helicobacter pylori, Chlamydia pneumoniae*, and cytomegalovirus have been suggested.[64,354]

The extent of lipoprotein incorporation into plaque depends on the concentration of lipids in the blood. Atherogenesis is positively associated with the concentration of total cholesterol and low-density lipoprotein (LDL) cholesterol, and negatively correlated with high-density (HDL) cholesterol. LDL cholesterol accumulates in vessel walls, where it becomes oxidized, stimulating other processes such as damage to the endothelium and the formation of foam cells. Behavioral stress stimulates increases in the concentration of cholesterol in some animal models.[334] Stress also stimulates total cholesterol and LDL cholesterol acutely in humans, although this response is due in part to changes in hemoconcentration, since plasma volume often decreases during stress, leading to increases in concentration without increased synthesis.[265,273] Long-term, episodic, naturalistic stressors—such as important academic examinations—have been found to alter lipid concentration in some studies, but not others.[265,289] However, it has proved difficult to demonstrate the effects of variations in work demands on lipid levels within-subjects.[240,264] Any such changes that take place might be due to alterations in dietary fat intake, since this also increases with workload in some individuals.[353]

Cross-sectional associations between lipids and job characteristics such as work demands and job control also have been inconsistent.[324] In the Whitehall II study of British civil servants, total cholesterol was not related to occupational grade, and differences in CHD risk associated with factors such as low job control were independent of cholesterol.[234,235] There were occupational grade differences in apolipoproteins A-1 and B, but these were explained quite substantially by concomitant variations in health-related behaviors such as smoking, exercise, and diet.[40] However, associations between high effort and low reward and elevated total and LDL cholesterol that are independent of lifestyle factors have been described in studies from Germany and Sweden.[279,342] Note that the well-established association between carbon disulphide and CHD may be mediated by the influence of this chemical on LDL cholesterol and blood pressure.[84]

The later stages of CAD and the development of acute ischemic syndromes are dominated by the process of thrombogenesis. As the disease progresses, arterial plaques characterized by thin, fibrous caps, substantial lipid accumulation, and a large number of macrophages are particularly vulnerable to disruption.[215] The disruption of unstable plaques is an important process in acute thrombosis, and complications are influenced by a number of factors such as catecholamine release and the concentration of fibrinogen.[116] These substances, in turn, affect platelet activation and other coagulation processes.

Fibrinogen plays an important role in the coagulation cascade, since it is converted to fibrin (a major constituent of thrombi) by thrombin. In conjunction with other hemostatic factors, fibrinogen promotes atherosclerosis by stimulating platelet aggregation and increasing blood viscosity, foam cell formation, and smooth muscle proliferation. It also may be important as an acute phase protein associated with inflammatory processes. Sjogren has suggested that occupational exposure to inhaled dust microparticles may provoke alveolar inflammation and the release of mediators such as fibrinogen.[345] Fibrinogen has been found prospectively to predict incidence of CHD.[244] Early studies relating work stress with fibrinogen concentration produced inconsistent findings.[233,254] The issue therefore was investigated more comprehensively in the Whitehall II study.[41] It was found that higher fibrinogen concentrations were associated with lower socioeconomic status in both men and women. Control over work, as assessed independently by managers, was inversely associated with fibrinogen concentration in both sexes. Fibrinogen also is associated with high effort and low reward at work.[342] Thus, it may be an important marker of the pathways through which work and other psychosocial factors influence CHD risk. Other hemostatic factors that are associated with work stress include tissue plasminogen activator (tPA), which regulates fibrinolysis. A study of Japanese middle-aged workers demonstrated that tPA was inversely associated with psychological job demands independently of standard risk factors.[158]

Currently, there is considerable interest in clinical research on the role of platelets in acute cardiac syndromes, with platelet activation and platelet size both as important parameters.[381] Platelets adhere to damaged endothelium, and their granules contain cytokines that stimulate the proliferation of monocytes and smooth muscle cells. Activated platelets also recruit further platelets into thrombi. No studies have been reported to date that relate platelet function with work characteristics. However, platelet activation as assessed by platelet factor 4 and beta-thromboglobulin is increased by acute emotional stress.[230,274] These acute responses probably are stimulated by catecholamine release. Cross-sectionally, associations between platelet activation and other psychosocial factors have been described. For example, Markovitz found that platelet activation in CHD patients was positively correlated with hostility scores,[232] and platelet responsivity is heightened among patients with clinical depression.[259] Both hostility and depression are factors that have been linked with increased CHD risk. It is possible, therefore, that the stimulation of thrombogenesis through enhanced platelet activation is another process that mediates psychosocial influence on cardiac events.

Current understanding of atherogenesis and thrombotic mechanisms highlights a number of pathways that are sensitive to stress-related neuroendocrine responses. Research linking these factors with the work environment is lacking. However, it is likely that much of the effort in gaining understanding of how the work environment affects CHD will be focused on these pathways over the next few years. This endeavor will be facilitated by the establishment of proxy measures of CHD, of which two of the most promising are carotid intima-medial wall thickness and plaque height. These measures can be taken noninvasively with high resolution carotid ultrasonography. Thickness of the carotid intima-mediated wall and height of carotid plaque are associated with CV risk factors and increased risk of CV events.[269] Progression in the development of carotid atherosclerosis over 4 years has been shown in Finnish men to be more rapid in those experiencing high demands and low economic rewards at work than in others with low demands and high rewards.[226] The integration of this index into population studies of other factors influencing atherogenesis will allow greater precision in prediction and understanding of mechanisms.

NEUROENDOCRINE MECHANISMS   *by Töres Theorell, MD, PhD*

Increasing awareness of the fact that most processes in the body are integrated in complicated CNS-end-organ interactions has had a profound impact on today's cardiology. The endocrine system could be regarded as an organ that is played upon by the brain. Overuse of it may cause many disturbances. "Chords" produced by the brain may be "harmonic" or "disharmonic." The effect of a short disharmonic chord may not be deleterious to the listeners (in our analogy: the body), but a long-lasting disharmonic one can disturb the whole audience.

Selye's hypothesis about the general adaptation syndrome (GAS) describes three different stages in the reaction to a situation that requires unusual energy mobilization:[332]

1. **Alarm**—an immediate reaction that the cortex of the brain is not aware of initially. Alarm causes arousal of some of the fast-reacting endocrine systems that are central in the mobilization of energy, such as the catecholamines adrenaline and noradrenaline.

2. **Defense**—a slightly slower reaction (within minutes) that is paralleled by cognitive processes. The cognitive functions include thoughts about how to handle the situation, immediate expectations, etc. The hormonal reactions in this phase aim at facilitating all aspects of the situation in which energy mobilization takes place. Release of fuel to the blood is the central aspect; lipids and glucose serve as fuel and are necessary in the energy production needed for muscular action (running or fighting). Several hormonal reactions ready the body to fight for a long time: the body becomes insensitive to pain, coagulation is facilitated (for the avoidance of excessive bleeding when injury occurs), retention of fluid and salt is facilitated (for the avoidance of excessive loss of plasma volume if sweating continues and there is no possibility to drink or to ingest salt), and some aspects of the immune system are activated. All of these components of the defense reaction are mirrored by physiological and endocrine processes that can be monitored in human beings.

According to Folkow, the defense reaction has "the greatest relevance for the cardiovascular system."[97] In its classical manifestation, it is an integrated cognitive-hemodynamic-metabolic response preparing the organism to physically cope with threat or challenge. Components of the defense response include sympathetic, adrenergically-mediated increased cardiac output with blood flow directed to the vasodilated skeletal muscles, heart, and brain; higher CNS suppression of baroreceptor vagal activity, yielding simultaneously increased heart rate; efferent renal SNS activation leading to decreased renal blood flow with lowered glomerular filtration rate, increased sodium retention, and increased blood volume, and activation of the renin-angiotensin system and antidiuretic hormone secretion; insulin resistance, to insure adequate glucose to the brain; and platelet activation, in anticipation of injuries.[78,97,166] Obviously, the defense reaction may lead to adaptation (phase 2 of Selye's GAS), which represents a successful reaction to the environment, and the energy mobilization calms down. But the same reaction also may be unsuccessful and result in defeat or loss of control,[142] which could be regarded as an alternative stage:

3. **Exhaustion**—either the end stage of an unsuccessful GAS, or the defeat phase of Henry's theory.[142] During this phase the limitations of the organism are shown and there is a breakdown of adaptation. There are several new concepts that partly overlap this one, such as burnout and vital exhaustion (psychologically defined) and chronic fatigue syndrome (physiologically defined).

A long-lasting physiological adaptation is associated with disturbances of the hypothalamic-hypophyseal-adrenocortical axis. The defense and defeat reactions may alternate and coexist in real life, and in vulnerable hearts this may have cardiodeleterious effects (see Chapter 4).

The GAS according to Selye is an example of **response stereotypy.**[205] One of the strongest critics of Selye's theory has been John Mason,[237] whose main point was that there is no such general phenomenon as the GAS. Every individual and every situation is unique. Mason's idea could be regarded as an argument for **response specificity,**[199] in which every individual/situation combination induces a unique set of endocrine reactions. Of course, both stereotyped and specific responses occur.

One of Mason's central concepts was **anabolism**, which corresponds to endocrine processes stimulating growth, restoration, and replacement of worn-out tissues. Unfortunately, anabolism, which is necessary for long-term survival, is inhibited by long-lasting energy mobilization. In line with Mason's reasoning, energy mobilization (in its extreme form, **catabolism**) and anabolism could be regarded as the two most essential concepts in the organization of our knowledge of endocrine processes of relevance to the interplay between psychosocial work environment and CVD.

Acute Energy Mobilization

There is a profound difference between acute and long-lasting mobilization of energy. The acute process has been studied extensively in experiments. It is characterized by initial release of the catecholamines adrenaline and noradrenaline (NA) to the blood, followed within minutes by release of glucocorticosteroids and mineralocorticosteroids. This is a necessary sequence of events if the organism is to survive in a critical situation, and absence or attenuation of it is accordingly evidence of a disturbance.

CATECHOLAMINES

Assessment Issues.   In preventive and clinical cardiology, it is possible to measure the catecholamines in urine and blood. The reader should be aware of the difficulties in this area.[123,149]

• Plasma catecholamine determinations: When measuring catecholamines in blood, remember that the fluctuations are so rapid that casual measurements may be meaningless. Furthermore, venipuncture induces pain, which immediately results in elevated catecholamine levels. Such an elevation is, of course, induced by a situation that is irrelevant to the relationship between the psychosocial work environment and CVD. One possibility is to measure the blood catecholamines by means of a venous catheter, which allows repeated blood sampling without repeated venipunctures. It is difficult, however, to make repeated samplings during work activities. To obtain a representative measurement of catecholamines during basal conditions, the physician may make the sampling after a resting period post insertion of a venous catheter.

The plasma NA concentration is to a large degree a reflection of muscular activity, which results in NA influx into the blood. Furthermore, NA reflects the activity in the SNS, which could react very differently in different parts of the body (e.g., specific reaction patterns in the gastrointestinal system, heart, and/or lungs). Therefore, plasma adrenaline (which is a weaker but "cleaner" indicator of mental stress than NA) frequently correlates more strongly with BP during restful conditions than does plasma NA.[370] Hjemdahl formulates this in the following way:

> *Plasma NA is a frequently used marker for sympathetic nerve activity in humans, but the data obtained are often misinterpreted due to lack of appreciation of the physiological determinants of the NA concentration measured. NA overflow from an organ gives a good reflection of nerve activity in that organ. However, sympathetic nerve activity is highly differentiated, particularly during stress, and conventional plasma NA levels (usually forearm venous samples) cannot be taken as an indication of "sympathetic tone" in the whole individual. NA is rapidly removed from the plasma, resulting in meaningless net veno-arterial concentration differences over organs unless its removal from arterial plasma is taken into account. In the forearm, for example, 40–50% of catecholamines are removed during one passage; about half of the NA in a venous sample is derived from the arm and half from the rest of the body. Therefore, conventional venous sampling overemphasizes local (mainly skeletal muscle) nerve activity.*[149]

With regard to adrenaline the physiologic background is different. Goldstein has formulated this in the following way:

> *Since the adrenal medulla secretes [epinephrine] EPI directly into the bloodstream, plasma EPI levels generally reflect neural outflow to the adrenal medulla. Thus, increments in adrenomedullary secretion of catecholamines resulting from manipulations of circulatory reflexes or from . . . administration of drugs correlate with increments in directly recorded adrenal nerve activity . . . however . . . plasma levels of adrenaline are very low in antecubital venous plasma of healthy volunteers at rest—as little as 3×10^{-11} mol/L. This contrasts with plasma levels of NE, which normally exceed 6×10^{-10} mol/L.*[123]

• Urinary catecholamine determinations: A useful approach is to measure catecholamines in urine. Urinary sampling of catecholamines is more suitable than plasma determinations for field studies. Hjemdahl has noted that urinary NE reflects arterial NE levels, and that changes in urinary EPI appear to reflect its secretion during stress, as well.[149]

The relevant measures are the amounts of excreted adrenaline and NA into the urine per time unit. To obtain such measurements, it is necessary to record the exact hours of urination and to collect all the urine during a given time period. This can be a difficult doctor-patient collaborative task, and it requires good preparation. The excretion of adrenaline and NA fluctuates during the 24-hour cycle. For adrenaline, the excretion during the most active part of the day is three times higher than that during deep sleep at night. Accordingly it is important to define the period of collection during the day. The shorter the period of collection, the more difficult it is for the patient to successfully collect during the defined period, although he or she could be instructed to drink water to increase urination.

The strength of the urinary measurement of catecholamines is that it reflects excretion over a defined period of time; it provides the physician with an integrated assessment of catecholamine excretion during several hours, for instance during an ordinary 8-hour working day. Early in the development of these assessments, it was proposed that work-free days should be compared with working days to minimize the effect of interindividual variation in basal excretion of catecholamines.[105] The assessment provides information about the intraindividual increase in catecholamines during working hours. Because of the marked diurnal variation in catecholamine output, corresponding hours during the work-free day and the working day should be compared.

There are several technical errors that may occur in the measurement of catecholamine excretion in the urine. Ingestion of certain kinds of food or fluids, for instance bananas and coffee, could influence the assessments. The urine must be
acidified to withstand the breakdown of catecholamines. Usually hydrochloric acid
is added in the aliquot before collection starts. If there is uncertainty regarding the
completeness or timing of the collection, the excretion could be related to the
amount of creatinine that is excreted. In summary, assessment of catecholamine excretion must be prepared carefully and in consultation with experts.

Empirical Findings On Work Stressors and Catecholamine Excretion.   The
classical work of Levi and Frankenhaeuser illustrated the usefulness of the assessment of urinary catecholamine excretion as an indicator of arousal in the workplace.[105,211] In additional studies, Fröberg, et al. showed that sleep deprivation caused
marked elevation of urinary adrenaline and NA urinary excretion, an observation
that has relevance to the growing scientific evidence that exposure to shiftwork increases the risk of developing MI.[112] Johansson, et al. and Lundberg and
Frankenhaeuser showed that monotonous, high-pressured work induces elevated
catecholamine excretion.[163,225] Rissler and Elgerot showed that a long-lasting period
of overtime work causes not only elevated excretion of adrenaline and NA but also a
delayed relaxation of the arousal function in the evening.[303] The overtime study indicated that it may take weeks before such a disturbance disappears after the end of
the overtime work.

Other experiments demonstrated that piece-rate work under high pressure induced marked elevation of urinary catecholamine excretion.[211] Field studies revealed
that Swedish city bus drivers had approximately twice the average level of adrenaline excretion compared to other occupational groups.[10] Urinary catecholamine excretion was shown to be rising as a function of traffic congestion among male Los
Angeles metropolitan bus drivers.[91] Frankenhaeuser, et al. found that a group of
working women had elevated catecholamine excretion after work when they were
confronted with the home situation.[108]

A study of male prison employees showed that the urinary excretion of adrenaline and NA was related to decision latitude: employees with a low degree of decision latitude had high catecholamine output, even after adjustment for body mass
index, coffee and alcohol drinking, and age.[132] The above-mentioned study of urinary excretion of adrenaline in bus drivers showed that drivers who reported job
strain (high psychological demands and low decision latitude) had a higher urinary
catecholamine output than others.[91]

CORTISOL

Metabolic (Catabolic) Effects of Cortisol on CVD.   The hypothalamo-pitu-
itary-adrenocortical axis (HPA) originates in the hypothalamus, which responds to
arousal situations by increasing the output of corticotrophic releasing factor (CRF).
CRF stimulates the pituitary to increase the output of adrenocorticotrophic hormone
(ACTH). ACTH, in turn, stimulates the adrenocortex to increase the output of those
corticosteroids that have an important role in the energy mobilizing process. The
HPA axis has to function well in terms of excitability—cortisol should increase in
situations that require energy mobilization—but it also must slow down once the sit-
uation has calmed. Cortisol inhibits the preceding steps in the chain—the release of
ACTH and CRF.[250]

Cortisol has been the most extensively studied of the corticosteroids with predominantly energy mobilizing function. It has both mineralocorticoid and glucocorticoid

effects, and it reacts less rapidly (within minutes) than catecholamines to a challenge. Accordingly, it is meaningful to study serum cortisol variations in real-life situations.

Cortisol is a counter-regulatory hormone that protects against insulin-induced hypoglycemia. Many of its effects facilitate the effects of other hormones that are important in energy mobilization and arousal. For instance, it enhances and prolongs the effects of epinephrine and glucagon, promotes hepatic gluconeogenesis and glycogen synthesis (glycogen then is acutely released in response to adrenaline and glucagon), and inhibits peripheral glucose utilization.[258] Physiologically, cortisol enhances the vascular reactivity to angiotensin II and NA.[258] It also promotes dyslipidemia by increasing very-low-density lipoprotein (VLDL) secretion and then enhances the transformation of VLDL to low-density lipoprotein.[39] It has been documented that cortisol stimulates vigilance and CNS arousal.

Cortisol Assessment. The plasma concentration of cortisol is not as rapidly fluctuating as that of catecholamines; thus, it is more meaningful to measure cortisol in plasma. The venipuncture itself causes an elevation of serum cortisol, but it takes several minutes, and therefore the use of a venous catheter is not necessary. Under normal conditions, a rising plasma cortisol level indicates a rising level of arousal. There is a marked circadian pattern, with high levels in the morning hours and gradually falling concentration during the mid-day and afternoon hours. Therefore, it is important to take hour of sampling into account when assessments are interpreted. Under most conditions it is favorable to measure the concentration in the morning. As with catecholamines, potential confounders include medication, smoking, alcohol, and food. Mostly free (not bound to protein) cortisol is measured.

Free cortisol also can be measured in urine (see precautions regarding urine collection of catecholamines, pages 141–142). Another method is saliva analysis. The saliva concentration of cortisol has been shown to reflect the free cortisol concentration in serum, and since repeated saliva samples can be collected more easily than repeated blood samples, the physician can study circadian variations of cortisol during real-life conditions. The patient can carry capillary tubes, which are inserted into the mouth for saliva collection many times during the day.[181]

• Empirical findings concerning work stressors and cortisol. The interpretation of the relationships between work stressors and cortisol excretion has been complicated by the fact that acute and long-term effects of stressors have been mixed. However, in normal healthy samples, short periods of stressful work do induce measurable elevations in plasma cortisol as well as urinary and salivary cortisol. For instance, studies of bus drivers have shown increasing cortisol excretion in relation to traffic peaks.[10] In a large study of prison employees, Härenstam and Theorell showed that employees in work sites with many psychosocial problems had higher plasma cortisol than other employees.[133]

• Empirical neuroendocrine findings in effort-distress or low control–high demand situations. The Effort-Distress Model (EDM) is based on performance of a monotonous task that requires much effort and vigilance, leading to arousal and substantial distress. This combination has been found to activate both the sympathoadrenomedullary and pituitary adrenocortical axes, while an enjoyable, self-paced task yields only a rise in urinary epinephrine.[100,106,109,224] Corroborative data from the worksite is provided by Timio and Gentili, who reported significantly elevated epinephrine, norepinephrine, and 11-hydroxycorticosteroid excretions among healthy metallurgists when performing paced assembly work with no control over work pace, compared to "ordinary work" outside the assembly line.[374] Experimental data on social interactions and conflicts in mice are quite coherent with these worksite and human laboratory observations. Henry and Stephens found that elicitation of the defense (fighting to achieve a dominant position) and the defeat (subordination) responses activated the sympathoadrenal and the pituitary adrenocortical systems, respectively.[142]

The EDM's distress and eustress reactions parallel the high demand-low control "job strain" situation (corresponding to distress) and high demand-high control "active job" situation (corresponding to eustress) when the Demand-Control Model is used as a framework. Of course, an important distinction is that the demand-control model focuses on the workplace environmental demands and constraints, whereas the EDM focuses on the individual's reaction to the laboratory environment.

Long-Lasting Energy Mobilization

Sustained exposure to situations that are uncontrollable, unrewarding, and demanding could induce repeated elevations of catecholamines and energy-mobilizing corticosteroids. Such iterative endocrine reactions by themselves may have profound effects on the CV system. The measurement of these endocrine reactions during long-lasting energy mobilization, however, is another matter. Scientific confusion existed in the literature before it was realized that the regulation of arousal can be disturbed if exposure to a psychosocial stressor is long-lasting. Some endocrine systems may be "set" on a higher activity level due to such exposure; for instance, the thyroid hormones may be elevated after long-lasting exposure to arousal in sensitive persons. However, cortisol regulation also may change.

Recently, Sluiter, et al. showed that long-distance truck driving with extremely long work hours causes a low excretion of adrenaline and noradrenaline as well as an abnormal cortisol circadian rhythm.[349] In the usual cortisol pattern, levels are high in the morning and start declining at 10 AM. Low levels are found before bedtime. In the long-distance truck drivers, the day after driving was characterized by low morning cortisol levels, which peaked after a couple of hours. This is an example of an early disturbance of the regulatory system. After even longer periods of arousing situations, however, more profound disturbances can arise. These more profound regulatory cortisol disturbances can take several forms, and they all have relevance to heart disease:

1. **Constantly elevated cortisol**, as in clinical depression. The normal inhibition of the drive in the HPA axis is not functioning.[317] Using symbolic language, this could be labeled "brake failure." Depression is an important risk factor with prognostic and therapeutic implications, particularly in rehabilitation after MI.

2. **Exhausted function**, as in the chronic fatigue syndrome (CFS). Cortisol levels are low, with very small variations, as though the HPA axis has stopped responding.[72] This could be labeled "accelerator failure," and it has relevance to the two psychologically defined concepts *vital exhaustion* and *burnout*. Vital exhaustion has been studied extensively in relation to heart disease risk.[192]

3. **Elevated sensitivity**, as in the post-traumatic stress disorder. If a subject has been exposed to extreme stress, such as torture and rape, serum cortisol concentration becomes markedly elevated for many weeks and months. This elevation may result in increasing numbers and sensitivity of cortisol receptors, so that only small amounts of cortisol are needed to induce marked effects. With such a disturbance, the arousal function shows marked fluctuations, in particular when the subject is reminded of the traumatic events that caused the disturbance.[47]

The HPA axis is associated with other functions. Hypothetically, an "exhausted" HPA axis function may be compensated for by overactivity in parallel systems. For instance, patients with CFS have shown elevated plasma concentration of NA. CFS also may be associated with overactivity in parts of the immune system, such as increased responsiveness of the natural killer cells and interleukins to physiologic stressors.[390] This overactivity may be part of the explanation why vital exhaustion is associated with a marked elevation of CV risk.

INHIBITION OF ANABOLISM

Michelson, et al. provide some mechanistic details to corroborate the downplaying of anabolic steroid synthesis in periods of crisis, "adaptive redirection of energy," showing that CRF inhibits LNRH, and that glucocorticoids suppress a number of sites in the reproductive endocrine axis—LNRH, gonadotropins, testosterone, and estradiol—as well as decrease the target tissue's response to these sex hormones.[250]

Accordingly, energy mobilization often is associated with inhibited anabolism. This inhibition can be measured by means of changes in testosterone in men. Interestingly, recent studies show that a disturbed cortisol rhythm, with low morning levels and small variations, is associated with low testosterone levels in men.[308] Theorell, et al. demonstrated that increasing job strain is associated with decreasing total plasma testosterone.[371] In a recent study of a police organization, Grossi, et al. found that police officers who lost their jobs because of a reorganization had relatively low plasma testosterone levels at the time of job loss, but the levels had increased 1 year later when most of them had new jobs.[127] Those with the most satisfactory jobs had the most pronounced increases in testosterone concentration. Serum lipids also had improved significantly, illustrating a pattern of CV risk factor improvement.

Stress-mediated elevations in plasma prolactin, as shown among nurses reporting high job strain[369] and among subway drivers with "person-under-train" incidents,[372] could be regarded as a manifestation of "passive coping,"[368] which also could suppress the reproductive endocrine axis via inhibition of LNRH.[65]

Rosmond and Bjorntorp have proposed that repeated arousal causing marked, iterative serum cortisol elevation is part of the etiology of the metabolic syndrome (which may include abdominal obesity, atherogenic lipid patterns, diabetes, and hypertension).[309] Part of the reason why long-term exposure to cortisol elevation is associated with decreased testosterone production and with the metabolic syndrome may be that the synthesis of energy-mobilizing steroids is favored over the synthesis of anabolic steroids. All the steroid hormones have the same sources. The downplaying of anabolic steroid synthesis may have phylogenetic reasons. In a period of crisis, reproduction has low priority.

OTHER HORMONES

Many hormones participate in the communication between brain and body. Due to space limitations, it is not possible to fully cover the effects of all of them. These processes and their interactions can be understood by understanding what a physiological reaction is. In this pursuit, the two dimensions that have been described, energy mobilization and anabolism, are helpful. Several other hormones are of relevance to the CV system.

Prolactin is a peptide that is released from the adenohypophysis. It is regulated by the dopamine and serotonin systems in the brain, both of which are important in mood regulation. Prolactin is important to the immune system (which is stimulated) and, at least in women, to BP regulation (high levels are associated with high BP). The plasma prolactin concentration increases in situations that induce passiveness and powerlessness in crisis situations, but decreases in situations that induce free-floating anxiety.[368] Increasing job strain in combination with depressed mood may induce marked plasma prolactin elevation in normal working men.[373] Marked elevations also have been observed in situations characterized by sudden, unexpected loss of control, such as when subway drivers are exposed to "person under train" accident situations[372] and when police officers lose their jobs due to reorganization.[127]

THE CARDIOVASCULAR METABOLIC SYNDROME
by Eigil Fossum, MD, Aud Høieggen, MD, Andreas Moan, MD, PhD, Morten Rostrup, MD, PhD, Sverre E. Kjeldsen, MD, PhD

The association between blood pressure (BP) and coronary heart disease may be caused by a concurrence of atherogenic biochemical abnormalities in hypertensive patients. These abnormalities—increased total cholesterol, triglycerides, glucose, insulin, and insulin resistance—form the cardiovascular metabolic (CVM) syndrome. There are numerous reports of **sympathetic nervous system** (SNS) over-activity in these patients, suggesting SNS overactivity as a pathophysiological link between high BP and this syndrome.[185]

The SNS and Hypertension
De Quatro and Chan[67] and others[183] identified increased SNS activity in patients with essential hypertension; increasing levels of plasma epinephrine and nor-epinephrine were associated with elevated BP and heart rate. Emotional stress provokes catecholamine release[79,313] and has been associated with CAD. Possibly, hypertensive subjects respond to environmental stimuli with larger sympathoadrenal responses than normal subjects.[85] Thus, elevated plasma epinephrine levels in hypertension may be a marker for an increased arousal reaction, with enhanced neurogenic activity of the type associated with the defense reaction.[148] Such arousal is caused by awareness of hypertension,[313] but is also a pathophysiological feature of essential hypertension.[314]

One of the main challenges in evaluating the pathophysiological role of the SNS in hypertension is the lack of equipment capable of measuring both the rapid oscillations of the system (within seconds) and the integrated SNS response, due to advanced differentiation of the SNS branches. In the clinical setting, heart rate and plasma catecholamines are widely used. Plasma catecholamines should be measured in arterial blood because they are subject to a peripheral arterial-venous extraction of approximately 50% at rest; thus, arterial epinephrine represents the epinephrine concentration to which the tissues are exposed. In addition, plasma catecholamine concentrations in peripheral venous blood may conceal important differences between hypertensive and normotensive groups.[186]

The concomitant increase in heart rate and BP together with reduced baroreceptor sensitivity is a characteristic feature of central nervous influence on CV adjustment,[96] and is compatible with a role of increased sympathetic tone, possibly combined with less parasympathetic inhibition of heart rate. The parasympathetic and sympathetic activities are coupled in a reciprocal, integrated response, so that an increase in the firing rate in one of these autonomic components is associated with a decrease in activity in the other branch.[171] The heart rate, therefore, may be an indicator of sympathetic tone. This notion is supported by studies showing significant positive correlations between plasma catecholamines and resting heart rate.[186]

The SNS and Metabolic Disturbances

The Oslo Study of Cardiovascular Diseases showed positive correlations among BP, serum cholesterol, triglycerides, and blood glucose levels.[208] In the Tecumseh study, those with "white coat" and sustained borderline hypertension had higher plasma triglycerides, insulin, and total cholesterol and lower values of high-density lipoprotein (HDL) cholesterol than the normotensive group.[170] Of the hypertensive subjects, 37% had a hyperkinetic circulation with increased cardiac output and raised plasma catecholamines. Plasma norepinephrine correlated positively and significantly with cholesterol, and heart rate correlated positively and significantly with fasting insulin, suggesting activation of the SNS as a pathophysiologic link between elevation of these CV risk factors. The Tromsø Study showed that heart rate correlated significantly with the progressive increase in age-adjusted levels of serum total cholesterol, non-HDL cholesterol, and triglycerides, as well as with a decrease in HDL cholesterol in both men and women.[36] There was a strong positive correlation between heart rate and BP, as also shown in other studies. These associations between heart rate and coronary risk factors remained significant when anthropometric and life-style factors were controlled.

The sympathetic activity influencing heart rate also may explain the association between heart rate and serum lipids.[36] Several lines of evidence suggest that the SNS may influence plasma lipid levels. Public speakers[361] and motor-racing drivers[360] have higher heart rates, plasma catecholamines, and triglycerides when active. α-Adrenergic antagonists lower very-low-density lipoprotein (VLDL) triglyceride concentrations and increase HDL cholesterol,[209] whereas β-adrenergic blockade gives the opposite effects.[182]

Catecholamines have cardiovascular and metabolic hormonal effects at concentrations slightly above low-normal resting levels;[55,350] even transiently and certainly chronically raised plasma catecholamine levels may cause biochemical abnormalities and deserve consideration as a pathophysiological feature of essential hypertension. Catecholamines may increase serum cholesterol concentrations by enhancing hepatic 3-hydroxy-3-methylglutaryl coenzyme A reductase activity and/or by decreasing receptor-mediated cellular binding and uptake of low-density lipoproteins. By stimulating α-adrenoceptors, catecholamines may decrease blood flow to peripheral vascular beds, thereby decreasing the activity of endothelial lipoprotein lipase. This enzyme is involved in the formation of HDL particles through catabolism of triglyceride-rich VLDLs.[82]

Epinephrine has a pronounced effect on raising hematocrit, even within the lower pathophysiological concentration range.[187] Hematocrit is the major determinant of whole blood viscosity,[150] which again, according to the Poiseuille-Hagen law, contributes to peripheral resistance. Accordingly, we recently showed a strong correlation between hematocrit and directly measured whole blood viscosity and insulin resistance in young normotensive men with hyper-reactive BP responses to mental stress.[150]

In recent years, hypercoagulability and reduced fibrinolysis have been added as an integrated entity of the cardiovascular metabolic syndrome.[3] Epinephrine activates blood platelets in vitro[267] and increases the number of circulating platelets.[187] Blood platelet count and function have been directly linked to cardiovascular mortality.[367]

Increased levels of circulating epinephrine secondary to SNS overactivity may there-fore explain both the metabolic disturbances and the hypercoagulability/platelet dys-function concomitantly present in the CVM syndrome.

The SNS and Insulin Resistance

Insulin resistance has been proposed as the metabolic link between the CVM syndrome and atherosclerotic CVD.[70,301] An increased sympathetic activity in hyper-tensive patients, directly by metabolic hormonal effects or indirectly and more chronically by inducing hemodynamic changes, may explain the association of in-sulin resistance and hypertension. Acutely, during low-rate infusion of epinephrine, even physiological concentrations cause intolerance to an oral glucose load and in-creased baseline glucose, mainly by interference with insulin action and not by inhi-bition of insulin secretion.[131] After an infusion of epinephrine that increased the peripheral venous concentration from 25 to 75 pg/ml, both plasma glucose and in-sulin levels increased significantly and remained high after 2 hours.[131] Inhibition of insulin secretion stems from stimulation of α-adrenergic receptors in the β cells in the pancreas,[290] but seems to be of importance only at supraphysiological levels of epinephrine. Insulin resistance in the liver and skeletal muscle is mediated by β-adrenergic receptors.

THE HEMODYNAMIC HYPOTHESIS OF INSULIN RESISTANCE

Julius, et al. suggested that the relationship between BP elevation and de-creased glucose extraction by skeletal muscle is secondary to hemodynamic factors; glucose delivery being a modulator of skeletal muscle glucose uptake.[168] We recently found a positive correlation between forearm blood flow and insulin sensitivity[103] and a negative correlation between peripheral vascular resistance and whole blood viscosity to insulin sensitivity[103,150] in young normotensive men with elevated BP re-sponses to mental stress. Pressure-induced restriction of the microcirculation may limit nutritional flow and thereby impair glucose uptake in the skeletal muscle. When epinephrine is infused intravenously, human forearm blood flow increases rather than decreases.[184] Therefore, acute effects of epinephrine, though inducing in-sulin resistance and glucose intolerance, are insufficient to explain the hemodynamic hypothesis.

However, repeated episodes of SNS overactivity may be different from the acute effects of epinephrine infusion and may lead to structural vascular changes that further aggravate both insulin resistance and hypertension.[168] High BP causes vascular hypertrophy, which is further enhanced by the trophic effects of the SNS.[134] The hypertrophy increases the α-adrenergic responsiveness of the vasculature,[83] which further accelerates the hypertrophy.[95] The same process may lead to vascular rarefaction and insulin resistance as its functional consequence. Chronic β-adrener-gic stimulation increases the size and number of fast-twitch muscle fibers, which are more insulin resistant than slow-twitch fibers. Furthermore, β-blockers aggravate whereas α-adrenergic antagonists ameliorate insulin resistance in hypertensive sub-jects, supporting the hemodynamic hypothesis of insulin resistance. β-Blockers de-crease blood flow and increase vascular resistance, whereas vasodilators increase flow and lower resistance.

The SNS and Hyper-Reactivity to Mental Stress

Since 1986, we have studied young men selected from the military draft proce-dure in Oslo. As attending is compulsory, these subjects comprise all 18-year-old

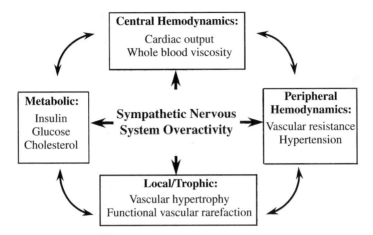

FIGURE 1. Overactivity in the sympathetic nervous system may directly or indirectly increase cardiac output, peripheral resistance, whole blood viscosity, glucose, insulin, and cholesterol, and may cause vascular hypertrophy and hypertension.

men without severe medical disorders, in the Oslo area. Ten percent of these men have a screening BP ≥ 140/90 mmHg.[313] They have normal ambulatory BP,[102,253] but are hyper-reactive to mental stress. BP values recorded during the draft procedure could be considered as "office" BP, or BP during an alert reaction.

In a series of protocols, we have documented that these men with elevated screening BP and hyper-reactivity to mental stress have metabolic disturbances resembling the pattern of the CVM syndrome. The insulin-resistant men have higher BP in response to an arithmetic challenge (mental stress test) than the insulin-sensitive men.[103] The men with the highest exercise BP responses have a significantly higher pre-exercise BP elevation (compared with ambulatory BP) than the men with the lowest exercise BP, as a mental stress response to the exercise test.[102] Rostrup, et al. showed that the psychological stress caused by awareness of hypertension increased resting BP, heart rate, and sympathetic responses to laboratory stressors.[311,312] The men selected from the higher screening BP levels, who were deliberately kept unaware of their BP status, were characterized with normal supine intra-arterial BP levels, but showed a hyper-reactive response in BP and heart rate to a mental arithmetic challenge.[314] These data support a link between high screening BP, specific hyper-reactivity to mental stress, and catecholamine sensitive coronary risk factors.

The SNS, Workplace Stress, and the Cardiovascular Metabolic Syndrome

In our studies demonstrating a close correlation between mental stress and the components of the CVM syndrome, including BP, we used a model of acute stress. Several authors have examined the effect of chronic stress related to the workplace.[91,107,211] Harenstam and Theorell found the urinary norepinephrine excretion to reflect self-reported work stress in a prison staff.[373] These results were supported by Gardell, who found higher levels of catecholamine excretion, triglycerides, BP, and self-reported work stress in bus drivers working in areas with heavy traffic compared with bus drivers working in suburbs.[118] Frohberg examined inter-shift differences and changes during shift-weeks on different shifts with regard to urinary cate-cholamine excretion and self-ratings of work stress and fatigue.[111]

The CVM syndrome, as an integrated entity, usually has not been investigated in epidemiologic studies of the workplace. However, in a prospective study of male, blue-collar workers by Siegrist, et al., the coincident occurrence of hyperlipidemia and hypertension was demonstrated empirically to have occupational psychosocial determinants.[343] A low prospect for being promoted was a significant multivariate predictor of high-risk coronary status. This association was independent of obesity, smoking, and individual characteristics of sustained anger and competitiveness.

The link between hypertension and CAD has been strongly documented in epi-demiologic studies. This association may not be casual, but may reflect a network of atherogenic biochemical abnormalities present in essential hypertension, added up as the cardiovascular metabolic syndrome. There are numerous reports of SNS over-activity in essential hypertension. Catecholamines may have metabolic hormonal ef-fects at concentrations slightly above low normal resting levels, and increased plasma catecholamines in hypertensive subjects may partly, or even fully, directly or indirectly, explain the metabolic disturbances constituting the cardiovascular meta-bolic syndrome. Because hypertensive subjects may respond to environmental stim-uli with larger sympathoadrenal responses than normal subjects, and emotional stress has been associated with CAD, catecholamines may be the crucial link be-tween stress and CVD. Environmental stress emanating from the workplace has been shown to activate the SNS. Thus, work stress may be considered a potential coronary risk factor.

REFERENCES

1. Allred EN, Bleecker ER, Chaitman BR, et al: Effects of carbon monoxide on myocardial ischemia. Environ Health Perspect 91:89–132, 1991.
2. Andersen IB, Jensen PL, Junker P, et al: The effects of moderate heat stress on patients with ischemic heart disease. Scand J Work Environ Health 4:256–272, 1976.
3. Andersen P: Hypercoagulability and reduced fibrinolysis in hyperlipidemia: Relationship to the metabolic cardio-vascular syndrome. J Cardiosvac Pharmacol 20 Suppl 8:S29–31, 1992.
4. Anderson DE, Dietz JR, Murphy P: Behavioral hypertension in sodium-loaded dogs is accompanied by sustained sodium retention. J Hypertens 5:99–105, 1987.
5. Andren L, Hansson L, Bjorkman M, Jonsson A: Noise as a contributory factor in the development of elevated arte-rial presure. A study of the mechanisms by which noise may raise blood pressure in man. Acta Medica Scandinavica 207:493–498, 1980.
6. Andren L, Lindstedt G, Bjorkman M, et al: Effect of noise on blood pressure and "stress hormones." Clin Sci 62:137–141, 1982.
7. Anonymous: The sixth report of the Joint National Committee on prevention, detection, evaluation, and treatment of high blood pressure. Arch Intern Med 157:2413–2446, 1997.
8. Appel LJ, Stason WB: Ambulatory blood pressure monitoring and blood pressure self-measurement in the diagno-sis and management of hypertension. Ann Intern Med 118:867–882, 1993.
9. Armstrong PW: Stable ischemic syndromes. In Topol EJ (ed): Textbook of Cardiovascular Medicine. Philadelphia, Lippincott-Raven, 1998, pp 333–364.
10. Aronsson G, Rissler A: Psychophysiological stress reactions in female and male urban bus drivers. J Occup Health Psychol 3:122–129, 1998.
11. Arstall MA, Wuttke RD, Arthur J, et al: The prevalence of ST segment depression on ambulatory electrocardio-graphic monitoring during daily life in high-risk asymptomatic police officers. J Cardio Risk 1:143–148, 1994.
12. Asmar R, Benetos A, Pannier B, et al: Prevalence and circadian variations of ST-segment depression and its con-comitant blood pressure changes in asymptomatic systemic hypertension. Am J Cardiol 77:384–390, 1996.
13. Assmussen E: Static (isometric) exercise: Cardiovascular respiratory and neural control mechanisms. Circ Res 48:I3–I10, 1981.
14. Atterhog JH, Eliasson K, Hjemdahl P: Sympathoadrenal and cardiovascular responses to mental stress, isometric handgrip and cold pressor test in asymptomatic young men with primary T wave abnormalities in the electro-cardiogram. Br Heart J 46:311–319, 1981.
15. Baba S, Nakamoto Y, Ueshima H, et al: Variations of blood pressures under regularly recurring stress in daily life and its relation to left ventricular hypertrophy in urban hypertensive men. J Hypertens 6:S695–S696, 1988.
16. Backman AL: Health survey of professional drivers. Scand J Work Environ Health 9:30–35, 1983.

17. Barry J, Selwin AP, Nabel EG: Frquency of ST segment depression produced by mental stress in stable angina pectoris from CAD. Am J Cardiol 61:989–993, 1988.
18. Bayes de Luna AJ, Soldevila JG, Vinolas Prat X: Do silent myocardial ischemia and ventricular arrhythmias interact to result in sudden death? Cardiol Clinics 10:449–459, 1992.
19. Belkic K: Methodology for detecting individuals at high risk for developing the acquired cardiovascular disorders. Master's Thesis, Center for Multidisciplinary Studies. Belgrade, University of Belgrade, 1984.
20. Belkic K: Light stress and the cardiovascular system: The glare pressor test. Ergonomics 29:563–568, 1986.
21. Belkic K: Psychosocial triggers of myocardial ischemia in women. Research Report to the Swedish Medical Research Council, 1995.
22. Belkic K, Emdad R, Theorell T: Occupational profile and cardiac risk: Possible mechanisms and implications for professional drivers. Int J Occup Med Environ Health 11:37–57, 1998.
23. Belkic K, Ercegovac D, Savic C, et al: EEG arousal and cardiovascular reactivity in professional drivers: The glare pressor test. Eur Heart J 13:304–309, 1992.
24. Belkic K, Gluhak M, Ugljesic M, et al: Ucestalost abnormalnosti arterijskog krvog pritiska i elektrokardiograma kod vozaca gradskog saobracajnog preduzeca Beograd (Prevalence of high blood pressure and electrocardiographic abnormalities among Belgrade mass transit drivers). Revija Rada 20:50–60, 1990.
25. Belkic K, Pavlovic S, Djordjevic M, et al: Determinants of cardiac risk in professional drivers. Kardiologija 13:145–149, 1992.
26. Belkic K, Savic C, Theorell T, et al: Mechanisms of cardiac risk among professional drivers. Scand J Work Environ Health 20:73–86, 1994.
27. Belkic KL, Mickovic L, Milic B, Savic S: Blood pressure and electrocardiographic changes elicited by the glare pressor test. Arch Environ Health 42:37–43, 1987.
28. Benson H, Gutmann MC: The relation of environmental factors to systemic arterial hypertension. In Eliot RS (ed): Stress and the Heart. Mt Kisco, Futura Publishing Co., 1974, pp 13–31.
29. Bhaghat K, Vallance P: Inflammatory cytokines impair endothelium-dependent dilation in human veins in vivo. Circulation 96:3042–3047, 1997.
30. Bhatt DL, James GD, Pickering TG, Devereux RB: Relation of arterial pressure level and variability to left ventricular geometry in normotensive and hypertensive adults. Blood Pressure Monitor 1:415–424, 1996.
31. Blake LM, Goldschlager N: Risk stratification of potential sudden death victims after myocardial infarction. Prim Cardiol 21:8–15, 1995.
32. Blankestijn PJ, Mann in't Veld AJ, Tulen J, et al: Support for adrenaline-hypertension hypothesis: 18-hour pressor effect after 6 hours adrenaline infusion. Lancet II:1386–1389, 1988.
33. Blumenthal JA, Jiang W, Waugh RA, et al: Mental stress-induced ischemia in the laboratory and ambulatory ischemia during daily life. Circulation 92:2102–2108, 1995.
34. Bohlin G, Eliasson K, Hjemdahl P, et al: Pace variation and control of work pace as related to cardiovascular, neuroendocrine, and subjective responses. Biol Psychol 23:247–263, 1986.
35. Boltwood MD, Taylor B, Burke MB, et al: Anger report predicts coronary artery vasomotor response to mental stress in atherosclerotic segments. Am J Cardiol 72:1361–1365, 1993.
36. Bonaa KH, Arnesen E: Association between heart rate and atherogenic blood lipid fractions in a population. The Tromsø Study. Circulation 86:394–405, 1992.
37. Borggrefe M, Fetsch T, Martinez-Rubio A, et al: Prediction of arrhythmia risk based on signal-averaged ECG in postinfarction patients. PACE 20:2566–2576, 1997.
38. Brod J, Fencl V, Hejl Z, Jirka J: Circulatory changes underlying blood pressure elevation during acute emotional stress (mental arithmetic) in normotensive and hypertensive subjects. Clin Sci 18:269–279, 1959.
39. Brown MS, Goldstein JL: The hyperlipoproteinemias and other disorders of lipid metabolism. In Wilson JD, Braunwald E, Isselbacher KJ, et al (eds): Harrison's Principles of Internal Medicine. New York, McGraw-Hill, Inc., 1991, pp 1814–1825.
40. Brunner EJ, Marmot MG, White IR, et al: Gender and employment grade differences in blood cholesterol, apolipoproteins and haemostatic factors in the Whitehall II study. Atherosclerosis 102:195–207, 1993.
41. Brunner EJ, Davey Smith GD, Marmot MG, et al: Childhood social circumstances and psychosocial and behavioral factors as determinants of plasma fibrinogen. Lancet 347:1008–1013, 1996.
42. Cardillo C, Kilcoyne CM, Cannon RO, Panza JA: Impairment of the nitric oxide-mediated vasodilator response to mental stress in hypertensive but not in hypercholesterolemic patients. J Am Coll Cardiol 32:1207–1213, 1998.
43. Cardillo C, Kilcoyne CM, Quyyumi AA, et al: Role of nitric oxide in the vasodilator response to mental stress in normal subjects. Am J Cardiol 80:1070–1074, 1997.
44. Carpeggiani C, Skinner JE: Coronary flow and mental stress: Experimental findings. Circulation 83:II90–II93, 1991.
45. Chaitman BR, Dahms TE, Byers S, et al: Carbon monoxide exposures of subjects with documented cardiac arrhythmias. Research Report, Health Effects Institute 52:1–26, 1992.
46. Chaney RH, Arndt S: Comparison of cardiovascular risk in maximal isometric and dynamic exercise. South Med J 76:464–467, 1983.
47. Charney DS, Deutch AY, Krystal JH, et al: Psychobiological mechanisms of posttraumatic stress disorder. Arch Gen Psychiatry 50:294–330, 1993.
48. Charvat J, Dell P, Folkow P, Folkow B: Mental factors and cardiovascular disease. Cardiologia 44:124–141, 1964.
49. Chatterjee K: Recognition and management of patients with stable angina pectoris. In Goldman L, Braunwald E (eds): Primary Cardiology. Philadelphia, WB Saunders Co., 1998, pp 234–256.
50. Chau N, Mallion J, de Gaudemaris R, et al: 24-hour ambulatory blood pressure in shift workers. Circulation 80:341–347, 1989.

51. Chauhan A, Mullins PA, Taylor G, et al: Effect of hyperventilation and mental stress on coronary blood flow in syndrome X. Br Heart J 69:516–524, 1993.

52. Chen CJ, Hsueh Y-M, Lai M-S, et al: Increased prevalence of hypertension and long-term arsenic exposure. Hypertension 25:53–60, 1995.

53. Chobanian AV, Dzau VJ: Renin angiotensin system and atherosclerotic vascular disease. In Fuster V, Ross R, Topol EJ (eds): Atherosclerosis and Coronary Artery Disease. Philadelphia, Lippincott-Raven, 1996, pp 237–242.

54. Christenfeld N, Gerin W, Linden W, et al: Social support effects on cardiovascular reactivity: Is a stranger as effective as a friend? Psychosom Med 59:388–398, 1997.

55. Clutter WE, Bier DM, Shah SD, Cryer PE: Epinephrine plasma metabolic clearance rates and physiological thresholds for metabolic and hemodynamic action in man. J Clin Invest 66:94–101, 1980.

56. Cobb LA: The mechanisms, predictors, and prevention of sudden cardiac death. In Hurst JW, Logue RB, Rackley CE, et al (eds): The Heart. New York, McGraw-Hill, 1990, pp 604–614.

57. Cobb S, Rose RM: Hypertension, peptic ulcer, and diabetes in air traffic controllers. JAMA 224:489–492, 1973.

58. Cocco G, Iselin HU: Cardiac risk of speed traps. Clin Cardiol 15:441–444, 1992.

59. Cooper RS, Rotimi CN, Ward R: The puzzle of hypertension in African-Americans. Scientific American 280:36–43, 1999.

60. Corley KC, Mauck HP, O'Schiel F: Cardiac responses associated with yoked-chair shock avoidance in squirrel monkeys. Psychophysiology 12:439–444, 1975.

61. Corley KC, O'Shiel F, Mauck HP: Myocardial degeneration and cardiac arrest in squirrel monkeys. Physiologic and psychologic correlates. Psychophysiology 14:322–328, 1977.

62. Cupples LA, Gagnon DR, Kannel WB: Long- and short-term risk of sudden coronary death. Circulation 85 Suppl I:I11–I18, 1992.

63. Dahms TE, Younis LT, Wiens RD, et al: Effects of carbon monoxide exposure in patients with documented cardiac arrhythmias. J Am Coll Cardiol 21:442–450, 1993.

64. Danesh J, Peto R: Risk factors for coronary heart disease and infection with *Heliobacter pylori*: Meta-analysis of 18 studies. BMJ 316:1130–1132, 1998.

65. Daniels GH, Martin JB: Neuroendocrine regulation and diseases of the anterior pituitary and hypothalamus. In Wilson J (ed): Harrison's Principles of Internal Medicine, 1991, pp 1655–1678.

66. de Faire U, Lindvall K, Nilsson B: Noninvasive ambulatory 24th blood pressure and basal blood pressures predict development of sustained hypertension from borderline state. Am J Hypertens 6:149–155, 1993.

67. De Quatro V, Chan S: Raised plasma catecholamines in some patients with primary hypertension. Lancet I 7755:806–809, 1972.

68. Deedewania PC, Nelson JR: Pathophysiology of silent myocardial ischemia during daily life. Hemodynamic evaluation of simultaneous electrocardiographic and blood pressure monitoring. Circulation 82:1296–1304, 1990.

69. Deedwania PC, Carbajal EV: Role of myocardial oxygen demand in the pathogenesis of silent ischemia during daily life. Am J Cardiol 70:19f–24f, 1992.

70. DeFronzo RA: Insulin resistance: The metabolic link between noninsulin-dependent diabetes mellitus, obesity, hypertension, dyslipidemia, and atherosclerotic cardiovascular disease. Curr Opin Cardiol 5:586–593, 1990.

71. Delaney KA, Goldfrank LR: Hot and cold work environments. In Rom WN (ed): Environmental and Occupational Medicine. Philadelphia, Lippincott-Raven, 1998, pp 1389–1401.

72. Demitrack MA, Dale JK, Straus SE, et al: Evidence for impaired activation of the hypothalamic-pituitary-adrenal axis in patients with chronic fatigue syndrome. J Clin Endocrinol Metab 73:1224–1234, 1991.

73. Devereux RB: Importance of left ventricular mass as a predictor of cardiovascular morbidity in hypertension. Am J Hypertension 2:650–654, 1989.

74. Devereux RB, Pickering TG, Harshfield GA, et al: Left ventricular hypertrophy in patients with hypertension: Importance of blood pressure to regularly recurring stress. Circulation 68:476–479, 1983.

75. Devereux RB, Roman MJ: Hypertensive cardiac hypertrophy: Pathophysiologic and clinical characteristics. In Laragh JH, Brenner BM (eds): Hypertension: Pathophysiology, Diagnosis, and Management. New York, Raven Press, Ltd., 1995, pp 409–432.

76. Deyanov C, Mincheva L, Hadjiolova I, Ivanovich E: Study on the level of blood pressure and prevalence of arterial hypertension depending on the duration of occupational exposure to industrial noise. Cent Eur J Occup Environ Med 1:109–116, 1995.

77. Di Marco JP: Coronary artery spasm, silent ischemia and cardiac arrest. N Engl J Med 32:1490–1491, 1992.

78. DiBona GF, Kopp UC: Neural control of renal function: Role in human hypertension. In Laragh JH, Brenner BM (eds): Hypertension: Pathophysiology, Diagnosis, and Management. New York, Raven Press, Ltd., 1995, pp 1349–1358.

79. Dimsdale J, Moss J: Plasma catecholamines in stress and exercise. JAMA 243:340–342, 1980.

80. Drayer JIM, Weber MA, DeJong JL: Blood pressure as a determinant of cardiac left ventricular muscle mass. Arch Intern Med 143:90–92, 1983.

81. Duan Y-F, Winters RW, McCabe PM, et al: Modulation of neuronal firing in the medullary solitary complex by electrical stimulation of the hypothalamic defense and vigilance areas in rabbits. Brain Research 643:218–226, 1994.

82. Eckel RH: Lipoprotein lipase. A multifunctional enzyme relevant to common metabolic diseases. N Engl J Med 320:1060–1068, 1989.

83. Egan B, Panis R, Hinderliter A, Schork N, Julius S: Mechanism of increased alpha-adrenergic vasoconstriction in human essential hypertension. J Clin Invest 80:812–817, 1987.

84. Egeland GM, Burkhart GA, Schnorr TM, et al: Effects of exposure to carbon disulphide on low density lipoprotein cholesterol concentration and diastolic blood pressure. Br J Ind Med 49:287–293, 1992.

85. Eliasson K, Hjemdal P, Kahan T: Circulatory and sympathoadrenal responses to stress in borderline and established hypertension. J Hypertens 1:131–139, 1983.

86. Eliot RS: Stress and the Major Cardiovascular Disorders. Mt. Kisco, Futura Publishing Co., 1979.
87. Eliot RS, Buell JC: Role of emotions and stress in the genesis of sudden death. J Am Coll Cardiol 5:95B–98B, 1985.
88. Emdad R, Belkic K, Theorell T, et al: Electrocortical responses to ecologically relevant visual stimuli among professional drivers with and without cardiovascular disease. Integr Physiol Behav Sci 31:96–111, 1996.
89. Epstein SE, Quyyumi AA, Bobow RO: Sudden cardiac death without warning. N Engl J Med 321:320–323, 1989.
90. Erikssen J, Johansen AH, Rodahl K: Coronary heart disease in Norwegian sea-pilots: Part of the occupational hazard? Acta Med Scand 645 Suppl:79–83, 1981.
91. Evans GW, Carrere S: Traffic congestion, perceived control, and psychophysiologic stress among urban bus drivers. Appl Psychology 76:658–663, 1991.
92. Every NR, Parsons L, Hlatky MA, et al: Use and accuracy of state death certificates for classification of sudden cardiac deaths in high-risk populations. Am Heart J 134:1129–1132, 1997.
93. Fogari R, Zoppi A, Vanasia A, Marasi G, Villa G: Occupational noise exposure and blood pressure. J Hypertens 12:475–479, 1994.
94. Folkow B: Sympathetic nervous control of blood pressure: Role of primary hypertension. Am J Hypertens 2:103S–111S, 1989.
95. Folkow B: Physiological aspects of primary hypertension. Physiol Rev 62:347–503, 1982.
96. Folkow B: Psychosocial and central nervous influence in primary hypertension. Circulation 76:10–19, 1987.
97. Folkow B: Autonomic nervous system in hypertension. In Swales JD (ed): Textbook of Hypertension. London, Blackwell Scientific Publications, 1994, pp 427–438.
98. Folkow B: Cardiovascular structural adaptation: Its role in the initiation and maintenance of primary hypertension. Clinical Science and Molecular Medicine 55 (Suppl 4):IV3–IV22, 1978.
98a. Folkow B, Grimby G, Thulesius O: Adaptive structural changes of the vascular walls in hypertension and their relation to the control of the peripheral resistance. Acta Physiol Scand 44:255–272, 1958.
99. Folkow B, Schmidt T, Uvnas-Moberg K: Stress, Health, and the Social Environment. James P. Henry's Ethological Approach to Medicine. Acta Physiologica Scandinavica 161 Suppl 640, 1997.
100. Forsman L: Individual and group differences in psychophysiological responses to stress with emphasis on sympathetic-adrenal medullary and pituitary-adrenal cortical responses. Department of Psychology, University of Stockholm, 1983.
101. Forsyth RP: Blood pressure responses to long-term avoidance schedules in the unrestrained rhesus monkey. Psychosom Med 31:300–309, 1969.
102. Fossum E, Hoieggen A, Moan A, et al: Insulin sensitivity is related to physical fitness and exercise blood pressure to structural vascular properties in young men. Hypertension 33:781–786, 1999.
103. Fossum E, Hoieggen A, Moan A, et al: Relationship between insulin sensitivity and maximal forearm blood flow in young men. Hypertension 32:838–843, 1998.
104. Frankenhaeuser M: The sympathetic-adrenal and pituitary-adrenal response to challenge: Comparison between the sexes. In Dembroski TM, Schmidt TH, Blomchen G (eds): Biobehavioral Bases of Coronary Heart Disease. Basel, Karger, 1983, pp 91–105.
105. Frankenhaeuser M: Psychoneuroendocrine approaches to the study of stressful person-environment transactions. In Selye H (ed): Selye's Guide to Stress Research, Vol. 1. New York, Von Nostrand Reinhold, 1980.
106. Frankenhaeuser M: Challenge-control interaction as reflected in sympathetic-adrenal and pituitary-adrenal activity: Comparison between the sexes. Scand J Psychol Suppl 1:158–164, 1982.
107. Frankenhaeuser M, Johansson G: On the psychophysiologic consequences of understimulation and overstimulation. In Levi L (ed): Society, Stress, and Disease. Vol. 4: Working Life. New York, Oxford University Press, 1981.
108. Frankenhaeuser M, Lundberg U, Fredrikson M, Melin B: Stress on and off the job as related to sex and occupational status in white-collar workers. Department of Psychology, University of Stockholm, 1987.
109. Fredriksson M, Sundin O, Frankenhaeuser M: Cortisol excretion during the defence reaction in humans. Psychosom Med 47:313–319, 1985.
110. Freeman JL, Nixon PGF, Sallabank P, et al: Psychological stress and silent myocardial ischemia. Am Heart J 114:447–482, 1987.
111. Froberg JE, Karlsson CG, Levi L: Shift work. A study of catecholamine excretion, self-ratings and attitudes. Studia Laboris Salutis 11:10–20, 1972.
112. Froberg JE, Karlsson CG, Levi L, Lidberg L: Circadian rhythms of catecholamine excretion, shooting range performance and self-ratings of fatigue during sleep deprivation. Biol Psychol 2:175–188, 1975.
113. Frohlich ED, Chobanian AV, Devereux RB, et al: The heart in hypertension. New Engl J Med 327:998–1008, 1992.
114. Fujimoto T, Peter T, Hamamoto H, Mandel WJ: Electrophysiologic observations on ventricular tachyarrhythmias following reperfusion. Am Heart J 105:201–209, 1983.
115. Furchgott R, Zawadzki J: The obligatory role of endothelial cells in the relaxation of arterial smooth muscle by achetylcholine. Nature 288:373, 1980.
116. Fuster V, Fallon JT, Nemerson Y: Coronary thrombosis. Lancet 348:s7–s10, 1996.
117. Gabbay FH, Krantz DS, Kop WJ, et al: Triggers of myocardial ischemia during daily life in patients with coronary artery disease: Physical and mental activities, anger and smoking. J Am Coll Cardiol 27:585–592, 1996.
118. Gardell B, Aronsson G, Barklof K: The working environment for local public transport personnel. Stockholm, The Swedish Work Environment Fund, 1983.
119. Genes N, Vaur L, Renault M, Cambou JP, Danchin N: Rythme circadien des infarctus du myocarde en France: Resultats de l'etude USIK (Circadian patterns of myocardial infarction in France: Results in the USIK study). La Presse Medicale 26:603–608, 1997.
120. Gerin W, Litt MD, Deich J, Pickering TG: Self-efficacy as a moderator of perceived control effects on cardiovascular reactivity: Is enhanced control always beneficial? Psychosom Med 57:390–397, 1995.

121. Gerin W, Pieper C, Pickering TG: Anticipatory and residual effects of an active coping task on pre- and post-stress baselines. J Psychosom Res 38:139–149, 1994.
122. Gilmore JP: Physiology of Stress, Stress, and the Heart. Mt. Kisco, Futura Publishing Co., 1974, pp 69–89.
123. Goldstein DS: Stress, Catecholamines, and Cardiovascular Disease. New York, Oxford University Press, 1995.
124. Goldstein DS: Plasma catecholamines in essential hypertension: An analytical review. Hypertension 5:86–89, 1983.
125. Gottdiener JS, Krantz DS, Howell RH, et al: Induction of silent myocardial ischemia with mental stress testing: Relation to the triggers of ischemia during daily life activity and to ischemic functional severity. J Am Coll Cardiol 24:1645–1651, 1994.
126. Green MS, Schwartz K, Harari G, Najenson T: Industrial noise exposure and ambulatory blood pressure and heart rate. J Occup Med 33:879–883, 1991.
127. Grossi G, Theorell T, Jurisso M, Setterlind S: Psychophysiological correlates of organizational change and threat of unemployment among police inspectors. Integr Physiol Behav Sci 34:30–42, 1999.
128. Grover RF, Reeves JT, Rowell LB, et al: The heart and environmental factors: The influence of environmental factors on the cardiovascular system. In Hurst JW, Logue RB, Rackley CE, et al (eds): The Heart. New York, McGraw-Hill, 1990, pp 1630–1644.
129. Guyton AC: Textbook of Physiology, 8th ed. Philadelphia, Saunders, 1991.
130. Harenstam AB, Theorell TPG: Work conditions and urinary excretion of catecholamines: A study of prison staff in Sweden. Scand J Work Environ Health 14:257–264, 1988.
131. Hamburg S, Hendler R, Sherwin RS: Influence of small increments of epinephrine on glucose tolerance in normal humans. Ann Intern Med 93:566–568, 1980.
132. Harenstam A, Theorell T: Work conditions and urinary excretion of catecholamines: A study of prison staff in Sweden. Scand J Work Environ Health 14:257–264, 1988.
133. Harenstam A, Theorell T: Cortisol elevation and serum GT in response to adverse job conditions—How are they interrelated? Biol Psychology 31:157–171, 1990.
134. Hart MN, Heistad DD, Brody MJ: Effect of chronic hypertension and sympathetic denervation on wall/lumen ratio of cerebral vessels. Hypertension 2:419–428, 1980.
135. Haskell WL, Brachfeld N, Bruce RA, et al: Determination of occupational working capacity in patients with ischemic heart disease. J Am Coll Cardiol 14:1016–1042, 1989.
136. Hayashi T, Kobayashi Y, Yamaoka K, Yano E: Effect of overtime work on 24-hour ambulatory blood pressure. J Occup Environ Med 38:1007–1011, 1996.
137. HDFP: Race, education, and prevalence of hypertension: The Hypertension Detection and Followup Program Cooperative Group. Am J Epidemiol 106:351–361, 1977.
138. Heathers GP, Yamada KA, Pogwizd SM: The contribution of alpha and beta-adrenergic mechanisms in the genesis of arrhythmias during myocardial ischaemia and reperfusion. In Kulbertus HE, Franck G (eds): Neurocardiology. Mount Kisco, Futura Publishing, 1988, pp 143–178.
139. Henry JP: Psychosocial stress and hypertension. The relevance of animal studies. In Swales JD (ed): Textbook of Hypertension. London, Blackwell Scientific Publications, 1994, pp 633–639.
140. Henry JP, Cassell: Psychological factors in essential hypertension. Am J Epidemiology 90:171–200, 1969.
141. Henry JP, Liu Y-y, Nadra WE, et al: Psychosocial stress can induce chronic hypertension in normotensive strains of rats. Hypertension 21:714–723, 1993.
142. Henry JP, Stephens PM: Stress, Health, and the Social Environment: A Sociobiologic Approach to Medicine. New York - Heidenberg - Berlin, Springer-Verlag, 1977.
143. Hertz-Piccioto I, Croft J: Review of the relation between blood lead and blood pressure. Epidemiol Rev 15:352–373, 1993.
144. Hietanen E: Cardiovascular responses to static exercise. Scand J Work Environ Health 10:397–402, 1984.
145. Higgins CB, Vatner SF, Braunwald E: Parasympathetic control of the heart. Pharmacol Rev 25:119–155, 1973.
146. Hines EA, Brown GE: The cold pressor test for measuring the reactibility of the blood pressure: Data concerning 571 normal and hypertensive subjects. Am Heart J 11:1–9, 1936.
147. Hirai A, Takata M, Mikawa M, et al: Prolonged exposure to industrial noise causes hearing loss but not high blood pressure: A study of 2124 factory laborers in Japan. J Hypertension 9:1069–1073, 1991.
148. Hjemdahl P: Plasma catecholamines as markers for sympathoadrenal activity in human hypertension. Pharmacol Toxicol 63 Suppl 1:27–31, 1988.
149. Hjemdahl P: Plasma catecholamines—Analytical challenges and physiological limitations. Baillieres Clin Endocrinol Metab 7:307–353, 1993.
150. Hoieggen A, Fossum E, Moan A, et al: Whole-blood viscosity and the insulin-resistance syndrome. J Hypertens 16:203–210, 1998.
151. Holbrook JH: Tobacco. In Wilson JD, Braunwald E, Isselbacher KJ, et al (eds): Harrison's Principles of Internal Medicine. New York, McGraw-Hill, Inc., 1991, pp 2158–2161.
152. Hollenberg NK, Williams GH, Adams DF: Essential hypertension: Abnormal renal vascular and endocrine responses to mild psychological stimulus. Hypertension 3:11–17, 1981.
153. Homs E, Marti V, Guindo J, et al: Automatic measurement of corrected QT interval in Holter recordings: Comparison of its dynamic behavior in patients after myocardial infarction with and without life-threatening arrhythmias. Am Heart J 134:181–187, 1997.
154. Houdas Y, Deklunder G, Lecroart JL: Cold exposure and ischemic heart disease. Int J Sports Med 13 Suppl 1:S179–181, 1992.
155. Huikuri HV: Heart rate dynamics and vulnerability to ventricular tachyarrhythmias. Ann Med 29:321–325, 1997.
156. Igarashi Y, Yamzoe M, Tamura Y, et al: Clinical characteristics and possible role of coronary artery spasm in syncope and/or aborted sudden death. Jpn Circ J 54:1477–1485, 1990.

157. Ironson G, Taylor CB, Boltwood M, et al: Effects of anger on left ventricular ejection fraction in coronary artery disease. Am J Cardiol 70:281–285, 1992.
158. Ishizaki M, Tsuritani I, Noborisaka Y, et al: Relationship between job stress and plasma fibrinolytic activity in male Japanese workers. Int Arch Occup Environ Health 68:315–320, 1996.
159. Iwasaki K, Sasaki T, Oka T, Hisanaga N: Effect of working hours on biological functions related to cardiovascular system among salesmen in a machinery manufacturing company. Ind Health 36:361–367, 1998.
160. Jain D, Burg M, Soufer R, et al: Prognostic implications of mental stress-induced silent left ventricular dysfunction in patients with stable angina pectoris. Am J Cardiol 76:31–35, 1995.
161. James GD, Schlussel YR, Pickering TG: The association between daily blood pressure and catecholamine variability in normotensive working women. Psychosom Med 55:55–60, 1993.
162. James MA, Hones JU: Systolic wall stress and ventricular arrhythmias: The role of acute change in BP in the isolated working rat heart. Clin Sci 79:499–504, 1990.
163. Johansson G, Aronsson G, Lindstrom BO: Social psychological and neuroendocrine stress reactions in highly mechanized work. Ergonomics 21:583–599, 1978.
164. Jones RD, Winter DP: Two case reports of deaths on industrial premises attributed to 1,1,1-trichloroethane. Arch Environ Health 38:59–61, 1983.
165. Julius S: Controversies in the research on hemodynamic mechanisms in the development of hypertension. In Sambhi M (ed): Fundamental Fault in Hypertension. Boston, Martinus Nijhoff, 1984, pp 264–275.
166. Julius S: The defense reaction—A common denominator of coronary risk and blood pressure in neurogenic hypertension? Clin Exper Hypertens 17:375–386, 1995.
167. Julius S, Amerena J, Smith S, Petrin J: Autonomic nervous and behavioral factors in hypertension. In Laragh JH, Brenner BM (eds): Hypertension: Pathophysiology, Diagnosis, and Management. New York, Raven Press, Ltd., 1995, pp 2557–2569.
168. Julius S, Gudbrandsson T, Jamerson K, et al: The hemodynamic link between insulin resistance and hypertension. J Hypertens 9:983–986, 1991.
169. Julius S, Li L, Brant D, Krause L, Buda AJ: Neurogenic pressor episodes fail to cause hypertension, but do induce cardiac hypertrophy. Hypertension 13:422–429, 1989.
170. Julius S, Mejia A, Jones K, et al: "White coat" versus "sustained" borderline hypertension in Tecumseh, Michigan. Hypertension 16:617–623, 1990.
171. Julius S, Schork M, Schork A: Sympathetic hyperactivity in early stages of hypertension: The Ann Arbor data set. J Cardiovasc Pharmacol 12 Suppl 3:S121–129, 1988.
172. Kaplan NM: Systemic hypertension. Mechanisms and diagnosis. In Braunwald E (ed): Heart Disease. A Textbook of Cardiovascular Medicine. Philadelphia, WB Saunders Co., 1997, pp 807–839.
173. Karagueuzian HS, Mandel WJ: Electrophysiologic mechanisms of ischemic ventricular arrhythmias: Experimental and clinical correlations. In Mandel WJ (ed): Cardiac Arrhythmias: Their Mechanisms, Diagnosis, and Management. Philadelphia, JB Lippincott Co., 1995, pp 563–603.
174. Karagueuzian HS, Wit AL: Studies on ventricular arrhythmias in animal models of ischemic heart disease: What can we learn? In Kulbertus HE, Wellens HJJ (eds): Sudden Death. The Hague, Martinus Nijhoff, 1980, pp 69–88.
175. Kaski JC, Crea F, Nihoyannopoulos P, et al: Transient myocardial ischaemia during daily life in patients with syndrome X. Am J Cardiol 58:1242–1247, 1986.
176. Kavanagh T, Matosevic V: Assessment of work capacity in patients with ischaemic heart disease: Methods and practices. Eur Heart J 9 Suppl L:67–73, 1988.
177. Kawano T, Okabe M, Arakawa K: Cold pressor test and variant angina. Angiology 34:429–435, 1983.
178. Kerber RE, Miller RA, Najjar SM: Myocardial ischemia effects of isometric, dynamic, and combined exercise in coronary artery disease. Chest 67:388–394, 1975.
179. Kirby D, Pinto JMB, Hottinger S, et al: Behavioral arousal enhances inducibility and rate of ventricular tachycardia. Am J Physiol 261:H1734–H1739, 1991.
180. Kirschbaum C, Helhammer D: Salivary cortisol in psychobiological research: An overview. Neuropsychobiology 22:150–169, 1989.
181. Kirschbaum C, Helhammer D: Salivery cortisol in psychoneuroendocrine research: Recent developments and applications. Psychoneuroendocrinology 19:313–333, 1994.
182. Kjeldsen SE, Eide I, Leren P, Foss OP: Effect on high density lipoprotein cholesterol of atenolol and oxprenolol in patients with mild essential hypertension. Clin Sci 63:463s–465, 1982.
183. Kjeldsen SE, Flaaten B, Eide I, et al: Evidence of increased peripheral catecholamine release in patients with long-standing, untreated essential hypertension. Scand J Clin Lab Invest 42:217–223, 1982.
184. Kjeldsen SE, Petrin J, Weder AB, Julius S: Contrasting effects of epinephrine on forearm hemodynamics and arterial plasma norepinephrine. Am J Hypertens 6:369–375, 1993.
185. Kjeldsen SE, Rostrup M, Moan A, et al: The sympathetic nervous system may modulate the metabolic cardiovascular syndrome in essential hypertension. J Cardiovasc Pharm 20 Suppl 8:S32–S39, 1992.
186. Kjeldsen SE, Schork NJ, Leren P, Eide IK: Arterial plasma norepinephrine correlates to blood pressure in middle-aged men with sustained essential hypertension. Am Heart J 118:775–781, 1989.
187. Kjeldsen SE, Weder AB, Egan B, et al: Effect of circulating epinephrine on platelet function and hematocrit. Hypertension 25:1096–1105, 1995.
188. Kleiman NS: Angina pectoris in patients with normal coronary angiograms. In Willerson JT, Cohn JN (eds): Cardiovascular Medicine. New York, Churchill Livingstone, 1995, pp 375–389.
189. Kleinman MT, Davidson DM, Vandagriff RB, et al: Effects of short-term exposure to carbon monoxide in subjects with coronary artery disease. Arch Environ Health 44:361–369, 1989.
190. Koepke JP, Jones S, DiBona GF: Stress increases renal nerve activity and decreases sodium excretion in Dahl rats. Hypertension 11:334–338, 1988.

191. Kohn M, Schooler C: An inquiry into the impact of social stratification. Norwood, NJ, Ablex, 1983.
192. Kop WJ, Hamulyak K, Pernot C, Appels A: Relationship of blood coagulation and fibrinolysis to vital exhaustion. Psychosomatic Medicine 60:352–358, 1998.
193. Kopka L, Mazurek K, Zawadzka-Bartczak E: Sinus node arrest and asystole from vaso-vagal phenomena during lower body negative pressure in a healthy pilot. Aviat Space Environ Med 67:572–575, 1996.
194. Kozena L, Frantik E, Horvath M: Cardiovascular reaction to job stress in middle-aged train drivers. Int J Behav Med 5:281–294, 1998.
195. Krantz DS, Kop WJ, Santiago HT, Gottdiener JS: Mental stress as a trigger of myocardial ischemia and infarction. Cardiology Clinics 14:271–287, 1996.
196. Kristal-Boneh E, Melamed S, Harari G, Green MS: Acute and chronic effects of noise exposure on blood pressure and heart rate among industrial employees. Arch Environ Health 50:298–304, 1995.
197. Kristensen TS: Cardiovascular diseases and the work environment. A critical review of the epidemiologic literature on chemical factors. Scand J Work Environ Health 15:245–265, 1989.
198. La Rovere MT, Schwartz PJ: Baroreflex sensitivity as a cardiac and arrhythmia mortality risk stratifier. PACE 20:2602–2613, 1997.
199. Lacey JH: Individual differences in somatic response patterns. J Comp Physiol Psychol 43:338–350, 1950.
200. Lacy E, O'Connor DT, Schmid-Schonbein GW: Plasma hydrogen peroxide production in hypertensives and nor-motensive subjects at genetic risk of hypertension. J Hypertens 16:291–303, 1998.
201. Laflamme N, Brisson C, Moisan J, et al: Job strain and ambulatory blood pressure among female white-collar workers. Scand J Work Environ Health 24:334–343, 1998.
202. Landsbergis PA, Schnall PL, Deitz D, et al: The patterning of psychological attributes and distress by "job strain" and social support in a sample of working men. J Behav Med 15:379–405, 1992.
203. Lanza GA, Pedrotti P, Pasceri V, et al: Autonomic changes associated with spontaneous coronary spasm in patients with variant angina. J Am Coll Cardiol 28:1249–1256, 1996.
204. Lauwers P, Aelvoet W, Sneppe R, Remion M: Effect of car driving on the electrocardiogram of patients with my-ocardial infarction and an ECG at rest devoid of dysrhythmia and repolarisation abnormalities. Acta Cardiol 28:27–43, 1973.
205. Lazarus RS: Psychological Stress and the Coping Process. New York, McGraw-Hill, 1966.
206. LeHeuzey JY, Guize L: Cardiac prognosis in hypertensive patients. Incidence of sudden death and ventricular ar-rhythmias. J Am Coll Cardiol 81:65–68, 1988.
207. Lennerlof L: Learned helplessness at work. In Johnson JV, Johansson G (eds): The Psychosocial Work Environment: Work Organization, Democratization, and Health. Essays in Memory of Bertil Gardell. Amityville, Baywood Publishing Co., Inc., 1991.
208. Leren P, Askevold EM, Foss OP, et al: The Oslo Study: Cardiovascular disease in middle-aged and young Oslo men. Acta Med Scand Suppl 588:1–38, 1975.
209. Leren P, Foss OP, Helgeland A, et al: Effect of propranolol and prazosin on blood lipids. The Oslo Study. Lancet 2:4–6, 1980.
210. Lerman Y, Winkler E, Tirosh MS, et al: Fatal accidental inhalation of bromochlorodifluoromethane. Hum Exp Toxicol 10:125–128, 1991.
211. Levi L: Stress and distress in response to psychosocial stimuli. Acta Med Scand 191 Suppl 528, 1972.
212. Levi L: Preventing Work Stress. Reading, Addison-Wesley Publishing Co., 1981.
213. Levy M: Time dependency of the autonomic interactions that regulate heart rate and rhythm. In Zipes DP, Jalife J (eds): Cardiac Electrophysiology From Cell to Bedside. Philadelphia, WB Saunders Co., 1995, pp 454–459.
214. Levy D, Garrison RJ, Savage DD, et al: Prognostic implications of echocardiographically determined left ventricu-lar mass in the Framingham Heart Study. New Engl J Med 322:1561–1566, 1990.
215. Libby P, Schoenbeck U, Mach F, et al: Current concepts in cardiovascular pathology: The role of LDL cholesterol in plaque rupture and stabilization. Am J Med 104:14S–18S, 1998.
216. Light KC, Koepke JP, Obrist PA, Willis PW: Psychological stress induces sodium and fluid retention in men at high risk for hypertension. Science 220:429–431, 1983.
217. Light KC, Turner JR, Hinderliter AL: Job strain and ambulatory work blood pressure in healthy young men and women. Hypertension 20:214–218, 1992.
218. Linden W: What do arithmetic stress tests measure? Protocol variations and cardiovascular responses. Psychophysiology 28:91–102, 1991.
219. Littler WA, Honour AJ, Sleight P: Direct arterial pressure and electrocardiogram during motor car driving. Brit Med J 2:273–277, 1973.
220. Lown B: Sudden cardiac death: Biobehavioral perspective. Circulation 76 Suppl I:I186–I195, 1987.
221. Lown B: Role of higher nervous activity in sudden cardiac death. Jpn Circ J 54:581–602, 1990.
222. Lown B, deSilva RA, Reich P, et al: Psychophysiologic factors in sudden cardiac death. Am J Psychiatry 137:1325–1335, 1980.
223. Lown B, Verrier RL: Neural activity and ventricular fibrillation. N Engl J Med 294:1165–1170, 1976.
224. Lundberg U, Frankenhaeuser M: Pituitary-adrenal and sympathetic-adrenal correlates of distress and effort. J Psychosom Res 24:125–130, 1984.
225. Lundberg U, Frankenhaeuser M: Psychophysiological reactions to noise as modified by personal control over noise intensive. Biol Psychol 6:51–60, 1978.
226. Lynch J, Krause N, Kaplan GA, et al: Workplace demands, economic reward, and progression of carotid athero-sclerosis. Circulation 96:302–307, 1997.
227. Majewski H, Hedler L, Starke K: The noradrenaline release rate in the anesthetized rabbit: Facilitation by adrena-line. Naunyn-Schmiederberg's Archives of Pharmacology 321:20–27, 1982.

228. Majewski H, Rand MJ: Prejunctional b-adrenoceptors as sites of action for adrenaline in stress-linked hypertension. J Cardiovasc Pharmacol 10 (Suppl 4):S41–S44, 1987.
229. Majewski H, Tung LH, Rand MJ: Adrenaline-induced hypertension in rats. J Cardiovasc Pharmacol 3:1979–1985, 1981.
230. Malkoff SB, Muldoon MF, Zeigler ZR, Manuck SB: Blood platelet responsivity to acute mental stress. Psychosom Med 55:477–482, 1993.
231. Mancia G: The sympathetic nervous system in hypertension. J Hypertension 15:1553–1565, 1997.
232. Markovitz JH: Hostility is associated with increased platelet activation in coronary heart disease. Psychosom Med 60:586–591, 1998.
233. Markowe HL, Marmot MG, Shipley MJ, et al: Fibrinogen: A possible link between social class and coronary heart disease. Br Med J 291:1312–1314, 1985.
234. Marmot MG, Bosma H, Hemingway H, et al: Contribution of job control and other risk factors to social variations in coronary heart disease incidence. Lancet 350:235–239, 1997.
235. Marmot MG, Davey Smith DG, Stansfeld S, et al: Health inequalities among British civil servants: The Whitehall II study. Lancet 337:1387–1393, 1991.
236. Maseri A, Chierchia S, L'Abbate A, et al: Role du spasme dans l'angine de poitrine, l'infarctus du myocarde et la mort subite (The role of spasm in angina pectoris, myocardial infarction and sudden death). Arch Mal Coeur 75:701–716, 1982.
237. Mason JW: A review of psychoendocrine research on the pituitary-adrenal-cortical system. Psychosom Med 30:576, 1968.
238. Matthews KA, Manuck SB, Saab P: Cardiovascular responses of adolescents during naturally occurring stressors and their behavioral and psychophysiological predictors. Psychophysiology 23:198–209, 1986.
239. McCabe PM, Duan Y-F, Winters RW, et al: Comparison of peripheral blood flow patterns associated with the defense reaction and the vigilance reaction in rabbits. Physiol Behavior 56:1101–1106, 1994.
240. McCann B, Warnick G, Knopp R: Changes in plasma lipids and dietary intake accompanying shifts in perceived workload and stress. Psychosom Med 52:97–108, 1990.
241. McCunney RJ, Meyer JD: Occupational exposure to noise. In Rom WN (ed): Environmental and Occupational Medicine. Philadelphia, Lippincott-Raven Publishers, 1998, pp 1345–1357.
242. McLenachan JM, Dargie HJ: A review of rhythm disorders in cardiac hypertrophy. Am J Cardiol 65 Suppl G:G42–G50, 1990.
243. McManus BM, Fleury TA, Roberts WC: Fatal catecholamine crisis in pheochromocytoma: Curable cause of cardiac arrest. Am Heart J 102:930–932, 1981.
244. Meade TW: Haemostatic function and arterial disease. Br Med Bull 50:755–775, 1994.
245. Mehta D, Curwin J, Gomes A, Fuster V: Sudden death in coronary artery disease. Circulation 96:3215–3223, 1997.
246. Mendall MA, Patel P, Asante M, et al: Relation of serum cytokine concentrations to cardiovascular risk factors and coronary heart disease. Heart 78:273–277, 1998.
247. Menkes MS, Matthews KA, Krantz DS, et al: Cardiovascular reactivity to the cold pressor test as a predictor of hypertension. Hypertension 14:524–530, 1989.
248. Messerli FH, Grodzicki T: Hypertension, left ventricular hypertrophy, ventricular arrhythmias, and sudden death. Eur Heart J 13 Suppl D:66–69, 1992.
249. Messerli FH, Nunez BD, Ventura HO, et al: Overweight and sudden death. Increased ventricular ectopy in cardiopathy of obesity. Arch Int Med 147:1725–1728, 1987.
250. Michelson D, Licinio J, Gold PW: Mediation of the stress response by the hypothalamo-pituitary-adrenal axis. In Friedman MJ, Charney DS, Deutch AY (eds): Neurobiological and Clinical Consequences of Stress. New York, Lippincott-Raven, 1995.
251. Milkovic-Krause S: Noise-induced hearing loss and blood pressure. Int Arch Occup Environ Health 62:259–260, 1990.
252. Miller PF, Light KC, Bragdon EE, et al: Beta-endorphin response to exercise and mental stress in patients with ischemic heart disease. J Psychosom Res 37:455–465, 1993.
253. Moan A, Nordby G, Rostrup M, et al: Insulin sensitivity, sympathetic activity, and cardiovascular reactivity in young men. Am J Hypertens 8:268–275, 1995.
254. Moller L, Kristensen TS: Plasma fibrinogen and ischaemic heart disease risk factors. Arteriosclerosis and Thrombosis 11:344–350, 1991.
255. Morikawa Y, Nakagawa H, Miura K, et al: Relationship between shift work and onset of hypertension in a cohort of manual workers. Scand J Work Environ Health 25:100–104, 1999.
256. Muller JE, Ludmer PL, Willich SN, et al: Circadian variation in the frequency of sudden cardiac death. Circulation 75:131–138, 1987.
257. Muller JE, Stone PH, Turi ZG, et al: Circadian variation in the frequency of onset of acute myocardial infarction. N Engl J Med 313:1315–1322, 1985.
258. Munck A, Naray-Fejes-Toth A: Glucocorticoid action. In De Groot LJ, Besser M, Burger HG, et al (eds): Endocrinology. 3rd ed. Philadelphia, WB Saunders Co., 1995, pp 1642–1667.
259. Musselman DL, Tomer A, Manatunga AK, et al: Exaggerated platelet reactivity in major depression. Am J Psychiat 153:1313–1317, 1996.
260. Nabel EG, Ganz P, Gordon JB, et al: Dilation of normal and constriction of atherosclerotic coronary arteries caused by the cold pressor test. Circulation 77:43–52, 1988.
261. Natelson BH, Chang Q: Sudden death. A neurocardiologic phenomenon. Neurol Clin 11:293–308, 1993.
262. Neill WA, Duncan DA, Kloster F, Mahler DJ: Response of the coronary circulation to cutaneous cold. Am J Med 56:471–476, 1974.
263. National Heart Lung and Blood Institute: Fact Book Fiscal Year 1996. Bethesda, MD, U.S. Dept of Health and Human Services, National Institutes of Health, 1997.

264. Niaura R, Herbert PN, Saritelli AL, et al: Lipid and lipoprotein responses to episodic occupational and academic stress. Arch Intern Med 151:2172–2179, 1991.
265. Niaura R, Stoney CM, Herbert PN: Lipids in psychological research: The last decade. Biol Psychol 34:1–43, 1992.
266. Novo S, Barbagallo M, Abrignani MG, et al: Increased prevalence of cardiac arrhythmias and transient episodes of myocardial ischemia in hypertensives with left ventricular hypertrophy but without clinical history of coronary heart disease. Am J Hypertension 10:843–851, 1997.
267. O'Brien JR: Some effects of adrenaline and anti-adrenaline compounds on platelets in vitro and in vivo. Nature 200:763–764, 1963.
268. Odemuyiwa O, Malik M, Farrell T, et al: Comparison of the predictive characteristics of heart rate variability index and left ventricular ejection fraction for all-cause mortality, arrhythmic events, and sudden death after acute myocardial infarction. Am J Cardiol 68:434–439, 1991.
269. O'Leary DH, Polak JF, Kronmal RA, et al: Carotid-artery intima and media thickness as a risk factor for myocardial infarction and stroke in older adults. New Engl J Med 340:14–22, 1999.
270. Oparil S, Chen YF, Berecek KH, et al: The role of the central nervous system in hypertension. In Laragh JH, Brenner BM (eds): Hypertension: Pathophysiology, Diagnosis, and Management. New York, Raven Press, Ltd., 1995, pp 713–740.
271. Opherk D, Mall G, Zebe H: Reduction of coronary reserve: A mechanism for angina pectoris in patients with hypertension and normal coronary arteries. Circulation 69:1–7, 1984.
272. Patel MB, Steewart HM, Loud AV, et al: Altered function and structure of the heart in dogs with chronic elevation in plasma norepinephrine. Circulation 84:2091–2100, 1991.
273. Patterson SM, Krantz DS, Gottdiener JS, et al: Prothrombotic effects of environmental stress: Changes in platelet function, hematocrit, and total plasma protein. Psychosom Med 57:592–599, 1995.
274. Patterson SM, Matthews KA, Allen MT, Owens JF: Stress-induced hemoconcentration of blood cells and lipids in healthy women during acute psychological stress. Health Psychol 14:319–324, 1995.
275. Pauletto P, Scannapieco G, Pessina AC: Sympathetic drive and vascular damage in hypertension and atherosclerosis. Hypertension 17 Suppl III:III75–III81, 1991.
276. Pepine CJ: Coronary angiography and cardiac catheterization. In Topol EJ (ed): Textbook of Cardiovascular Medicine. Philadelphia, Lippincott-Raven Publishers, 1998, pp 1935–1956.
277. Perloff D, Sokolow M, Cowan R: The prognostic value of ambulatory blood pressure. JAMA 249:2792–2798, 1983.
278. Perloff D, Sokolow M, Cowan R, Juster RP: Prognostic value of ambulatory blood pressure measurements: Further analyses. J Hypertension 7 (Suppl 3):S3–S10, 1989.
279. Peter R, Alfredsson L, Hammar N, et al: High effort, low reward, and cardiovascular risk factors in employed Swedish men and women: Baseline results from the WOLF study. J Epidemiol Community Health 52:540–547, 1998.
280. Peter R, Siegrist J: Chronic work stress, sickness absence, and hypertension in middle managers: General or specific sociological explanations? Social Sci Med 45:1111–1120, 1997.
281. Peters ML, Godaert GL, Ballieux RE, et al: Cardiovascular and endocrine responses to experimental stress: Effects of mental effort and controllability. Psychoneuroendocrinology 23:1–17, 1998.
282. Peters RW, McQuillan S, Resnick SK, Gold MR: Increased Monday incidence of life-threatening ventricular arrhythmias: Experience with a third-generation implantable defibrillator. Circulation 94:1346–1349, 1996.
283. Philipp T: Sympathetic nervous activity in essential hypertension: Activity and reactivity. J Cardiovasc Pharmacol 10 (Suppl 4):S31–S36, 1987.
284. Pichard A, Gorlin R, Smith H, et al: Coronary flow studies in patients with left ventricular hypertrophy of the hypertensive type: Evidence for an impaired coronary vascular reserve. Am J Cardiol 47:547, 1981.
285. Pickering TG: Ambulatory Monitoring and Blood Pressure Variability. London, Science Press, 1991.
286. Pickering TG: The effects of environmental and lifestyle factors on blood pressure and the intermediary role of the sympathetic nervous system. J Hum Hypertension 11 (Suppl 1):S9–S18, 1997.
287. Pickering TG: Psychosocial stress and hypertension. B: Clinical and experimental evidence. In Swales JD (ed): Textbook of Hypertension. London, Blackwell Scientific Publications, 1994, pp 641–654.
288. Pieper C, LaCroix AZ, Karasek RA: The relation of psychosocial dimensions of work with coronary heart disease risk factors: A meta-analysis of five United States data bases. Am J Epidemiol 129:483–494, 1989.
289. Pollard T, Steptoe A, Canaan L, et al: The effects of academic examination stress on eating behavior and blood lipid levels. Int J Behav Med 2:299–320, 1995.
289a. Pollard TM, Ungpakorn G, Harrison GA, Parkes KR: Epinephrine and cortisol responses to work: A test of the models of Frankenhaeuser and Karasek. Annals of Behavioral Medicine 18:229–237, 1996.
290. Porte D: A receptor mechanism for the inhibition of insulin release by epinephrine in man. J Clin Invest 46:86–94, 1967.
291. Poulter NP, Sever PS: Low blood pressure populations and the impact of rural-urban migration. In Swales JD (ed): Textbook of Hypertension. London, Blackwell Scientific Publications, 1994, pp 22–35.
292. Previtali M, Klersy C, Salerno J, et al: Ventricular tachyarrhythmias in Prinzmetal's variant angina: Clinical significance and relation to the degree and time course of S-T segment elevation. Am J Cardiol 52:19–25, 1983.
293. Pringle SD, Dunn FG, Tweddel AC, et al: Symptomatic and silent myocardial ischaemia in hypertensive patients with left ventricular hypertrophy. Br Heart J 67:377–382, 1992.
294. Prisant LM, Carr AA: Ambulatory blood pressure monitoring and echocardiographic left ventricular wall thickness and mass. Am J Hypertension 3:81–89, 1990.
295. Pucheu S, La Croix H, Tonet JL, et al: Ventricular arrhythmias. In MacFarlane PW, Veitch Lawrie TD (eds): Comprehensive Electrocardiology. New York, Pergamon Press, 1989, pp 961–998.
296. Rabkin SW, Mathewson FAL, Tate RB: Chronobiology of cardiac sudden death in men. JAMA 44:1357–1358, 1980.

297. Ragland D, Winkelby MA, Schwalbe J, et al: Prevalence of hypertension in bus drivers. Int J Epidemiol 16:208–214, 1987.
298. Ragland DR, Greiner BA, Holman BL, Fisher JM: Hypertension and years of driving in transit vehicle operators. Scand J Soc Med 25:271–279, 1997.
299. Raizner AE, Chahnine RA, Ishimori T, et al: Provocation of coronary artery spasm by the cold pressor test. Circulation 62:925–932, 1981.
300. Ravogli A, Trazzi S, Villani A, et al: Early 24-hour blood pressure elevation in normotensive subjects with parental hypertension. Hypertension 16:491–497, 1990.
301. Reaven GM: Banting lecture: Role of insulin resistance in human disease. Diabetes 37:1595–1607, 1988.
302. Ridker PM, Cushman M, Stampfer MJ, Tracy RP: Inflammation, aspirin, and the risk of cardiovascular disease in apparently healthy men. New Engl J Med 336:973–979, 1997.
303. Rissler A, Elgerot A: Stressreacktioner vid overtidsarbete (Stress reactions during overtime work). Stockholm, Department of Psychology, University of Stockholm, 1978.
304. Robertson D, Johnson GA, Robertson RM, et al: Comparative assessment of stimuli that release neuronal and adrenomedullary catecholamine in man. Circulation 59:637–642, 1979.
305. Robinson CC, Kuller LH, Perper J: An epidemiologic study of sudden death at work in an industrial county, 1979–1982. Am J Epidemiol 128:806–820, 1988.
306. Rosenman KD: Occupational heart disease. In Rom WN (ed): Environmental and Occupational Medicine. Philadelphia, Lippincott-Raven Publishers, 1998, pp 733–741.
307. Rosenstock L, Cullen MR: Clinical Occupational Medicine. Philadelphia, WB Saunders, 1986.
308. Rosmond R, Bjorntorp P: The interactions between hypothalamic-pituitary-adrenal axis activity, testosterone, insulin-like growth factor I, and abdominal obesity with metabolism and blood pressure in men. Int J Obesity Rel Metab Disorders 22:1184–1196, 1998.
309. Rosmond R, Dallman MF, Bjorntorp P: Stress-related cortisol secretion in men: Relationship with abdominal obesity and endocrine, metabolic and hemodynamic abnormalities. J Clin Endocrinol Metab 83:1853–1859, 1998.
310. Ross R: Atherosclerosis—an inflammatory disease. New Engl J Med 340:115–126, 1999.
311. Rostrup M, Ekeberg O: Awareness of high blood pressure influences on psychological and syapthetic responses. J Psychosom Research 36-2:117–123, 1992.
312. Rostrup M, Kjeldsen SE, Eide IK: Awareness of hypertension increases blood pressure and sympathetic responses to cold pressor test. Am J Hypertens 3:912–917, 1990.
313. Rostrup M, Mundal HH, Westheim A, Eide I: Awareness of high blood pressure increases arterial plasma catecholamines, platelet noradrenaline, and adrenergic responses to mental stress. J Hypertens 9:159–166, 1991.
314. Rostrup M, Westheim A, Kjeldsen SE, Eide I: Cardiovascular reactivity, coronary risk factors and sympathetic activity in young men. Hypertension 22:891–899, 1993.
315. Rozanski A, Bairey N, Krantz DS, et al: Mental stress and the induction of silent myocardial ischemia in patients with coronary artery disease. N Engl J Med 318:1005–1012, 1988.
316. Rozanski A, Krantz DS, Bairey CN: Ventricular responses to mental stress testing in patients with coronary artery disease. Pathophysiological implications. Circulation 83 Suppl II, 1991.
317. Rubin RT: Neuroendocrine aspects of primary endogenous depression I. Cortisol secretory dynamics in patients and matched control subjects. Arch Gen Psychiatry 44:328–336, 1987.
318. Sambhi MP, Weil MH, Udhoji VN: Pressor response to norepinephrine in humans before and after corticosteroids. Am J Physiol 103:961–963, 1962.
319. Sawada Y: Reproducible increases in blood pressure during intermittent noise exposure: Underlying haemodynamic mechanisms specific to passive coping. Eur J Appl Physiol Occup Physiol 67:367–374, 1993.
320. Schatzkin A, Cupples A, Heeren T, et al: Epidemiology of sudden unexpected death: Risk factors for men and women in Framingham. Am Heart J 107:1300–1306, 1984.
321. Schiffer F, Hartley LH, Schulman CL, Abelmann WH: Evidence for emotionally-induced coronary arerial spasm in patients with angina pectoris. Br Heart J 44:62–66, 1980.
322. Schlesinger Z, Barzilay J, Stryjer D, Almog CH: Life-threatening "vagal reaction" to emotional stimuli. Israel J Med Sci 13:59–61, 1977.
323. Schnall PL, Devereux RB, Pickering TG, Schwartz JE: The relationship between job strain, workplace diastolic blood pressure, and left ventricular mass index: A correction [letter; comment]. JAMA 267:1209, 1992.
324. Schnall PL, Landsbergis PA, Baker D: Job strain and cardiovascular disease. Annu Rev Public Health 15:381–411, 1994.
325. Schnall PL, Landsbergis PA, Schwartz J, et al: A longitudinal study of job strain and ambulatory blood pressure: Results from a three-year follow-up. Psychosom Med 60:697–706, 1998.
326. Schnall PL, Pieper C, Schwartz JE, et al: The relationship between job strain, workplace diastolic blood pressure, and left ventricular mass index. Results of a case-control study [published erratum appears in JAMA 1992 Mar 4;267(9):1209]. JAMA 263:1929–1935, 1990.
327. Schnall PL, Schwartz JE, Landsbergis PA, et al: Relation between job strain, alcohol, and ambulatory blood pressure. Hypertension 19:488–494, 1992.
328. Schwartz JE, Warren K, Pickering TG: Mood, location and physical position as predictors of ambulatory blood pressure and heart rate: Application of a multi-level random effects model. Ann Behav Med 16:210–220, 1994.
329. Schwartz JE, Pickering TG, Landsbergis PA: Work-related stress and blood pressure: Current theoretical models and considerations from a behavioral medicine perspective. J Occup Health Psychol 1:287–310, 1996.
330. Schwartz PJ, Zaza A, Locati E, et al: Stress and sudden death: the case of the long QT syndrome. Circulation Suppl:II-71–II-80, 1991.
331. Seligman M: Helplessness—On Depression, Development, and Death. San Francisco, Freeman, 1975.
332. Selye H: The Physiology and Pathology of Exposure to Stress. Montreal, ACTA Press, 1950.

333. Sen S, Tarazi RC, Khairallah P, Bumpus M: Cardiac hypertrophy in spontaneously hypertensive rats. Circ Res 35:775–781, 1974.

334. Servatius RJ, Ottenweller JE, Gross JL, Natelson BH: Persistent plasma cholesterol elevations are produced by one or three stressor exposures in rats fed a normal laboratory diet. Physiol Behav 53:1101–1104, 1993.

335. Sheehan FH, Epstein SE: Determinants of arrhythmic death due to coronary spasm: Effect of preexisting coronary artery stenosis on the incidence of reperfusion arrhythmia. Circulation 65:259–264, 1982.

336. Sheldahl LM, Wilke NA, Dougherty S, Tristani FE: Cardiac responses to combined moderate heat and exercise in men with coronary artery disease. Am J Cardiol 70:186–191, 1992.

337. Sheldahl LM, Wilke NA, Tristani FE, Kalbfleisch JH: Responses of patients after myocardial infarction to carrying a graded series of weight loads. Am J Cardiol 52:698–703, 1983.

338. Shepherd JT, Blomquist CG, Lind AR, et al: Static (isometric) exercise: Retrospection and introspection. Circ Res Suppl 48:1–179, 1981.

339. Sheps DS, Ballenger MN, DeGent G, et al: Psychophysical responses to a speech stressor: Correlation of plasma beta-endorphin levels at rest and after psychological stress with thermally measured pain threshold in patients with coronary artery disease. J Am Coll Cardiol 25:1499–1503, 1995.

340. Sheridan DJ, Penkoske PA, Sobel BE, Corr PB: Alpha-adrenergic contributions to dysrhythmia during myocardial ischemia and reperfusion in cats. J Clin Invest 65:161–171, 1980.

341. Siegrist J: Adverse health effects of high-effort/low-reward conditions. J Occup Health Psychol 1:27–41, 1996.

342. Siegrist J, Peter R, Cremer P, Seidel D: Chronic work stress is associated with atherogenic lipids and elevated fibrinogen in middle aged men. J Intern Med 242:149–156, 1997.

343. Siegrist J, Peter R, Georg W, et al: Psychosocial and biobehavioral characteristics of hypertensive men with elevated atherogenic lipids. Atherosclerosis 86:211–218, 1991.

344. Singer DH, Baumgarten CM, Ten Eick RE: Cellular electrophysiology of ventricular and other dysrhythmias: Studies on diseased and ischemic heart. In Sonnenblick EH, Lesch M (eds): Sudden Cardiac Death. New York, Grune & Stratton, 1981, pp 13–72.

345. Sjogren B: Occupational exposure to dust: Inflammation and ischaemic heart disease. Occup Environ Med 54:466–469, 1997.

346. Skantze HB, Kaplan J, Pettersson K, et al: Psychosocial stress causes endothelial injury in cynomolgus monkeys via beta 1-adrenoceptor activation. Atherosclerosis 136:153–161, 1998.

347. Skinner JE: Regulation of cardiac vulnerability by the cerebral defense system. J Am Coll Cardiol 5:88B–94B, 1985.

348. Skinner JE, Lie JT, Entman ML: Modification of ventricular fibrillation latency following coronary artery occlusion in the conscious pig: The effects of psychological stress and beta-adrenergic blockage. Circulation 51:656–667, 1975.

349. Sluiter JK, van der Beek AJ, Frings-Dresen MH: Work stress and recovery measured by urinary catecholamines and cortisol excretion in long-distance coach drivers. Occup Environ Med 55:407–413, 1998.

350. Staten MA, Matthews DE, Cryer PE, Bier DM: Physiological increments in epinephrine metabolic rate in humans. Am J Physiol 253:E322–330, 1987.

351. Steptoe A, Cropley M, Joekes K: Job strain, blood pressure, and response to uncontrollable stress. J Hypertens 17:193–200, 1999.

352. Steptoe A, Vogele C: Methodology of mental stress testing in cardiovascular research. Circulation Suppl II 83:II14–II24, 1991.

353. Steptoe A, Wardle J, Lipsey Z, et al: The effects of life stress on food choice. In Murcott A (ed): The Nation's Diet. London, Longman, 1998, pp 29–42.

354. Strachan DP, Carrington D, Mendall MA, et al: Relation of *Chlamydia pneumoniae* serology to mortality and incidence of ischaemic heart disease over 13 years in the Caerphilly prospective heart disease study. Br Med J 318:1035–1040, 1999.

355. Struijker-Boudier HAJ: Vascular growth and hypertension. In Swales JD (ed): A Textbook of Hypertension. London, Blackwell Scientific Publications, 1994, pp 200–213.

356. Surawicz B: Ventricular fibrillation. Am J Cardiol 28:268–287, 1971.

357. Swynghedauw B, Delcayre C, Cheav SL, et al: Biological basis of diastolic dysfunction of the hypertensive heart. Eur Heart J 13 Suppl D:2–8, 1992.

358. Taccola A, Assandri J, Gotti GB: Dynamic electrocardiographic findings in a precision casting factory. Med Lav 70:215–222, 1979.

359. Tafalla RJ, Evans GW: Noise, physiology and human performance: The potential role of effort. J Occup Health Psychol 2:148–155, 1997.

360. Taggart P, Carruthers M: Endogenous hyperlipidemia induced by emotional stress of racing driving. Lancet 1:363–366, 1971.

361. Taggart P, Carruthers M, Somerville W: Electrocardiogram, plasma catecholamines and lipids, and their modification by oxyprenolol when speaking before and audience. Lancet 2:341–346, 1973.

362. Taggart P, Gibbons D, Somerville W: Some effects of motor-car driving on the normal and abnormal heart. Br Med J 4:130–134, 1969.

363. Taggart P, Parkinson P, Carruthers M: Cardiac responses to thermal, physical, and emotional stress. Br Med J 3:71–76, 1972.

364. Talbott E, Helmkamp J, Matthews K, Kuller L, et al: Occupational noise exposure, noise-induced hearing loss, and the epidemiology of high blood pressure. Am J Epidemiol 121:501–514, 1985.

365. Talbott EO, Gibson LB, Burks A, et al: Evidence for a dose-response relationship between occupational noise and blood pressure. Arch Environ Health 54:71–78, 1999.

366. Ten Eick RE, Baumgarten CM, Singer DH: Ventricular dysrhythmias: Membrane basis of current, channels, gates and cables. In Sonnenblick EH, Lesch M (eds): Sudden Cardiac Death. New York, Grune & Stratton, 1981, pp 73–104.

367. Thaulow E, Erikssen J, Sandvik L, et al: Blood platelet count and function are related to total and cardiovascular death in apparently healthy men. Circulation 84:613–617, 1991.
368. Theorell T: Prolactin—a hormone that mirrors passiveness in crisis situations. Integr Physiol Behav Sci 27:32–38, 1992.
369. Theorell T, Ahlberg-Hulten G, Jodko M, et al: Influence of job strain and emotion on blood pressure in female hospital personnel during work hours. Scand J Work Environ Health 19:313–318, 1993.
370. Theorell T, Hjemdahl P, Ericsson F, et al: Psychosocial and physiological factors in relation to blood pressure at rest—a study of Swedish men in their upper twenties. J Hypertens 3:591–600, 1985.
371. Theorell T, Karasek RA, Eneroth P: Job strain variations in relation to plasma testosterone fluctuations in working men—a longitudinal study. J Intern Med 227:31–36, 1990.
372. Theorell T, Leymann H, Jodko M, et al: "Person-under train" incidents: Medical consequences for subway drivers. Psychosom Med 54:480–488, 1992.
373. Theorell T, Perski A, Akerstedt T, et al: Changes in job strain in relation to changes in physiological states—a longitudinal study. Scand J Work Environ Health 14:189–196, 1988.
374. Timio M, Gentili S, Pede S: Free adrenaline and noradrenaline excretion related to occupational stress. Br Heart J 42:471–474, 1979.
375. Tofler GH: Triggering and the pathophysiology of acute coronary syndromes. Am Heart J 134:S55–S61, 1997.
376. Torp-Pedersen C, Kober L, Elming H, Burchart H: Classification of sudden and arrhythmic death. PACE 20:2545–2552, 1997.
377. Turkkan JS, Harris AH, Goldstein DS: Do chronically repeated episodes cause sustained elevations in blood pressure? In Weiss SM, Matthews KA, Detre T, Graef JA (eds): Stress, Reactivity, and Cardiovascular Disease, NIH Publication NO. 84-2698, 1984, p 237.
378. Tzivoni D, Stern S: Complementary role of ambulatory electrocardiographic monitoring and exercise testing in evaluation of myocardial ischemia. Cardiol Clin 10:461–466, 1992.
379. Ugljesic M, Belkic K, Boskovic S, et al: Porast arterijskog krvnog pritiska tokom rada i profil rizika kod stresogenih profesija: novinari i vozaci gradskog saobrcaja (Increased arterial blood pressure during work and risk profile among high-stress occupations: journalists and city mass transit drivers). Kardiologija 13:150–154, 1992.
380. van Amelsvoort LGPM: Coronary heart disease among truck drivers. Report of the International Workshop on the Epidemiology of Coronary Heart Disease among European Truck Drivers. Bilthoven, European Commission, 1995.
381. Van der Loo B, Martin JF: Megakaryocytes and platelets in vascular disease. Baillieres Clin Haematol 10:109–123, 1997.
382. Vandevoir D, Gournay M: Coronary and vascular pathology in dynamite workers. Phlebologie 42:223–232, 1989.
383. Verdecchia P, Porcellati C, Schillaci G, et al: Ambulatory blood pressure: An independent predictor of prognosis in essential hypertension. Hypertension 24:793–801, 1994.
384. Verdecchia P, Schillaci G, Guerrieri M, et al: Circadian blood pressure changes and left ventricular hypertrophy in essential hypertension. Hypertension 16:528–536, 1990.
385. Verdun di Cantogno L, Dallerba R, Teagno PS, et al: Urban traffic noise, cardiocirculatory, and coronary risk factors. Acta Otolaryng Suppl 339:55–63, 1976.
386. Verrier RL: Neural factors and ventricular electrical instability. In Kulbertus HE, Wellens HJJ (eds): Sudden Death. The Hague, Martinus Nijhoff, 1980, pp 137–155.
387. Waldron I, Nowatarski M, Freimer M, et al: Cross-cultural variation in blood pressure: A qualtitative analysis of the relationship of blood pressure to cultural characteristics, salt consumption, and body weight. Soc Sci Med 16:419–430, 1982.
388. Warren JV: Monday morning sudden death. Transactions of the American Clinical and Climatological Association 99:10–16, 1987.
389. Wellens HJJ, Vermeulan A, Durrer D: Ventricular fibrillation occurring on arousal from sleep by auditory stimuli. Circulation 46:661–665, 1972.
390. Wemm KM Jr, Trestman RL: The effects of a laboratory stressor on natural killer cell function in chronic fatigue syndrome patients (letter). Psychosomatics 32:470–471, 1991.
391. Wenger NK: Occupation and cardiovascular disease. In Hurst W, Schlant R, Rackley CE, et al (eds): The Heart. New York, McGraw-Hill Services Company, 1990, pp 1666–1669.
392. Whelton PK, He J, Klag MJ: Blood pressure in Westernized populations. In Swales JD (ed): Textbook of Hypertension. London, Blackwell Scientific Publications, 1994, pp 11–21.
393. White HD: Unstable angina. Ischemic syndromes. In Topol EJ (ed): Textbook of Cardiovascular Medicine. Philadelphia, Lippincott-Raven, 1998, pp 365–393.
394. Whitworth JA, Gordon D, Andrews J, Scoggins BA: The hypertensive effect of synthetic glucocorticoids in man: Role of sodium and volume. J Hypertens 7:535–549, 1989.
395. Williams GH, Dluhy RG: Diseases of the adrenal cortex. In Wilson JD, Brauwald E, Isselbacher KJ, et al (eds): Harrison's Principles of Internal Medicine. New York, McGraw-Hill, 1991, pp 1713–1735.
396. Williams JK, Vita JA, Manuck SB, et al: Psychosocial factor impact in vascular responses of coronary arteries. Circulation 84:2146–2153, 1991.
397. Willich SN, Goldberg RJ, Maclure M, et al: Increased onset of sudden cardiac death in the first 3 hours after awakening. Am J Cardiol 70:65–68, 1992.
398. Willich SN, Linderer T, Wegscheider K, et al: Increasing morning incidence of myocardial infarction in the ISAM Study: Absence with prior beta-adrenergic blockade. Circulation 80:853–858, 1989.
399. Willich SN, Lowel H, Lewis M, et al: Weekly variation of acute myocardial infarction: Increased Monday risk in the working population. Circulation 90:87–93, 1994.

400. Willich SN, Maclure M, Mittleman M, et al: Sudden cardiac death support for a role of triggering in causation. Circulation 87:1442–1450, 1993.
401. Winkleby MA, Ragland DR, Fisher JM, Syme SL: Excess risk of sickness and disease in bus drivers: A review and synthesis of epidemiological studies. Int J Epidemiol 17:255–262, 1988.
402. Wit AL, Rosen MR: Cellular electrophysiological mechanisms of cardiac arrhythmias. In MacFarlane PW, Veitch Lawrie TD (eds): Comprehensive Electrocardiology. New York, Pergamon Press, 1989, pp 801–841.
403. Wolf S: Sudden death and the oxygen-conserving reflex. Am Heart J 71:840–841, 1966.
404. Yamasaki F, Schwartz JE, Gerber LM, et al: Impact of shift work and race/ethnicity on the diurnal rhythm of blood pressure and catecholamines. Hypertension 32:417–423, 1998.
405. Yasue H, Kugiyama K: Coronary spasm: Clinical features and pathogenesis. Int Med 36:760–765, 1997.
406. Yasue H, Omote S, Takizawa A, Nagao M: Coronary artery spasm in ischemic heart disease and its pathogenesis. A review. Circulation Research 52:1145–1152, 1983.
407. Yeung AC, Vekshtein VI, Drantz DS, et al: The effects of atherosclerosis on the vasomotor responses of coronary arteries to mental stress. N Engl J Med 325:1551–1556, 1991.
408. Yokoyama E, Teru S, Mijake T, et al: Health care of truck drivers with reference to blood pressure control. Nihon Univ J Med 27:225–238, 1985.
409. Zhou D, Kusnecov AW, Shurin MR, et al: Exposure to physical and psychological stressors elevates plasma inter-leukin 6: Relationship to the activation of hypothalamic-pituitary-adrenal axis. Endocrinology 133:2523–2530, 1993.
410. Zipes DP, Gilmour RF, Martinus JB, Ruffy R: Autonomic nervous system and sudden death. In Kulbertus HE, Wellens HJJ (eds): Sudden Death. The Hague, Martinus Nijhoff, 1980, pp 156–162.
411. Zipes DP, Inoue H: Autonomic neural control of cardiac excitable properties. In Kulbertus HE, Franck G (eds): Neurocardiology. Mount Kisco, Futura Publishing, 1988, pp 59–84.

MEASUREMENT OF PSYCHOSOCIAL WORKPLACE EXPOSURE VARIABLES

SELF-REPORT QUESTIONNAIRES   *by Paul Landsbergis, PhD, and Töres Theorell, MD, PhD*

Despite differences in the ways workplace CVD risk factors—psychosocial, chemical, physical, and schedule-related—are measured, basic similarities exist. All require assessment of the duration, intensity, and frequency of exposure. To assess duration of exposure (or cumulative exposure), "detailed work history records [are] virtually essential. . . . where job mobility occurs frequently."[16] A job-exposure matrix is necessary when individual data are not available (or for more objective measures of psychosocial factors). Data in such a matrix can be provided at broader or narrower levels of aggregation, i.e., broad occupational categories or specific job titles in specific companies or work areas. For more detail on physical and chemical exposure assessment, we refer the reader to basic texts in occupational epidemiology[16] and industrial hygiene.[18]

Research and debate have been spurred by efforts to develop more objective measures and other measurement issues. First, should one use occupation-specific measures, or measures that can be generalized across occupations? Second, which aspects of work should be measured: job characteristics (e.g., demands, control), role characteristics, organizational climate, hours, or broader systems of work organization (e.g., lean production)? Third, are the characteristics a property of the individual, job, job title, occupation, or organization? Fourth, which questionnaires based on which theories best measure psychosocial exposures associated with an increased risk of CVD?

Here, we do not focus on measuring the perception of stress. Due to adaptation, people working in a stressful job may not report feelings of stress. For example, in the Cornell blood pressure (BP) study, job strain (high job demands plus low job decision latitude) was not associated with perceived anxiety or distress.[63] Nor do we examine interactions between personality and the work environment. Rather, we focus on **job stressors**—the large number of environmental conditions at work "thought to impact on the health and well-being of the worker."[43]

Occupation-Specific Versus General Measures

One approach to developing job stressor questionnaires has been to ask questions *specific* to a particular occupation or a workplace, for example, nurses,[27] teachers,[85] or bus drivers.[9,59,109] Such measures provide rich, detailed information, especially for intervention efforts[43] designed to identify and change specific features of the work environment associated will ill health. For example, in the San Francisco bus driver study, back and neck pain were associated with a number of job conditions such as equipment problems, too many passengers, problems with supervisors, not maintaining the run schedule, long or odd hours, having been "written-up" for rule violations, serious traffic or road problems, and poor access to restrooms on the line.[59] Interestingly, a sum score of such job conditions was found to be inversely associated with hypertension (when measured by job stressor questionnaire in 1983–85), or not associated with hypertension (when measured in 1993–95). Such findings highlight the need to also employ more objective measures of job stressors.

Since job-specific questionnaires cannot be used to compare job stressors across different occupations, an alternative approach has been to measure generic or *global* job characteristics, such as demands, control, and social support, using language general enough to apply to a variety of occupations.[9,56,69,91] This approach is less useful for intervention studies because questions are more "remote from actual work experiences."[43] It has been essential, however, to the development of theories of job stress, such as the demand-control model and the effort-reward model, which have enabled researchers to document associations between job characteristics and CV outcomes across occupations (see Chapters 2 and 3).

A recent innovative approach uses occupation-specific questions (useful for workplace interventions), which are based on general questions.[10] The Occupational Stress Index (OSI) can be tailored to specific occupations, thus allowing comparison among occupations of the stress burden faced by workers.

Measuring Job Characteristics:
Questionnaires and Theoretical Models

The global job stressor questionnaires focus, for the most part, on characteristics of individuals' jobs (Table 1), rather than on systems of work organization. Only occasional questions ask about broader issues such as employee influence over departmental or employer policies or procedures, representative influence through labor organizations, or promotion prospects. Similarly, few questionnaires measure systems of management, such as electronic monitoring or piece-rate pay systems, or new systems of work organization, such as lean production, total quality management, cellular or modular manufacturing, or patient-focused care.[62] These new work systems may have dramatic impacts on task-level job characteristics; research suggests that some systems increase job stressors.[62]

Modern job stress assessment "was given tremendous impetus by research conducted at the University of Michigan in the early 1960s."[43] Questionnaires were developed to measure factors such as role ambiguity, workload, role conflict, responsibility for persons or things, participation, and social relations. The Michigan researchers hypothesized that stress is greatest when there is a misfit between a person's abilities and work demands, or a person's motives and the work environment's "supplies" to satisfy these motives.[15] This Person-Environment (P-E) Fit model focuses on individuals' subjective perceptions of the work environment, and incorporates a variety of perceived and objective stressors, feedback loops, and the potential moderating effects of personality factors, nonwork factors, and demographic measures. However, this model has "demonstrated limited ability to predict what objective work conditions are likely to result in stress."[7]

NIOSH has developed an extensive questionnaire to measure job stressors, based, in part, on the University of Michigan questionnaire.[72] Over 100 questions, included in 20 scales with high internal consistency, ask about stressors in the work

TABLE 1. Content of Questionnaires Used to Measure Job Stressors in Studies of CVD

	Core JCQ	Full JCQ	DCQ	WOM	Whitehall	ERI	OSI
			(No. of Questions)				
Psychological Job Demands							
Time pressure, workload	4	5	5	2	4	2	3
Conflicting demands	1	1					1
Intense concentration		1					1
Interruptions		2				1	1
Increasing demands						1	
Responsibility						1	2
High demand							19
Avoidance/disaster potential							5
Conflict/uncertainty							8
Job Decision Latitude/Control							
Skill discretion	6	6	4	3	6		5
Decision-making authority	3	3	2	8	9		3
Underload							8
Strictness							6
Skill underutilization	2	2					4
Status inconsistency						1	
Work group decision authority		3					
Formal authority		2					
Union/representative influence		3					
Social Support							
Supervisor support	4	5			4		
Coworker support	4	6		4	2		
General support						1	1
Respect						3	
Unfair treatment						1	
Job Insecurity							
General job insecurity	3	4				2	
Skill obsolescence		1					
Promotion prospects		1				2	
Physical Demands							
General physical loading	1	1				1	
Isometric load		2					
Aerobic load		2					
Noxious Exposures/Aversiveness				7			7
Income						1	
TOTAL	28	50	11	24	25	17	74

JCQ = Job Content Questionnaire; DCQ = Swedish Demand-Control Questionnaire; WOM = Swedish Work Organization Matrix; ERI = Effort-Reward Imbalance; OSI = Occupational Stress Index

Notes: This table does not include the 29 questions from the ERI intrinsic effort scale, because intrinsic effort is considered to be a personality trait. The number of OSI questions does not total to 58 since the same items may be used to form more than one scale.

Adapted from Karasek R, Brisson C, Kawakami N, et al: The Job Content Questionnaire: An instrument for internationally comparative assessments of psychosocial job characteristics. J Occup Health Psychol 3:322–355, 1998; with permission.

environment. While the NIOSH questionnaire (and the earlier P-E Fit questionnaire) have been used in numerous studies examining self-reported psychological strain outcomes (e.g., anxiety, depression) and job dissatisfaction, they rarely have been used to study CV outcomes.

Since the 1960s, ". . . a plethora of questionnaires, scales, interview schedules and other stress measurement devices have emerged and evolved. . . . choosing a measurement tool poses a bewildering challenge."[43] Hurrell, et al. point out that many of these questionnaires have good reliability and construct validity, and therefore are potentially useful for studying working conditions related to CVD.[43] Here, we focus on the questionnaires that have been widely used in studies of CVD to describe working conditions (see Table 1).

JOB CONTENT QUESTIONNAIRE

The core questions of the Job Content Questionnaire (JCQ)[53,56] are taken from the U.S. Quality of Employment Surveys (QES), administered to nationally representative samples of employed individuals in 1969, 1972, and 1977. The "core JCQ" is based on 27 psychosocial questions included in the three QES. The "full JCQ" (version 1.1) was developed in 1985 by adding eight additional QES items and 14 new questions. A 1995 update (version 1.5) included pilot versions of a set of questions addressing the global economy. JCQ scale scores for any sample can be compared to national U.S. scale averages by job title, sex, and industry code.

The JCQ has been widely used in North America, Europe, and Japan, and reliability information contained in Table 2 is based primarily on six major studies from the U.S., Canada, the Netherlands, and Japan.[53] The means and standard deviations of scales are similar across the six studies, and internal consistency tends to be similar across populations (average Cronbach's α for women is .73 and for men is .74). The alpha coefficients are generally acceptable ($\alpha > .70$), however, the five-item psychological demands scale is only borderline (average $\alpha = .63$), and the three-item job insecurity scale has low reliability ($\alpha < .60$) for two of the three studies for which data are available. Studies using the JCQ typically have employed a response format based on intensity, i.e., ranging from "strongly agree" to "strongly disagree."

To obtain the JCQ: www.uml.edu/Dept/WE/jcq.htm

SWEDISH DEMAND-CONTROL QUESTIONNAIRE

The Swedish Demand-Control Questionnaire (DCQ), a shortened and modified version of the JCQ, was introduced in 1988[99] and has been used in a number of epidemiologic studies. It contains only six questions assessing decision latitude (two on decision authority and four on intellectual discretion). These scales have adequate internal consistency ($\alpha = .75–.80$ for demands and $\alpha = .76–.77$ for latitude).[97] There is also a social support scale; however, it is oriented toward the atmosphere in the worksite, while the JCQ social support questions are more objective and instrumental in nature. Response options are frequency-based (i.e., "how often"). The DCQ and the JCQ appear to be very similar.

A recent study explored the validity of some of the most crucial questions in the DCQ by asking subjects to describe in their own words what they mean by their responses to the standardized questionnaires. According to a content analysis, the questions dealing with psychological demands and decision latitude have similar meaning to both healthcare personnel and workers who deal with "things" in their daily work.[2]

To obtain the DCQ: e-mail Tores.Theorell@ipm.ki.se

TABLE 2. Internal Consistency Reliability of Main Questionnaire Scales Used to Measure Job Stressors in CVD Studies

Scale	Questionnaire	# of Items	Reference	Cronbach's Alpha
Psychological demands				
Psychological demands	JCQ	9	Karasek, 1998	.72 (men), .71 (women)
Psychological demands	JCQ	5	Karasek, 1998	.63 (men), .63 (women)
Psychological demands	JCQ	5	Original analyses-Cornell WSBPS	.70–.74
Psychological demands	DCQ	5	Theorell, 1996	.75 (men), .81 (women)
Psychological demands	WOM	2	Johnson, 1993	.60
Job demands	Whitehall	4	Bosma, 1997	.67
Extrinsic effort	ERI	6	Rothenbacher, 1998	.76
Extrinsic effort	ERI	6	Vrijkotte, 1999	.76
High demand	OSI	19	Belkic, 1995b; 1996	.80
Extrinsic time pressure	OSI	5	Belkic, 1995b, 1996	.54
Avoidance/serious consequences	OSI	5	Belkic, 1995b; 1996	.67
Conflict/uncertainty	OSI	8	Belkic, 1995b; 1996	.80
Job decision latitude				
Skill discretion	JCQ	6	Karasek, 1998	.73 (men), .75 (women)
Skill discretion	JCQ	6	Original analyses-Cornell WSBPS	.72–.80
Decision authority	JCQ	3	Karasek, 1998	.68 (men), .68 (women)
Decision authority	JCQ	3	Original analyses-Cornell WSBPS	.77–.81
Organizational influence	JCQ	3	Landsbergis, 1994	.62
Job decision latitude	JCQ	9	Karasek, 1998	.81 (men), .82 (women)
Job decision latitude	JCQ	9	Original analyses-Cornell WSBPS	.81–.83
Job decision latitude	DCQ	6	Theorell, 1996	.76 (men), .77 (women)
Work control	WOM	12	Johnson, 1993	.75
Job control	Whitehall	15	Bosma, 1997	.84
Underload	OSI	8	Belkic, 1995b; 1996	.62
Strictness	OSI	6	Belkic, 1995b; 1996	.41
Social support				
Supervisor support	JCQ	4	Karasek, 1998	.84 (men), .84 (women)
Supervisor support	JCQ	4	Original analyses-Cornell WSBPS	.87–.89
Co-worker support	JCQ	4	Karasek, 1998	.75 (men), .77 (women)
Co-worker support	JCQ	4	Original analyses-Cornell WSBPS	.67–.72
Social support	Whitehall	6	Bosma, 1997	.79
Job insecurity				
Job insecurity	JCQ	3	Karasek, 1998	.61 (men), .58 (women)
Job insecurity	JCQ	3	Original analyses-Cornell WSBPS	.46–.77
Extrinsic reward				
Extrinsic reward	ERI	11	Rothenbacher, 1998	.81
Extrinsic reward	ERI	11	Vrijkotte, 1999	.82
Hazardous exposures				
Hazardous exposure	WOM	7	Johnson, 1993	.71
Noxious exposure	OSI	7	Belkic, 1995b; 1996	.67
TOTAL OSI	General OSI	58	Belkic, 1995b; 1996; Emdad, 1998	.81
	Professional driver OSI*	27	Belkic, 1996	.84

* Variable items only for Cronbach alpha   JCQ: Job Content Questionnaire; ERI: Effort-Reward Imbalance Questionnaire; OSI: Occupational Stress Index; DCQ: Swedish Demand-Control Questionnaire; WOM: Swedish Work Organization Matrix; WSBPS: Work Site Blood Pressure Study

SWEDISH WORK ORGANIZATION MATRIX

Researchers in Sweden also developed an elaborate instrument, the Work Organization Matrix (WOM), for imputing job title averages of job characteristics to study subjects.[4,38,50,51] It is based on questions from the nationally representative Level of Living surveys administered in Sweden in 1977. The WOM is not directly related to the JCQ and has only two items on job demands. However, its work-control scale includes some questions that go beyond task-level influence, and ask about influence over selection of supervisor and coworkers, and planning of vacations. As in the JCQ, internal consistency values are higher for the work-control scale (α = .75) than for the psychological job-demands scale (α = .60).[50] The response format is "yes/no" for the job-demands items and "often/sometimes/never" for the work-control items.

WHITEHALL JOB CHARACTERISTICS QUESTIONNAIRE

Researchers conducting the Whitehall study of British civil servants adapted the JCQ for their study[13] by adding questions on decision authority and changing to a response format based on frequency (a 4-point scale ranging from "often" to "never"). They found higher internal consistency for their job-control scale (α = .84) than for the job-demands scale (α = .67). A slightly shorter version of the Whitehall questionnaire has been used by researchers in the Copenhagen Heart Study.[74]

To obtain the Whitehall Questionnaire: Dr. Amanda Nicholson, Department of Epidemiology & Public Health, University College London, 1-19 Torrington Place, LONDON WC1E 6BT, Tel 0171-391-1684, e-mail amandan@public-health.ucl.ac.uk

EFFORT-REWARD IMBALANCE QUESTIONNAIRE

The effort-reward imbalance (ERI) model of work stress expands some of the concepts described in the previous questionnaires (see Table 1). Siegrist, et al. define threatening job conditions as a "mismatch between high workload (high demand) and low control over long-term rewards."[92] *Extrinsic effort* is defined very similarly to job demands in the JCQ, DCQ, WOM, and Whitehall, although in some studies it includes piecework and shiftwork. Low *reward* refers to low "esteem reward" (similar to lacking social support), low income, and poor job security/career opportunities (i.e., layoffs, undesirable change, poor promotion prospects, and work not adequately reflecting education level [status inconsistency]).[91,92] Response options in the current version of the questionnaire are "agree" or "disagree," and if "agree" is chosen, the level of distress—ranging from "very" to "not at all" on a 4-point scale—is requested. The internal consistencies of the extrinsic effort scale (α = .76) and the reward scale (α = .81–.82) are good.[82,104]

The ERI model emphasizes broader aspects of job control than the JCQ, DCQ, WOM, or Whitehall questionnaires. However, Karasek and Theorell's model was not intended to restrict the concepts of demands and control to task-level measures.[54] The core JCQ and the DCQ were derived from specific U.S. and Swedish surveys and therefore created post hoc. However, the full JCQ contains items and scales that measure income and aspects of low job security/career opportunities.[56] Roughly 9 of the 14 concepts employed by Siegrist and Peter to measure extrinsic effort and low reward are contained in the JCQ.[91] Many researchers have chosen to use only two of the core JCQ scales (14 items measuring decision latitude and workload demands) due to limited space and time constraints; however, the full JCQ includes a broader set of measures. In addition, the *life course perspective* of work task control developed by Johnson using the WOM [Johnson, 1996] reflects job security/career opportunities.[96] In a study of Swedish men, dichotomous measures of ERI and job strain were mildly correlated (r = .21).[79]

To obtain the ERI questionnaire: Johannes Siegrist, e-mail siegrist@uni-dusseldorf.de

OCCUPATIONAL STRESS INDEX

The Occupational Stress Index (OSI) incorporates essential elements of the job demands-control model, as well as other formulations of how stress leads to CVD, such as features of work in high-risk occupations.[9–11,21,22] The OSI is reflective of a cognitive ergonomic-neurophysiologic approach (see Chapter 3). The factors are organized into a two-dimensional matrix with the stress dimensions (underload, high demand, strictness, extrinsic time pressure, noxious physical exposures, threat-avoidant characteristics, and conflict/uncertainty) along the horizontal axis. The levels of human information transmission—sensory input, central decision-making, and task execution—plus a general level, form the vertical axis.[107] Thus, each factor has a set of coordinates, localizing it to the type of stress and the level at which it affects the worker. The OSI contains 58 items, including more specific questions than standard job stressor questionnaires, and thus can be useful as a diagnostic tool for intervention strategies. For example, the OSI operationalizes the specific elements that contribute to psychological demand and thus can discriminate professional drivers from control subjects (building tradesworkers and subway guard attendants); job demands-control measures (e.g., DCQ) often cannot.[8] In addition to the general OSI (Cronbach's α = 0.81), a version specific to professional drivers has been developed (Cronbach's α = 0.84),[9] and an OSI for physicians is being developed. Each of the seven subscales of the OSI have shown acceptable internal consistency reliability (see Table 2), with the exception of "strictness" and "extrinsic time pressure." The OSI also emphasizes stressful aspects of work that have disaster potential or "life and death" consequences, such as are experienced by professional drivers, air traffic controllers, healthcare workers, and sea pilots. Response options vary, but are usually on a 3-point scale, and include intensity and frequency.

To obtain the OSI: Karen Belkic, Center for Social Epidemiology, Room 202, 1528 6th St., Santa Monica, CA 90401, 310-319-6595, e-mail kbelkic@hsc.usc.edu

OTHER MEASURING TOOLS

The NIOSH generic job stress instrument also contains items on cognitive demands, role conflict, role ambiguity, responsibility for people, and threat of violence or injury.[72] Jackson and colleagues have examined monitoring demands (e.g., undivided attention, keeping tract of processes, concentrating all the time, reacting quickly to prevent problems arising), problem-solving demands, and production responsibility. Some researchers have suggested adding "emotional demands" (items about death, sickness, human suffering, aggressive and awkward patients or clients).[12,17] Borg and Kristensen, in Danish national studies also have examined sensorial job demands (attention, need for precision, intensity), cognitive demands, and the demand for suppressing one's emotions.[12] However, none of these studies have examined CVD outcomes.

Jackson, et al. differentiate control over scheduling/pacing of tasks ("timing control") from control over the process by which tasks are performed ("method control").[45] In addition to expanding the concept of job control to work group or organizational policies or procedures (as in the full JCQ or the NIOSH questionnaire) and to long-term job security/career opportunities (as in the ERI), the full JCQ begins to measure aspects of job control exercised collectively.[47] Such collective control, e.g., through a union collective bargaining agreement, may be an important means for employees (particularly lower socioeconomic status employees) to exercise task control, increase income, achieve job security, improve promotion prospects, and minimize undesirable change.

The JCQ, DCQ, WOM, ERI, OSI, and NIOSH instruments also contain questions on physical demands and hazardous physical or chemical exposures. The association of these characteristics with job strain or ERI rarely has been examined and, in fact, may confound or modify the effect of job strain on CVD risk.

To obtain the NIOSH questionnaire: Joseph J. Hurrell, Jr., NIOSH Division of Surveillance, Hazard Evaluations and Field Studies, Mail Stop R12, 4676 Columbia Parkway, Cincinnati, OH 45226, 513-841-4428, e-mail jjh3@NIOSHE1.em.cdc.gov

Formulations of Job Strain

Job Demands and Job Decision Latitude.   The interaction between job demands and job decision latitude, which defines job strain, has been operationalized primarily in four ways.[64,84] (1) The most common procedure applies a quadrant approach, identifying employees who are above the median on demands and below the median on latitude as "high strain". The determination is made by dichotomizing self-reports of demands and latitude at either the sample medians or national medians/means. (2) A newer approach (used in seven studies with positive results[64,84]) creates a continuous, independent variable—demands divided by latitude. (3) Eight studies have employed a multiplicative interaction term partialled for main effects (demands × latitude, controlling for demands and latitude). However, the interaction term significantly improved the variance explained by the model beyond what could be obtained with only the main effects in only four of those studies.[37,39,48,64] (4) Exploratory graphical approaches examine interaction effects and thresholds (non-linear effects). For example, demands and latitude have been divided into tertiles or quartiles, and patterns of heart disease risk examined across the resulting nine[48] or 16[52] exposure cells.

Main effects often were not reported in the studies utilizing quadrant or quotient terms. (A number of studies have examined the main effects of job demands and job decision latitude, finding some significant associations.[84]) Therefore, we cannot determine whether such formulations model interaction or the sum of two main effects. In the Cornell Work Site Blood Pressure Study (WSBPS), all four formulations of job strain were significantly associated with elevated ambulatory SBP, and the quadrant term was a significant predictor of SBP controlling for the main effects of demands and latitude. However, associations with DBP and risk of mild hypertension appeared to be more appropriately modeled as the sum of two significant main effects.[64] True interaction effects frequently are difficult to detect due to a lack of statistical power.[55,83]

Thresholds.   If a population threshold exists for the effect of job strain, the proportion of subjects exceeding this threshold typically varies across nonpopulation based samples. For example, if only 10% of a given sample is experiencing "high" (biologically relevant) job strain, but 25% is classified as "high strain" using the quadrant definition, misclassification and a dilution of the effect estimate occurs. One approach for exploring possible thresholds, or nonlinear or nonmonotonic dose-response curves, is to dichotomize a continuous exposure variable at various points and plot the resulting odds ratios or mean differences.[106] In the Cornell WSBPS, a significant effect of job strain (using the demands/latitude quotient term) on work and home ambulatory BP was seen at cutpoints beginning at about the upper tertile of the distribution of job strain, and this effect increased in magnitude as the cutpoints increased. Another strategy used in the Cornell study was to define as high strain the group defined by the lowest tertile of decision latitude and the highest tertile of demands (6.5% of the sample). This group had work SBP about 10 mmHg higher than those in low demand or in high latitude groups. Using national means for decision latitude and demands to define the high strain group (8% of the sample) also resulted in larger effect sizes, 11.5 mmHg SBP and 4.1 mmHg DBP. Therefore, in this sample, there was evidence of both a threshold of effect for job strain, and increasing effects at higher levels (or "doses") above the threshold.[64]

Social Support. Workplace social support has been examined in conjunction with the job strain model in several studies of CVD. Some evidence exists for a social support main effect,[23,48] although null results also have been reported.[4,6,51,69] Some studies have found an interaction—a buffering by social support of the effects of job strain.[6,23,58,51] A third approach, used in one study with positive findings,[49] does not try to disentangle main effects and interaction, but simply hypothesizes that socially isolated, high-strain work ("iso-strain") carries the highest risk. This approach was proposed since iso-strain is a univariate measure, "a more parsimonious instrument for measuring and analyzing workplace conditions."[49]

Cumulative Exposure. In most studies, exposure to job strain was measured at only one point in time; thus, the effect of duration of exposure could not be assessed. *Current* exposure may be an inadequate measure of *cumulative* exposure since people gain skills with time and age, may be promoted, or may select out of high strain jobs. (In the U.S. QES there is evidence of an inverse association between age and job strain.) In the first 3 years of the Cornell WSBPS, test-retest reliability of the decision-latitude and job-demand scales was fairly high (both $r = 0.64$). However, 22% of participants changed their (dichotomous) job strain status in 3 years—resulting in a more than 50% turnover in the initial high-strain group. Therefore, complete work histories were collected from Cornell study participants. Six questions from the JCQ were asked about each past job held by 379 study participants. Internal consistency of the three two-item scales was high for workload demands ($\alpha = .81$), but borderline for job decision latitude ($\alpha = .62$) and workplace social support ($\alpha = .63$). Two items were added to increase the reliability of the latitude scale. Among the 255 participants who answered all four latitude items, scale reliability increased to $\alpha = .83$. In preliminary analyses, job strain during the 5 years prior to Time 1 is associated with Time 1 work and home SBP among men > 44 years of age and men with ≤ 14 years of education, independent of Time 1 job strain. For example, men > 44 years of age who report job strain at Time 1 *and* job strain during at least 3 of the 5 years prior to Time 1 have ambulatory SBP about 14 mmHg higher than men with neither exposure. The measure of job strain during the past 5 years had a modest association with Time 1 job strain (kappa = .24).

Johnson, et al., using the Swedish WOM, found that low work control, in each 5-year cumulative exposure interval over the past 25 years, was associated with significant elevations of risk of CVD mortality among Swedish men, with relative risks ranging from 1.6 to 1.8.[51] However, exposure > 25 years was not associated with increased mortality, implying an induction period of 25 years or less.

IMPUTATION OF JOB CHARACTERISTICS SCORES
by Joseph Schwartz, PhD

Many datasets contain rich health information, but lack details about subjects' job characteristics or work situation. An example is the U.S. National Health and Nutrition Examination Surveys (NHANES), which provide physical exams to large numbers of individuals, and panels of experts adjudicate individual cases with respect to the presence or absence of a variety of diseases and conditions, including MI. It would be unfortunate if there were no way to use such studies to examine the relationship of working conditions and health.

Fortunately, most large health studies do contain information on a variety of related demographic characteristics, including participants' education, employment status, occupation, and, sometimes, industrial sector. There is a long tradition in sociology of using occupation to rank individuals along a hierarchical dimension of social status or prestige.[20,24,41,42,71,90] As a result, if a survey includes information on participants' occupations, coded according to a standard classification scheme such as that used by the U.S. Census, it usually is a straightforward process to translate the occupation codes into a measure of social status. While this has been useful for addressing questions pertaining to the relationship of socioeconomic status to health or disease, it has only marginal utility for addressing questions concerning the specific factors about work that may put individuals at increased risk for cardiovascular or other diseases. The ability to infer decision latitude, psychological job demands, and other specific characteristics on the basis of occupation would be helpful.

At least four linkage systems allow assigning of scores on a variety of job characteristics to individuals on the basis of their occupations. The oldest is based on the **Dictionary of Occupational Titles** (DOT).[100,101] Department of Labor experts defined 12,099 job titles and rated each according to 44 characteristics, subdivided into seven broad categories. Three "worker functions" summarize the job's complexity with respect to data (or information), people, and things (equipment). There are two measures of the average level of training required, one for general education and the other for specialized vocational training. Eleven skill areas, ranging from general intelligence to finger dexterity, are rated in terms of the amount required to perform the job at an average level. Ten temperaments describe various characteristics of jobs that workers may have to accommodate to; these include influencing others, repetitive or continuous tasks, performing under stress, and variety or change. Jobs are also rated in terms of five bipolar "interests," identifying which of two extreme preferences that an individual might hold would be more consistent with the job; for example, a preference for abstract/creative activities versus routine/concrete/organized activities. Finally, jobs are rated with respect to physical demands (six characteristics) and physical environment (seven characteristics).

The primary goal of the DOT has always been to facilitate the matching of workers to jobs by employment offices. Spenner was the first to use the detailed job titles to estimate the average characteristics of each three-digit census occupation category and suggest that these be linked to other datasets and used for research purposes.[94] Subsequently, the DOT variables were linked into one of the U.S. Census Bureau's nationally representative Current Population Surveys (n = approximately 55,000) using detailed job titles, and then the means of the 44 job characteristics for each 1970 census occupation category were computed. Using the resulting database (available from the Inter-university Consortium for Political and Social Research), it is possible to merge the occupation means into any existing dataset containing 1970 census occupation codes. Miller, et al. provide a thorough review of the strengths and weaknesses of the DOT.[70] No one has ever investigated the ability of these scores to predict CV functioning or disease.

The second linkage system was developed by Schwartz, Karasek, and Pieper[87] and is closely related to the **Job Content Questionnaire**. Using identical, or nearly identical, questions administered to three random samples of the U.S. labor market in 1969, 1972, and 1977 (Survey of Working Conditions, 1969; Quality of Employment Surveys, 1972, 1977[80]), eight subscales were constructed. These became the core of the JCQ.[56] Pooling the three surveys resulted in combined samples of approximately 3000 men and 1500 women. After combining some of the smaller census occupational categories, occupation-level means of the subscales were estimated and linked to the National Health Interview Survey and NHANES I study.* The analyses of the linked data were the first to document an association between job strain and MI prevalence in U.S. males.[57]

The third and fourth linkage systems were developed in Sweden. The first[3] is similar to that of Schwartz, et al. Employed male respondents to a national random sample of households rated their jobs on a number of psychosocial factors, including amount of overtime, shift work, hectic or monotonous pace, influence over work pace, contact with coworkers, and opportunity to learn new things. Responses to each question were dichotomized and the percentage of positive responses in each occupational group (n = 118 occupations, based on the Nordic version of the three-digit International Standard Classification of Occupations) was determined. Occupations were then classified as either having or not having each characteristic based on whether the proportion of positive responses (from individuals in that occupation) exceeded 50%. When these dichotomous occupation scores were linked to the 1970 or 1975 occupations of a sample of individuals who were born 1911–1935 and died 1974–1976, those individuals whose occupations were classified as hectic *and* providing either little influence over work pace or lack of opportunity to learn new things were 35–45% more likely to have died from MI.

The second Swedish linkage system was developed by Johnson and colleagues.[50] Using the responses to a random sample of the employed Swedish population (n = 12,084), scales measuring work control, psychological job demands, social support, physical demands, and exposure to hazards were constructed. As in the other linkage systems, the mean score for each scale was computed for each occupation (n = 261). This system was the first to be applied to work history data to assess the relationship between CV mortality and cumulative exposure to work-related psychosocial factors; low work control, especially in combination with low workplace social support, was associated with an increased risk of CV mortality.[51] In other studies, low work control was associated with incident MI in middle-aged men[99] and in both men and women.[38] For men in the latter study, the combination of low work control, high psychological job demands, and low social support was associated with the highest risk.

Occupation-based linkage systems for imputing psychosocial work characteristics have both advantages and disadvantages relative to the more common self-report questionnaires. The ability to impute or infer work characteristics to existing

---

* A second, parallel linkage system imputes job characteristic scores using not only an individual's occupation, but also several other demographic characteristics: education, age, race-ethnicity, marital status, and whether self-employed. Scores based on the two linkage systems are highly correlated. Separate linkage systems were developed for men and women.

datasets that contain information about subjects' occupations, but little or no information about other work characteristics, is beneficial. The other major advantage is that imputed scores are much less susceptible to self-report bias. First, they are based on the average of several self-reports; thus, individual biases tend to cancel each other out.* Second since linkage systems almost always are applied to datasets other than the one from which they were generated (for an exception, see Johnson and Stewart, 1993), the individuals who provided the self-reports are not the individuals in whom the relationship between health and work characteristics is assessed. This rules out the possibility that an observed relationship is due to **reverse causation**, such that those with a particular health condition are more likely (as a consequence of their disease) to report, for example, having less decision latitude or more job demands. The primary threat to the validity of an observed association is the possibility of **self-selection**, that those at higher risk (due to nonwork-related factors) are more likely to enter particular occupations. Of course, concern about selection bias is at least as applicable to findings from self-report data as to findings based on imputed work characteristics, and the goal of both types of analysis should be to try to statistically control for those nonwork-related risk factors that might influence occupational selection.

An additional strength of these linkage systems is that they are based on moderately large (1500–3000) to very large (> 10,000) representative national samples of the labor force. The representativeness of the original samples is critical to the validity of imputing job characteristics based on the occupation means in one sample to individuals in another sample. Another factor is the sample size of each occupation. Not surprisingly, the sample means of those occupations with more individuals are more accurate estimates of the occupations' true means than are the sample means of smaller occupations; the estimated precision of each sample mean is inversely proportional to the square root of the number of individuals in the sample with that occupation. Thus, most of the linkage systems do not impute means for those occupations for which the "parent" survey has fewer than three[3,87] or five[50] incumbents. Still, those occupation means that are based on 40 individuals will be twice as precise as those based on only 10. The degree of imprecision due to sampling variability, as reflected in the standard errors of the occupation means, is comparable to unreliability in multi-item scales and limits the generalizability of the estimated occupation means when they are imputed to other samples from the same population and time period.

Equally critical is the generalizability of the occupation means to other populations, subpopulations, or cohorts. These linkage systems have not been applied outside their country of origin, but they have been applied to geographically defined subpopulations[38] and to occupations held by individuals more than a decade before or after the occupational information was collected.[51] It is not clear to what extent the average work characteristics of an occupation in the mid-1970s reflect the characteristics of that occupation in the early 1990s; certainly some occupations have gone through substantial transformation while others have remained relatively stable. This issue is particularly important when a linkage system is applied to complete work histories to estimate cumulative exposure to hypothesized putative factors. In

---

* The possibility of a collective bias (or subjective perception) in the self-reports of individuals within specific occupations, based on shared experiences, professional organizations, and perhaps culture (e.g., police, skilled trades), cannot be ruled out. Such collective biases, to the extent they exist, are likely to be reflected in the occupation means of each of the linkage systems described above.

this situation, the same work characteristics are imputed to a job regardless of whether it was held during the 1950s or the 1980s.

The DOT-based linkage system is based on expert evaluations of occupations, performed by employees of the U.S. Department of Labor, while the other three linkage systems are based on self-reports of individuals in each occupation. The latter offers greater knowledge, but potential subjectivity. The expert observer's understanding of the work situation is more superficial because it usually is based on a limited period of observation. However, experts may be in a better position to make comparative assessments of jobs/occupations, due to training and experience of observing many jobs. They may be able to apply rating scales in a more consistent fashion than a set of individuals who each rate only their own job.

Certainly the greatest disadvantage of linkage systems is that they cannot characterize any of the variability among jobs within an occupation. All individuals in the same occupation are assigned identical scores for each job characteristic. This implicitly ignores all within-occupation heterogeneity, and certainly there is substantial variability among the multitude of jobs that are aggregated into one occupational category. Some of these differences are related to the company, specific supervisor, or coworkers, and maybe even characteristics of the incumbent. For example, a given job is likely to be less psychologically demanding for someone who is highly skilled and/or has cooperation and support from coworkers.

EXPERT-OBSERVER ASSESSMENT OF JOB CHARACTERISTICS   *by Birgit A. Greiner, PhD and Niklas Krause, MD, PhD*

A growing number of studies, including longitudinal studies, consistently show associations between occupational stressors and CVD morbidity and mortality. However, it is not clear to what extent the characteristics of the job or the individual's interpretation of the job situation, based on factors such as coping strategies and personality, contribute to this association, because stressors are usually measured by self-report. To disentangle the effects of the person from the effects of the job environment, it has been suggested that stressors be measured by different methods within one study.[26,33,60,89] For example, Kristensen suggested a "triangulation strategy" for CV research using self-rated measures of each individual, average measures (all workers with the same job title are given the average values of responses provided by workers with this particular job), and independent measures of job characteristics, (e.g., assessments by external experts).[60]

To date, most studies on CVD and work stressors are based on either **individual self-ratings** of the worker, or on the **average method** as a strategy to minimize the variation caused by individual differences. Schnall, et al. report that the average method usually yields lower associations between job strain and CVD than the individual self-ratings.[84] Does the individual appraisal of stress factors contribute more to the stress-health association than the actual work conditions? Such a conclusion would be premature, since the use of average measures based on job titles introduces a methodological problem that biases the association toward the null. Most occupational titles are crude, covering not only a wide range of occupations with different stressor levels but also a wide range of organizational settings that might affect stressors within even a single, narrowly defined occupation. A third method is the use of self-reported data averaged over several workers on the level of a particular job within one company—the **shared job strain concept**.[89] Averaging individual stressor measures within only one company ensures that measures apply to the same job and the same organizational setting. This method appears especially suitable for simple, blue-collar jobs in large companies where exactly the same task exists more than once. However, this method might be difficult to apply at the white-collar level due to a lack of identical jobs within one company.

Another measurement approach to minimize variation caused by the individual is the **external assessment** of working conditions. The advantage of such measures is that they are (ideally) not confounded with the personality of the worker, and the specific organizational setting of the job, as it affects job characteristics, can be taken into account.

Methods for External Assessment of Job Characteristics

Each method has a specific strategy for measurement "objectivization," intended to minimize or eliminate distortion of job characteristic data by individuals:

1. Archival data from company or insurance records. Objectivization is achieved by the *nonreactivity* of the measurement. Bias caused by worker reactivity to the measurement is excluded. However, the interpretation of archival data is limited, because the data usually provides only crude indicators of stress factors, which often are restricted to a specific occupational group (e.g., traffic density as a measure for demands in bus drivers, or number of incoming phone calls as a measure of demands in telephone operators). Additionally, archival data usually is collected for practical rather than scientific purposes; thus quality is limited due to inconsistent coding, lack of check for data entry mistakes, and empty data fields.

2. Assessment by external experts without inspection of the individual workstation. There is presently no widely accepted method for this assessment. In studies of state employees in England, experts have rated job conditions with regard to the crucial dimensions in the demand-control model (DCM).[76] Others used expert ratings based on the U.S. Dictionary of Occupational titles.[1,70a] The measurement objectivization of this method is achieved by benefiting from the knowledge of experts over a wide range of occupations, which *minimizes personal bias*. This method has the same limitations as the average method, due to the crude definition of job titles and the variety of organizational settings.

3. Supervisor or coworker assessments of individual jobs. Objectivization results from relying on the direct experience of supervisors and coworkers.[5,76,93,108] In this method, supervisors and colleagues serve as *quasi-observers* of *day-to-day working conditions*. The validity and reliability of such measures might be highly dependent on the closeness of the supervisors and colleagues to their subordinates and coworkers and their familiarity with the jobs to be rated. For example, North, et al. reported only moderate agreement between two supervisors rating the same job who were not the immediate supervisors.[76]

4. Worksite observations conducted by trained observers. This assessment occurs during regular working hours in the tradition of job analysis.[46] Actual job behaviors and working conditions are measured in *real time*, rather than retrospectively as in self-report. Observations can provide detailed quantitative and qualitative information about individual work tasks within different organizational settings, thereby allowing description of those workplace factors requiring modification to reduce stressors. Limitations of this method include nonobservability of mental processes; the restricted observation period, which makes the identification of rare events difficult; and the temptation for observers to base their ratings on worker behavior rather than on characteristics of the environment.[26]

Regardless of these potential biases, the interpretation of any type of expert rating is limited if different experts do not refer to the same concept about stress factors, but instead apply their individual concepts. If they do not have a mutual underlying theory, the same measurement problem that affects self-reports is transferred from the worker to the expert.

5. Theory-guided observational interview. This is a variation of worksite observation that might minimize bias.[77] It is performed at the worksite by an analyst who is trained in the application of the theoretical framework. (We avoid the term "observer" because the observational interview consists of more than just observation.) The analyst is the agent of the measurement objectivization by serving as a "translator" for observations and self-reports, and theory and definitions. Questions of the instrument are worded in expert language and addressed toward the analyst. The advantage of expert language, versus colloquial language used in self-reports, is that it can be more precise and can minimize subjective interpretation of the analyst. In theory-guided interviews, analysts are not restricted to obtain the necessary information by worksite observation only, but also can use self-reports and archival data (e.g., work schedules). In this method, the strength of *observational techniques* (real-time assessment) and *structured interviews* (worker as the expert of his/her job) and the advantage of *archival measures* (nonreactivity of measurement) can be combined. Observational interviews can gather information that is not available by observation alone, and information that is likely to be missed during the observational period (rare events) can be included in the analysis.

There is no commonly agreed upon procedure, and only a few theory-guided observational instruments have been developed and validated in epidemiologic studies with explicit health outcomes. One challenge for the development of these instruments is their applicability to a range of different occupations. This goal excludes the use of simple stressor event checklists, which usually are applicable only to narrowly defined occupational groups. Instead it requires the use of theoretical concepts that allow for a common definition of stress factors in a range of different jobs.

Theory-guided interviews have been used in CV research.[30,95] The job analysis instrument RHIA/VERA, used in a multimethod approach in CVD research[30] and in studies with other health outcomes,[32–34,61,65,68] is described on the following pages.

The Theory-Guided Observational Instrument RHIA/VERA

There are two tested versions of this instrument in German—one for blue-collar work[67] and one for white-collar work[66]—and an English version for the assessment of job characteristics in transit driving jobs.[31] Currently, a shortened version of the RHIA/VERA method is being used to assess the job characteristics of a subsample of the Whitehall Study.[29] Interrater reliability coefficients are very good for most dimensions.[33,34,66,67]

Theoretical Basis and Definitions

The theoretical basis is Action Regulation Theory. This theory conceptualizes psychological processes important for human action, such as planning, thinking, deciding, and motor regulation, in interaction with the environment.[25,35,36,102] Applied to the work situation, the unit of analysis is not the individual worker but the task—more precisely, the **mental structure of the work task**. This structure comprises the mentally regulated operations by which the worker carries out a job.

Two main dimensions for the analysis of work are assessed: level of requirements for skill utilization and work hindrances. The model conceptualizes hindrances as factors that potentially impair health, whereas high levels of skill utilization promote health and personality development.[19] Studies using the RHIA/VERA instrument show that hindrances are associated with impaired physical health or health complaints, whereas skill utilization is more strongly associated with mental health and active leisure-time activities.[65,68]

The **level of requirements for skill utilization** is defined as the degree of independent thinking, planning, and decision-making that is required from the worker to carry out the task. The instrument includes a 10-level scale with defined categories (Table 3). The lowest level of skill utilization is the application of preset rules without any latitude for independent thinking or planning. Medium levels require one or more decisions of the worker; high levels include complex strategy decisions that affect other workers. To categorize the task into one of these levels, the analyst has to become familiar with the content of the task as a first step of the analysis.

Hindrances (or stressors), the second main dimension, are defined as characteristics of the work task that hinder the action regulation processes due to poor technical or organizational design. The underlying cause of stressors is seen in restrictions of worker control, or "partialized" work.[77] Conditions are not considered stress factors if workers have the control to remove the hindrance so that it will not reappear in the future. Subdimensions of hindrance include work barriers, time pressure (a measure of the work pace), time binding (a measure of worker control over time handling), and monotonous conditions.[34] The main subdimension is *work bar-*

TABLE 3. Synopsis from RHIA/VERA Instrument for White-Collar Work: Levels of Skill Utilization

	Level 5 Introduction of New Work Processes
5	The worker is responsible for organizing conditions for the introduction of new work processes. Existing work processes *have to be combined* in a new way.
5R	The worker is responsible for organizing conditions for the introduction of new work processes. Existing work processes *are not changed* in a major way.
	Level 4 Coordination of Work Areas
4	The worker has to make at least two *strategy decisions* in areas of others and has to coordinate them.
4R	The worker has to make at least two strategy decisions and take strategy decisions in work areas of others into account without changing them.
	Level 3 Strategy Decision
3	The worker has to make *one strategy decision*, that is a plan about what needs to be decided. From there it is clear what needs to be done next.
3R	The worker has to make *more than one decision* within one work assignment.
	Level 2 Decision
2	Before or during the processing of an assignment the worker has to make *one decision*.
2R	It is necessary to *visualize* the work procedure before starting or during executing the assignment.
	Level 1 Rule Application
1	For processing of the assignment the *recognition* of the externally determined procedure is necessary.
1R	The assignments are always done in the same way with the same work means. The procedure is *fully externally determined*.

From Greiner B: Work analysis instrument to measure objective work stressors and skill utilization in white-collar work: RHIA-VERA, shortened version. (Original version by Leitner K, Lueders E, Greiner B, et al, Technical University of Berlin, 1993.) Translated from the German, edited, and revised by B. Greiner. Greifswald, University of Greifswald, 1999.

riers, defined as obstacles that hinder work performance. Barriers create a dilemma for the worker: the worker is required to perform the job a certain way, but the technical or organizational design of the job impedes performance. If this dilemma is associated with objective negative consequences for the worker, such as extra work or unsafe behavior, then, by definition, work barriers constitute a stressor. Barriers can be caused by technical or ergonomic problems, lack of tools or supplies, difficulties regarding the flow of work information, environmental factors, and organizational problems. These problems are not considered stressors if the worker is given partial or full control over them by the company, (for example, if the worker is explicitly allowed to lower the quality of work or to postpone deadlines without additional effort when the problem is present).

OVERLAP WITH THE DEMAND/CONTROL MODEL

Although based on a different theoretical background, the stressor dimensions described above overlap with the dimensions of the DCM. Barriers correspond with the "high-strain quadrant" in the DCM. They are conceptualized as work obstacles that require extra work and, therefore, put additional demands on the worker without the opportunity for efficient control. In contrast to the DCM, demands and control are not documented as two distinct dimensions in the assessment of barriers. Instead, the analyst evaluates each demand that could potentially constitute a barrier whether or not the specific demand can be controlled efficiently. In this way, the contextual factors that restrict control can be determined and described on a highly detailed level, helpful for job redesign. The concept of time pressure is comparable to the demand concept, especially to the aspect of work pace.

Thus, the RHIA/VERA approach provides a more differentiated picture than the Job Content Questionnaire via two dimensions: work barriers, as high demands that are posed on the worker due to work obstacles, time pressure, as a measure of work intensity under regular conditions due to an excessive amount of work per time unit. The dimension of skill utilization corresponds to the "learning axis" in the DCM that assumes a learning and personality development potential for the worker if he or she does work with high latitude.[54]

MEASURES OBTAINED

The analysis results in five quantitative measures.[34] Three measures reflect absolute numbers expressed in minutes per working day or week (work barriers as summary measures of extra work minutes spent to compensate for the obstacle, time pressure in minutes of detachment time, monotony in minutes of presence of this condition). Two measures are derived from scales with defined categories (time binding on a five-level scale, skill utilization on a 10-level scale). Rating scales (e.g., Likert scales) are not used to minimize the bias of subjective interpretation of the analyst. Furthermore, a detailed description of the task, stress factors, and skill utilization factors, and suggestions for work redesign to reduce stress (e.g., by increasing the decision latitude or other organizational solutions) are obtained.

PROCEDURE: THREE-PHASE MODEL TO OBSERVATIONAL INTERVIEW

The RHIA/VERA job analysis instrument provides the analyst with a protocol for interview and observation that includes definitions of work stressors and skill utilization, stressor classification, and stressor and skill utilization evaluation and quantification (Table 4). (1) In the **descriptive phase**, the observer describes in detail the required work result and work steps to achieve the result, including motor

TABLE 4. Three-Phase Assessment Model of the RHIA/VERA Procedure

Phase	Part of the Instrument	Function
1: Orientation		**Describe task, contrast with available resources**
	Work result: describe expected quantity and quality standards of work result; observed deviations from standards	Deviations from expected standards might indicate stress factors (time pressure or work barriers)
	Work means (resources): describe equipment, machinery, tools, technology, and work information used to accomplish task; use of resources	Contrast expected work result with available resources; determine potential barriers related to lack of resources
	Work context: count and describe potential barriers due to interruptions	Potential barriers are tested later in analysis—whether they are "true" barriers
	Work steps: describe sequence of steps necessary to accomplish task	Describe mental structure of task to determine stress factors and skill level
2: Reflection		**Detach from worker, objectify information, develop focus points**
	Identify missing or contradictory information: summarize information obtained during Phase 1	Helps analyst focus observational interview in evaluative phase and probe worker
	Indications for stressors: follow guidelines to formulate hypotheses about potential stress factors for each work step (tested in Phase 3)	Specific hypotheses about potential stress factors help analyst focus observation
3: Evaluation		**Describe and quantify stress factors and skill utilization; suggest work redesign**
	Skill utilization: definitions of levels and standardized questions for classification	Classification of task into one of 10 sub-levels
	Classification of barriers: provides definitions of different types	Potential barriers classified
	Barrier test: standardized questions to determine whether potential stress factors are "true" stress factors	Potential barriers rated if are barriers according to theoretical definition
	Summary of barriers: procedure to describe barriers and potential technical/organizational solutions, and to estimate frequency of barrier and duration of extra work	Description and quantification of barriers
	Time-binding: rating based on observed (and archival) information on a five-level scale	Quantification of time-binding
	Monotonous working conditions: standardized questions to determine whether monotonous conditions exist; for how long during task performance	Quantification of exposure to monotonous working conditions
	Time pressure: detachment periods are subtotaled; time saved by neglecting safety and quality standards and working overtime is subtracted	Quantification of time pressure

processes as well as decision and thinking processes (mental structure of the task). This is contrasted with a description of provided resources to achieve the result—such as hardware, software, machines, tools, and access to necessary information—and with contextual factors that might interfere with task performance, such as interruptions by persons and phone calls. (2) In the **reflective phase**, the information obtained by observation and interview is objectified. This requires the analyst to detach from the social situation with the worker by interrupting the observation for 30–60 minutes. During this period the analyst reflects on the obtained information, "translates" it into the concepts and definitions given in the observer manual, determines the missing pieces of information still to be gathered, and evaluates if the task can be done in the required way considering the available resources and the contextual situation. At the end of this phase, the analyst develops hypotheses about concrete stress factors to focus additional observations and questions. (3) In the **evaluative phase**, the analyst identifies, describes, and quantifies the hindrances and skill utilization factors. Discordance between observed and self-reported information may need to be probed and dissolved during the evaluative phase.

Multi-Method Approach in CVD Research

The RHIA/VERA method was used together with self-report measures in a study of hypertension in urban transit operators in San Francisco.[30,34] This occupational group is particularly interesting for studies on stress and BP for two reasons: they are a high-risk group for CVD morbidity and mortality,[58,81] and there have been several unexplained results in this group. For example, Netterstrom and Suadicani reported an excess risk of IHD for bus drivers in Denmark with low exhaustion and high job satisfaction and drivers who reported high variation in their job,[75] and Winkleby found an inverse association between self-reported stress and hypertension in the same San Francisco transit operator population.[109] (These unexplained findings have been attributed to possible distortions due to the use of self-report stressor measures. One potential explanation might be that individuals who cope with stress by denial underestimate stress factors. These individuals might be at high risk for hypertension.)

For a subsample of the San Francisco Transit Operator Health and Safety Study (SFTOS), a multimethod design was applied that included both self-report (perceived strain; stress factors) and job characteristics (stress factors) assessed by observational interview. The externally assessed measures were averaged on the level of the transit line across individuals, and self-report strain and stress factors were used on the level of the individual and on the level of line-specific average measures. There was a significant gradient between externally assessed barriers and hypertension and between externally assessed time pressure and hypertension after adjusting for several potential confounders.[30] This finding suggests validity of the externally assessed measures. Neither of the self-report measures (strain and stress) predicted hypertension. Averaging self-report measures for identical jobs (in this case identical transit lines) to cancel out individual variation did not substantially improve the association to the health outcome. The hypothesis that individuals who rate high on the externally assessed stress factors but low on self-report stress factors (possibly due to denial) were at the highest risk for hypertension was not confirmed. However, the sample size available to test this interaction was small.

Four general methodological issues can be researched with such a multimethod study. The first issue concerns the association between self-report stressor measures and externally assessed measures. In the SFTOS, associations between the externally assessed and self-report measures were low to moderate. Similar results were reported by others using supervisor ratings[5,76] or observational data.[89,110] This might indicate that both general measurement approaches capture different aspects of stress factors, particularly for demands. The correspondence between the expert-rated or imputed assessment and the self-reported estimate of different aspects of psychological demands usually is poorer than the correspondence for decision latitude.[76,88,99] In a study that used expert ratings (determined by an occupational healthcare team) of 4000 employees in several companies in Stockholm, the correspondence between expert ratings and self-reports was highest for decision latitude; the self-reports explained approximately 30–40% of the variation in the expert ratings.[40] Zapf differentiated between job characteristics that are more or less observable, dependent on one's own affective reaction, and stable over time.[99]

The second issue concerns the pattern of associations between stressor measures and the health outcome. If only externally assessed measures are associated with the outcome, questions about the validity of the self-reports can be raised. Alternatively, such a finding might indicate that both measurement approaches capture different, valid aspects of stressors, and that the aspect assessed by external measures is truly associated with the outcome. The reverse might be true, if only self-report measures predict the health outcome. A finding of both measures predicting the outcome independently, e.g., in a common regression model, suggests that both are describing different aspects of stressors and each one is important for the outcome. For example, in the Whitehall Study, both supervisor ratings and self-reports of low job control predicted new events of CHD[14] and sick leave rate.[76]

The third issue concerns individual variation in self-reports and expert assessments. If measures are confounded by individual perception of the worker, stressor measures averaged over the same job should be more predictive than individual measures. In a study of German blue-collar workers, the concept of "shared job strain" as a latent variable was introduced.[89] Shared job strain comprises symptoms that two workers with the same job have in common. If they share some variance, then the common aspect lies in the job. Job stressors were estimated by self-reports of two workers and two independent observers as indicators. In this study, the importance of "objective" job stressors was confirmed. Four job stressors explained two-thirds of the variance of shared job strain, whereas the trait model, which included individual worker variation, was not as predictive.

The fourth issue concerns the importance of measuring different concepts of stress with the same method. Stress can be either conceptualized as a "stress factor" (the environmental source of stress), or as "strain," understood here as perception of the severity of the stress factor. The concept more predictive of health outcome can be determined by holding the assessment method constant.

APPLICABILITY OF MULTIMETHOD APPROACHES

Several questions can be addressed by the parallel use of self-report and observational measures. The choice of the most suitable method for the external assessment of job characteristics—archival data, expert ratings, or observational interviews—depends on the research question, the nature of the job, and the sample. Observational interviews are time-consuming, and their use is recommended specifically for the following:

1. Researchers who are concerned about the validity of their self-report data and want to validate these data by contrasting them with other measures.[89] New information about work demands that are difficult to capture by self-reports is particularly helpful.[110] Validation by observational interview also may be necessary when social stereotypes about the stressfulness of particular jobs are likely to distort self-reports and coworker and supervisor ratings.

2. In studies with health outcomes potentially caused by repressive coping and denial (e.g., hypertension, alcohol abuse). Valid ratings for job characteristics might not be obtainable by self-reports from individuals with predominantly repressive coping. Comparing observational with self-report data and analyzing individuals with high discordance between the two can be interesting.

3. In companies with a large number of equal work tasks. One or two observational interviews can be conducted per work task and the same value assigned to all workers with identical jobs. In this way, the sample size can be increased greatly with just a few interviews.

4. For studies about occupational grade level and CV health. The skill utilization dimension provides a highly reliable measure of the skill level objectively required for carrying out the job and of the learning potential provided by the job. Mismatches between the worker's skills and the required skill level can be determined.

5. If researchers want detailed analyses of potential organizational and technical causes of stress factors for intervention purposes. Observational interviews expand upon information obtained by questionnaire and provide a basis for job redesign strategies.

CONCLUSIONS AND RECOMMENDATIONS   *by Paul Landsbergis, PhD, Birgit Greiner, PhD, Niklas Krause, MD, PhD, Joseph Schwartz, PhD, and Töres Theorell, MD, PhD*

It is important to determine whether it is primarily the objective characteristics of jobs or workers' subjective perceptions and evaluations of them (or both) that are most predictive of changes in BP or the development of CVD. This determination would allow more precise and valid theory and measurement, improving estimation not only of magnitude of effect, but also interaction, thresholds of effect, cumulative exposure, and induction periods—estimates which generally have had limited statistical power.

Self-report questionnaires tend to be inexpensive and easy to administer. When national occupational survey data is available, comparisons can be made between study participants and national averages of job characteristics by job title. Questionnaire limitations include the possibility of self-report bias, difficulties due to low literacy, and problems of transcultural validation (e.g., translation into the participants' native language). We recommend supplementing generic job stressor questionnaires with questions specific to the occupation(s) and target groups being studied. Specific data is particularly useful for intervention research and communicating study findings to participants. When study participants have identical job titles and the same employer, self-report measures averaged across that job title may reduce the likelihood of self-report bias.

Imputation of job characteristics scores does not suffer from the same problems as self reports, and they can be used in studies containing information on an individual's occupation but no details of work characteristics. The limitations of this method include the loss of within-occupation variability in work characteristics, the lack of precision of occupation means for small occupations, and the questionable generality of the occupation scores to subpopulations and other time periods.

External assessment of job characteristics can be time-consuming and expensive to conduct; however, this method is valuable in certain situations (see pages 182–183).

In general, we recommend multimethod strategies—convergent validation using as many of these approaches as possible. A number of important issues remain to be resolved through future research:

1. Assessment methods that integrate self-reported stressors with objective features of the job, such as the OSI, require further development and testing.[10]

2. The constructs of job demands and job control may require expansion to improve prediction of CVD, hypertension, and other health outcomes. Adding a measure of organizational influence to the task-level decision-latitude variable produced a stronger association with hypertension due to job strain in the Cornell study.[64] To what extent is "low job security and limited career opportunities" an important risk factor beyond task-level or even organizational level control, as suggested by the Whitehall study?[14] To what extent is control exercised collectively as important as individually exercised control in reducing job strain and CVD risk?[47] Similarly, is CVD risk associated with various alternative conceptualizations of psychological job demands, such as problem-solving, monitoring or emotional demands, or threat/disaster potential? Valid instruments are needed to measure global systems of work organization, such as lean production, and to apply to economically underdeveloped areas of the world. These factors can have dramatic effects on job characteristics.[62]

3. To what extent are current questionnaires valid for service occupations, women, ethnic minorities, older workers, and conditions of downsizing and new work systems?[43] The JCQ and other job stressor questionnaires need to be further tested in different populations, particularly non-Northern European racial/ethnic groups.

4. Periodic, detailed occupational surveys (such as the Quality of Employment Surveys) in the U.S., similar to those being conducted in Europe, are needed to determine job characteristics' time trends and current occupational averages.

5. Are certain survey or expert observer methods (or job stressor models) more predictive of certain health outcomes (e.g., CVD, work-related musculoskeletal disorders, or psychological strain outcomes) than others?

6. Are there differences in validity of external assessment and self-report assessment for different dimensions of job characteristics?

7. Do psychological constructs such as denial or repressive coping help to explain paradoxical results in stress research?[109] Does contrasting externally assessed measures with self-report measures and studying inconsistencies between the two on the level of the individual help to shed light on the role of repressive coping?

8. Are expert observer methods applied and used in cooperation with management and employees toward the goals of stress reduction and increased skill utilization,[103] or are they used predominantly to increase productivity?

9. How much do qualitative assessment methods (e.g., focus groups, interviews, and ethnographic observation), in conjunction with quantitative methods, improve our understanding of the social context of stress in a particular workplace and help us conduct and evaluate interventions?[73,78] Standardized interviews may better explore the objective components of psychological demands, decision latitude, and social support at work.[105] Qualitative assessment, especially in intervention studies, allows researchers to learn from employees about the context of stress, helps insure dissemination of results, and serves educational purposes for all participants.

10. To what degree can both employees and management be included in the development of assessment methods, and support the collection and interpretation of data?[44] Researchers have to maintain scientific standards in their study, but if studies are to lead to positive change in the workplace, employees and management must be involved. How can the balance between science and practical application be maintained?

REFERENCES

1. Adelmann P: Occupational complexity, control, and personal income: The relation to psychological well-being in men and women. J Appl Psychol 72:529–537, 1987.
2. Ahlberg-Hulten G: Psychological demands and decision latitude within healthcare work. Academic thesis. Stockholm, Sweden, Karolinska Institutet, 1999.
3. Alfredsson L, Karasek R, Theorell T: Myocardial infarction risk and psychosocial work environment: An analysis of the male Swedish working force. Soc Sci Med 16:463–467, 1982.
4. Alfredsson L, Spetz C, Theorell T: Type of occupation and near-future hospitalization for myocardial infarction and some other diagnoses. Int J Epidemiol 14:378–388, 1985.
5. Algera JA: "Objective" and perceived task characteristics as a determinant of reactions by task performers. J Occup Psychol 56:95–107, 1983.
6. Astrand NE, Hanson BS, Isacsson SO: Job demands, job decision latitude, job support, and social network factors as predictors of mortality in a Swedish pulp and paper company. Br J Ind Med 46:334–340, 1989.
7. Baker D: Occupational stress. In Levy BS, Wegman DH (eds): Occupational Health. Boston, Little, Brown & Co., 1995, pp 381–406.
8. Belkic K: Psychosocial triggers of myocardial ischemia in women. Research Report to the Swedish Medical Research Council, 1995b.
9. Belkic K, Emdad R, Theorell T, et al: Neurocardiac mechanisms of heart disease risk among professional drivers. Final report. Stockholm, Swedish Fund for Working Life, 1996.
10. Belkic K, Savic C, Theorell T, Cizinsky S: Work Stressors and Cardiovascular Risk: Assessment for Clinical Practice. Part I. Stockholm, National Institute for Psychosocial Factors and Health. Section for Stress Research, Karolinska Institute, WHO Psychosocial Center, 1995a.
11. Belkic K, Savic C, Theorell T, et al: Mechanisms of cardiac risk among professional drivers. Scand J Work Environ Health 20:73–86, 1994.
12. Borg V, Kristensen TG: Measurement of psychological job demands in the national Danish psychosocial study. Work, Stress, and Health '99. Baltimore, MD, 1999.
13. Bosma H, Marmot MG, Hemingway H, et al: Low job control and risk of coronary heart disease in Whitehall II (prospective cohort) study. Br Med J 314:558–565, 1997.
14. Bosma H, Stansfeld SA, Marmot MG: Job control, personal characteristics, and heart disease. J Occup Health Psychol 3:402–409, 1998.
15. Caplan RD, Cobb S, French JRP Jr, et al: Job demands and worker health. Pub. No. 75-168. Cincinnati, National Institute for Occupational Safety and Health, 1975.
16. Checkoway H, Pearce NE, Crawford-Brown DJ: Research Methods in Occupational Epidemiology. New York, Oxford University Press, 1989.
17. de Jonge J, Mulder MJGP, Nijhuis FJN: The incorporatio of different demand concepts in the job demand-control model: Effects on healthcare professionals. Soc Sci Med 48:1149–1160, 1999.
18. DiNardi SR: The occupational environment—its evaluation and control. Fairfax, VA American Industrial Hygiene Association, 1997.
19. Ducki A, Greiner B: Gesundheit als Entwicklung von Handlungsfahigeit - Ein "arbeitspsychologischer Baustein" zu einem allgemeinen. Gesundheitsmodell, Zeitchrift fur Arbeits - und Organisationsspycholgie 36:184–189, 1992.
20. Duncan PD: A socioeconomic index for all occupations. In Reiss AJ Jr (ed): Occupations and Social Status. New York, Free Press, 1961.
21. Emdad R, Belkic K, Theorell T, Cizinsky S: What prevents professional drivers from following physicians' cardiologic advice? Psychoth Psychosom 67:226–240, 1998.
22. Emdad R, Belkic K, Theorell T, et al: Work environment, neurophysiologic and psychophysiologic models among professional drivers with and without cardiovascular disease: Seeking an integrative neurocardiologic approach. Stress Med 13:7–21, 1997.
23. Falk A, Hanson BS, Isacsson SO, Ostergren PO: Job strain and mortality in elderly men: Social networks, support, and influence as buffers. Am J Public Health 82:1136–1139, 1992.
24. Featherman DL, Sobel M, Dickins D: A manual for coding occupations and industries into detailed 1970 categories and a listing of 1970-basis Duncan socio-economic scores. Working Paper 75-1. Madison, University of Wisconsin, Center for Demography and Ecology, 1975.
25. Frese M, Zapf D: Action as the core of work psychology: A German approach. In Triandis HC, Dunette MD, Hough LM (eds): Handbook of Industrial and Organizational Psychology. Palo Alto, CA, Consulting Psychologists Press, 1994, pp 183–224.
26. Frese M, Zapf D, Methological issues in the study of work stress: Objective vs. subjective measurement of work stress and the question of longitudinal studies. In Cooper CL, Payne R (eds): Causes, Coping, and Consequences of Stress at Work. New York, Wiley, 1988, pp 375–411.
27. Gray-Toft P, Anderson TG: The nursing stress scale: Development of an instrument. J Behav Assess 3:11–23, 1981.
28. Greiner B: Objective stress factors and task requirements in blue-collar and white-collar work: Example from Germany. Stress in the 90's: A changing workforce in a changing workplace. Washington, DC, American Psychological Association and the National Institute for Occupational Safety and Health, 1992.
29. Greiner B: Work analysis instrument to measure objective work stressors and skill utilization in white-collar work: RHIA-VERA, shortened version. (Original version by Leitner K, Leuders E, Greiner B, et al, Technical University of Berlin, 1993.) Greifswald, University of Greifswald, 1999.
30. Greiner BA: Contrasting objective and subjective measures of stress in regard to hypertension. Tel Aviv, Israel, Second International Conference on Work Environment and Cardiovascular Diseases, 1998.

31. Greiner BA: Instrument to determine occupational stress in transit driving tasks: Observer manual and response sheets. Unpublished, 1993.

32. Greiner BA, Krause N, Ragland DR, Fisher J: Objective stress factors, accidents, and absenteesim in transit operators: A theoretical framework and empirical evidence. J Occup Health Psychol 3:130–146, 1998.

33. Greiner BA, Leitner K: Assessment of job stress: The RHIA instrument. In Landau K, Rohmert W (eds): Recent Developments in Work Analysis. Philadelphia, Taylor & Francis, 1989, pp 53–66.

34. Greiner BA, Ragland DR, Krause N, et al: Objective measurement of occupational stress factors—An example with San Francisco urban transit operators. J Occup Health Psychol 2:325–342, 1997.

35. Hacker W: Action Regulation Theory and occupational psychology. Review of German empirical research since 1987. German J Psychol 18:91–120, 1994.

36. Hacker W: Activity: A fruitful concept in industrial psychology. In Frese M, Sabini J (eds): Goal Directed Behavior: The Concept of Action in Psychology. Hillsdale, Erlbaum, 1985, pp 262–284.

37. Hallqvist J, Diderischsen F, Theorell T, et al: Is the effect of job strain on myocardial infarction due to interaction between high psychological demands and low decision latitude? Results from Stockholm Heart Epidemiology Program (SHEEP). Soc Sci Med 46:1405–1415, 1998.

38. Hammar N, Alfredsson L, Johnson JV: Job strain, social support at work, and incidence of myocardial infarction. Occup Environ Med 55:548–553, 1998.

39. Haratani T, Kawakami N, Araki S: Job stress and cardiovascular risk factors in a Japanese working population. Cincinnati, OH, 9th International Symposium on Epidemiology in Occupational Health. 1992.

40. Hasselhorn HM, Hammar N, Alfredsson L, et al: Differences in the impact of self-rated and externally-rated job strain on risk factors for coronary heart disease. Work Stress and Health: Organization of work in a global economy. Baltimore, APA and NIOSH, 1998.

41. Hollingshead AB: Two-Factor Index of Social Position. New Haven, (privately printed), 1957.

42. Hollingshead AB: Four-Factor Index of Social Status. New Haven, Yale University, 1975.

43. Hurrell JJ, Nelson DL, Simmons BL: Measuring job stressors and strains: Where we have been, where we are, and where we need to go. J Occup Health Psychol 3:368–389, 1998.

44. Israel BA, Schurman SJ, House JS: Action research on occupational stress: Involving workers as researchers. Int J Health Services 19:135–155, 1989.

45. Jackson PR, Wall TD, Martin R, Davids K: New measures of job control, cognitive demand, and production responsibility. J Appl Psychol 78:753–762, 1993.

46. Jenkins GC, Nadler DA, et al: Standardized observations: An approach to measuring the nature of jobs. J Appl Psychol 60:171–181, 1975.

47. Johnson JV: Collective control: Strategies for survival in the workplace. Int J Health Services 19:469–480, 1989.

48. Johnson JV, Hall EM: Job strain, workplace social support, and cardiovascular disease: A cross-sectional study of a random sample of the Swedish working population. Am J Public Health 78:1336–1342, 1988.

49. Johnson JV, Hall EM, Theorell T: Combined effects of job strain and social isolation on cardiovascular disease morbidity and mortality in a random sample of the Swedish male working population. Scand J Work Environ Health 15:271–279, 1989.

50. Johnson JV, Stewart W: Measuring work organization exposure over the life course with a job-exposure matrix. Scand J Work Environ Health 19:21–28, 1993.

51. Johnson JV, Stewart W, Hall EM, et al: Long-term psychosocial work environment and cardiovascular mortality among Swedish men. Am J Public Health 86:324–331, 1996.

52. Karasek R, Baker D, Marxer F, et al: Job decision latitude, job demands, and cardiovascular disease: A prospective study of Swedish men. Am J Public Health 71:694–705, 1981.

53. Karasek R, Brisson C, Kawakami N, et al: The Job Content Questionnaire: An instrument for internationally comparative assessments of psychosocial job characteristics. J Occup Health Psychol 3:322–355, 1998.

54. Karasek R, Theorell T: Healthy Work: Stress, Productivity, and the Reconstruction of Working Life. New York, Basic Books, 1990.

55. Karasek RA: Control in the workplace and its health-related aspects. In Sauter SL, Hurrell JJ, Cooper CL (eds): Job Control and Work Health. New York, Wiley, 1989, pp 129–159.

56. Karasek RA, Gordon G, Pietroskovsky C, et al: Job Content Instrument: Questionnaire and User's Guide. Los Angeles/Lowell, MA, University of Southern California/University of Massachusetts, 1985.

57. Karasek RA, Theorell T, Schwartz JE, et al: Job characteristics in relation to the prevalence of myocardial infarction in the U.S. Health Examination Survey and the Health and Nutrition Examination Survey. Am J Public Health 78:910–918, 1988.

58. Kompier MAJ, di Martino V: Review of bus drivers' occupational stress and stress prevention. Stress Med 11:253–262, 1995.

59. Krause N, Ragland DR, Greiner BA, et al: Psychosocial job factors associated with back and neck pain in public transit operators. Scand J Work Environ Health 23:179–186, 1997.

60. Kristensen TS: The demand-control-support model: Methodological challenges for future research. Stress Med 11:17–26, 1995.

61. Laflamme L, Friedrich P: Patterns in tasks demands and in occupational accidents: A relationship investigated in the Swedish sawmill industry. Solna, Sweden, National Institute of Occupational Health (Arbetsmiljoeinstitutet), Division of Social and Organizational Psychology, 1993.

62. Landsbergis PA, Cahill J, Schnall P: The impact of lean production and related new systems of work organization on worker health. J Occup Health Psychol 4:108–130, 1999.

63. Landsbergis PA, Schnall PL, Deitz D, et al: The patterning of psychological attributes and distress by "job strain" and social support in a sample of working men. J Behav Med 15:379–405, 1992.

64. Landsbergis PA, Schnall PL, Warren K, et al: Association between ambulatory blood pressure and alternative formulations of job strain. Scand J Work Environ Health 20:349–363, 1994.
65. Leitner K: Auswirkungen von Arbeitsbedingungen auf die psychosoziale Gesundheit. Zeitschrift fuer Arbeitswissenchaft 2:98–108, 1993.
66. Leitner K, Lueders E, et al: Analyse psychischer Anforderungen und Belastungen in der Bueroarbeit. Das Rhia/Vera Buero-Verfahren. Goettingen, Hoegrefe, 1993b.
67. Leitner K, Volpert W, et al: Analyse psychischer Belastung in der Arbeit. Das RHIA-Verfahren und Handbuch. Koeln, TUEV Rheinland, 1987.
68. Lueders E: Die intergrierte Analyse gesundheitsforderlicher und-beeintraechtigender Merkmale von Arbeitsbedingungen mit dem RHIA/VERA-Buero-Verfahren. Zeitschrift fuer Arbeitswissenchaften 48:36–43, 1994.
69. Marmot MG, Bosma H, Hemingway H, et al: Contribution of job control and other risk factors to social variations in coronary heart disease incidence. Lancet 350:235–239, 1997.
70. Miller AR, Treiman DJ, Cain PS, Roos PA: Work, Jobs, and Occupations: A Critical Review of the Dictionary of Occupational Titles. Washington DC, National Academy Press, 1980.
70a. Muntaner C, Nieto FJ, Cooper L, et al: Work organization and atherosclerosis: Findings from the ARIC study. Atherosclerosis Risk in Communities. Am J Prev Med 14:9–18, 1998.
71. Nam CB, Terie EW: 1980-Based Nam-Powers occupational status scores. Working Paper Series 88-48, Center for the Study of Population, Florida State University, 1988.
72. National Institute for Occupational Safety and Health: NIOSH generic job stress questionniare. Cincinnati, NIOSH, 1997.
73. Neale MS, Singer JA, Schwartz GE: A systems assessment of occupational stress: Evaluating a hotel during contract negotiations. In Riley AW, Zaccaro SJ (eds): Occupational Stress and Organizational Effectiveness. New York, Praeger, 1987, pp 167–203.
74. Netterstrom B, Kristensen TS, et al: Angina pectoris, job strain, and social issues: A cross-sectional study of employed urban citizens. Int J Behav Med 5:312–322, 1998.
75. Netterstrom B, Suadicani P: Self-assessed job satisfaction and ischemic heart disease mortality: A 10-year followup of urban bus drivers. Int J Epidemiol 22:51–56, 1993.
76. North FM, Syme L, Feeney A, et al: Psychosocial work environment and sickness absence among British civil servants: The Whitehall II Study. Am J Public Health 86:332–340, 1996.
77. Oesterreich R, Volpert W: Task analysis for work design on basis of action regulation theory. Economic and Industrial Democracy 7:503–527, 1986.
78. Patton MQ: How to Use Qualitative Methods in Evaluation. Newbury Park, Sage, 1987.
79. Peter R: Comparative analysis of the effort-reward embalance model and the job strain model: Preliminary results from a Swedish case-control study. Socioeconomic variations in cardiovascular disease in Europe: The impact of the work environment and lifestyle (The Heart at Work Network). London, University College of London, Department of Epidemiology and Public Health, 1997, pp 102–104.
80. Quinn R, Staines G: The 1977 Quality of Employment Survey. Descriptive statistics with comparison data from the 1969–70 and 1972–73 surveys. Ann Arbor, Survey Research Center, Institute for Social Research, 1979.
81. Ragland D, Winkelby MA, Schwalbe J, et al: Prevalence of hypertension in bus drivers. Int J Epidemiol 16:208–214, 1987.
82. Rothenbacher D, Peter R, Bode G, et al: Dyspepsia in relation to *Heliobacter pylori* infection and psychosocial work stress in white collar employees. Am J Gastroenterol 93:1443–1449, 1998.
83. Rothman KJ, Greenland S: Modern Epidemiology. Philadelphia, Lippincott-Raven, 1998.
84. Schnall PL, Landsbergis PA, Baker D: Job strain and cardiovascular disease. Annu Rev Public Health 15:381–411, 1994.
85. Schonfeld I: Psychological distress in a sample of teachers. J Psychol 123:321–338, 1990.
86. Schwartz: Original analyses–Cornell worksite study. 1999.
87. Schwartz JE, Pieper C, Karasek RA: A procedure for linking psychosocial job characteristic data to health surveys. Am J Public Health 78:904–909, 1988.
88. Semmer N, Zapf D: Validity of various methods of measurements in job analysis. In Landau K, Rohmert W (eds): Recent Developments in Job Analysis. London, Taylor & Francis, 1989, pp 67–78.
89. Semmer N, Zapf D, Greif S: Shared job strain: A new approach for assessing the validity of job stress measurements. J Occup Organiz Psychol 69:293–310, 1996.
90. Siegel PM: Prestige in the American Occupational Structure. University of Chicago, 1971.
91. Siegrist J, Peter R: Measuring effort-reward imbalance at work: Guidelines. Dusseldorf, University of Dusseldorf, 1996.
92. Siegrist J, Peter R, Junge A, et al: Low status control, high effort at work, and ischaemic heart disease: Prospective evidence from blue-collar men. Soc Sci Med 31:1127–1134, 1990.
93. Spector PE, Jex SM: Relations of job characteristics from multiple data sources with employee affect, absence, turnover intentions, and health. J Appl Psychol 76:46–53, 1991.
94. Spenner KI: Occupational characteristics and classification systems: New uses of the Dictionary of Occupational Titles in social research. Soc Methods Res 9:239–264, 1980.
95. Stark H, Enderlein G, et al: Stress am Arbeitspltazz und Herz-Kreislauf-Krankheiten. Bremerhaven, Verlag fuer neue Wissenschaft CmbH, 1998.
96. The Heart at Work Network: Socioeconomic variations in cardiovascular disease in Europe: The impact of the work environment and lifestyle. London, University College of London, Department of Epidemiology and Public Health, 1997.

97. Theorell T: The demand-control-support model for studying health in relation to the work environment: An interactive model. In Orth-Gomer K, Schneiderman N (eds): Behavioral Medicine Approaches to Cardiovascular Disease Prevention. Mahway, NJ, Erlbaum, 1996.

98. Theorell T, Perski A, Akerstedt T, et al: Changes in job strain in relation to changes in physiological states—A longitudinal study. Scand J Work Environ Health 14:189–196, 1988.

99. Theorell T, Tsutsumi A, Hallqvist J, et al: SHEEP Study Group: Decision latitude, job strain, and myocardial infarction. Am J Public Health 88:382–388, 1998.

100. U.S. Department of Labor: Dictionary of Occupational Titles, 4th ed. Washington DC, U.S. Government Printing Office, 1977.

101. U.S. Department of Labor: Handbook for Analyzing Jobs. Washington DC, U.S. Government Printing Office, 1972.

102. Volpert W: The model of the hierarchical-sequential organization of action. In Hacker W, Volpert W, von Cranach M (eds): Cognitive and Motivational Aspects of Action. Amsterdam, North-Holland, 1982, pp 35–51.

103. Volpert W, Koetter W, Gohde H-E, Weber W: Psychological evaluation and design of work tasks: Two examples. Ergonomics 32:881–890, 1989.

104. Vrijkotte TGM, van Doornen LJP, de Geus EJC: Work stress and metabolic and hemostatic risk factors. Submitted, 1999.

105. Waldenstrom M, Theorell T, Ahlberg-Hulten G, et al: Assessment of psychological and social current working conditions in the Music-Norrtalje Study. Division of Occupational Health, Department of Public Health Sciences. Stockholm, Karolinska Institutet, 1999.

106. Wartenberg D, Northridge M: Defining exposure in case-control studies: A new approach. Am J Epidemiol 133:1058–1071, 1991.

107. Welford AT: The measurement of sensory-motor performance: Surbery and reappraisal of twelve years' progress. Ergonomics 3:189–230, 1960.

108. Wells J: Objective job conditions, social support, and perceived stress among blue-collar workers. J Occup Behav 3:79–94, 1982.

109. Winkleby MA, Ragland DR, Syme SL: Self-reported stressors and hypertension: Evidence of an inverse association. Am J Epidemiol 127:124–134, 1988.

110. Zapf D: Selbst-und Fremdbeobachtung in der psychologischen Arbeitsanalyse. Goettingen, Hogrefe, 1989.

ASSESSMENT OF THE CARDIOVASCULAR SYSTEM AT THE WORKPLACE

OBTAINING A CVD HISTORY: OBSTACLES AND CHALLENGES
by Peter Schnall, MD, and Karen Belkić, MD, PhD

In the process of ascertaining the cause of an illness (i.e., making the diagnosis) the medical history plays a key role, as the information obtained from the patient informs the analytic process and shapes subsequent questioning. This exchange leads to an ongoing iterative process which, hopefully, results in an intervention intended to correct the problem. The key to the success of this endeavor for the physician is to obtain complete and accurate information from the patient(s) regarding symptoms and other related historical information such as past history of exposures.[45]

There are unfortunately, a number of reasons, many of which are not under the control of the clinician, as to why this is easier said than done. The person being interviewed may be unaware of his or her condition, or may feel anxious over the symptoms or illness and frightened of the possible diagnosis with its implications for future health. Denial may dominate the person's responses if there is a general fear of life-threatening illness, or if there are other possible negative consequences of a diagnosis. All of these factors may interfere with the doctor-patient relationship.

The health professional must be aware that employees may fear losing their jobs under certain circumstances as the result of a visit to a physician. This obstacle is of greatest concern in the work setting. In fact, doctors often function as "gatekeepers," especially in their role of evaluating an individual's fitness for work. Working people usually are well aware of this function and may act in what they perceive to be "their own best interest." The individual's need to continue working may hamper a frank admission of symptoms or conditions which could compromise employability. The physician needs to be acutely aware of the complex social relationships among the patient, clinician, and employer, as well as of societal expectations. The perception that the clinician is acting in the interests of the company can have a chilling effect on the patient. Ethical issues involving confidentiality are raised by this gatekeeping function[141] (see Chapters 8, 9, and 10).

Limitation on clinician's time, especially in primary care settings, represents yet another impediment to obtaining an adequate history. Accurate history-taking requires that the clinician first and foremost establish a rapport with the patient. The interview must be conducted in an environment that is conducive to developing a trusting relationship. The clinician must communicate an interest in the person and a willingness to listen. Time constraints undermine this entire process.

A mix of open-ended and directed questions are needed to get a complete history. The physician's need to collect both qualitative and quantitative data is somewhat akin to the work of an anthropologist. However, too many open-ended questions may waste time and increase the physician's sense of urgency, which can be counterproductive. Questions that are too directed may miss key symptoms, or give the patient the impression that the physician is not truly interested. The latter often is discovered when the physician learns of a key symptom late in the diagnostic process, and the patient comments, "Well, you didn't ask me."

Issues Specific to CVD History-Taking in the Workplace

CV symptoms may be quite prominent and direct the physician quickly in the direction of a relevant diagnosis, e.g., complaint of angina in patients with CAD. There are, of course, standard questions for use by the physician in pursuing a diagnosis of a specific form of CVD. (Chapter 8 outlines an approach to taking a clinical occupational work history as it relates to the CV system.)

However, under- and over-reporting of symptoms is frequent in CV illness—the issue of false positives and false negatives. Employees with chest pain may be quick to conclude they have cardiac disease, requiring the physician to rule out specific heart problems (false positives). As stated by Jennison: "Exaggerated reporting of symptoms might be a way of protesting against a hazardous environment. . . . Under-reporting, which is probably more common, may result from a lack of awareness of symptoms, denial, or fear of being replaced or dismissed from the workplace."[61] The clinician should be alert to the possibility that denial of cardiac symptoms may be especially likely among those very persons whose occupations show high cardiac risk. This denial has been reported, for example, among professional drivers.[12]

In addition, asymptomatic CVD (false negatives) is widespread and, with more sensitive and improved diagnostic techniques, increasingly recognized. Disease processes such as hypertension and myocardial ischemia frequently are asymptomatic or have very subtle symptoms. In high-risk occupations, the clinician should inquire carefully for nonspecific symptoms and maintain a high level of vigilance for complaints of fatigue, malaise, and sleep disturbances. Furthermore, while job strain is implicated in the etiology of hypertension in many studies, subjects frequently do not report psychological or physiologic symptoms even while they report jobs characterized by high demands and little control.[130] Another potential piece of information from the history that should alert the clinician is a job change to avoid work stressors; this could be a clue to the presence of subclinical disease. A notable example is the high cardiac risk seen among persons who have recently switched out of night shiftwork.[95]

The History-Taking and Public Health

An awareness that specific occupations may contribute to the development of certain CV illness can be helpful in both early detection and prevention of serious illness. The presence of symptoms among substantial numbers of people at a workplace may be the first clue to lead the astute clinician to analyze and identify clusters of CV illness related to that workplace (see Chapter 10). Recognition of such clusters of symptoms should motivate the clinician to screen the worksite for the presence of cardionoxious factors, such as job strain. Detection of specific workplace stressors as well as physiologic abnormalities, such as increased prevalence of high blood pressure, aids in the diagnosis of potentially unhealthy worksites.

BLOOD PRESSURE MEASUREMENT: CASUAL, SELF-MEASURED, AND AMBULATORY MONITORING
by Thomas G. Pickering, MD, DPhil

High blood pressure (BP) is one of the major risk factors for CVD, and also contributes to the morbidity of renal disease and diabetes. The relationship between BP and disease is continuous, so that even small elevations can be considered potentially harmful. While it is accepted that the average level of BP over time (often referred to as the true BP) is responsible for much of the damage, it is likely, but unproven, that transient increases of BP also contribute. In addition, there is a pronounced diurnal rhythm of pressure, which is increasingly recognized to be of pathological significance.

Until relatively recently, the vast majority of BP measurements were made using a mercury or aneroid sphygmomanometer in a laboratory or clinic setting, which limited both the number of readings that could be taken and their ecological validity. Thus, measurements made at the worksite were few and far between. The introduction of the techniques of ambulatory monitoring and self-measurement with digital devices has completely revolutionized our ability to measure BP at the workplace and in other settings while subjects go about their normal daily activities. Research using these techniques has shown that BP is highest for many people while they are at work.

Basic Techniques of BP Measurement

THE AUSCULTATORY METHOD

Conventionally, the gold standard in clinical practice has been measurements made with the Korotkoff sound technique by a physician using a mercury sphygmomanometer. However, although hypertension can be identified only by measuring the BP, this popular method is notoriously unreliable. There are three main reasons for this: inaccuracies in the methods, some of which are avoidable; the inherent variability of BP; and the tendency for BP to increase in the presence of a physician (the so-called white coat effect). The Korotkoff sound method tends to give values for systolic pressure (SP) that are lower than the intra-arterial pressure, and diastolic values that are higher, but there is no obvious superiority of phase 5 over phase 4.[22] The official recommendations of organizations such as the American Heart Association is to use the fifth phase.[113]

Some of the major causes of a discrepancy between the conventional clinical measurement of BP and the true BP are listed in Table 1. A number of factors may lead to inaccuracies with the Korotkoff sound technique:

TABLE 1.   Comparison of Features of Three Techniques for BP Measurement

Features	Conventional	Monitor Type Electronic (Self-)	Ambulatory
Use for screening	Yes	Possibly	No
Use for BP changes	Limited	Days/weeks	24 hours
No. of subjects	Large	Small	Small
No. of readings	Small	Large	Large
Cost	Low	Low-moderate	High

Cuff Size. The size of the cuff relative to the diameter of the arm is critical. A typical mistake is to use a cuff that is too small, resulting in an overestimation of the pressure.[93] In general, error can be reduced by using a large, adult-sized cuff for all except the skinniest arms. The British Hypertension Society recommends that if the arm circumference exceeds 33 cm, a large adult cuff should be used (width 12.5–13 cm, length 35 cm).[114]

Arm Position. BP measurements also are influenced by the position of the arm.[98] There is a progressive increase in the pressure of about 5–6 mmHg as the arm is moved down from the horizontal to vertical position.

Observer Error and Observer Bias. These are important sources of error when conventional sphygmomanometers are used. Differences in auditory acuity between observers may lead to consistent errors, and digit preference is common, with most observers recording a disproportionate number of readings ending in 5 or 0.[111] The average BP values recorded by trained individual observers have been found to vary by as much as 5–10 mmHg.[44] The level of pressure that is recorded also may be profoundly influenced by behavioral factors related to the effects of the observer on the subject, the best known of which is the presence of a physician. Other factors that can influence the pressure that is recorded include the race and sex of the observer.[94]

Rate of Cuff Inflation and Deflation. The rate of inflation has no significant effect on BP,[72] but very slow rates of deflation (2 mmHg/second or less) diminish the intensity of the Korotkoff sounds, resulting in slightly higher diastolic pressures (DPs). The generally recommended deflation rate is 2–3 mmHg/second.

Technical Sources of Error. There usually are fewer technical errors when a mercury column is used than when a semiautomatic method is applied. The column should be positioned approximately at the level of the heart; the mercury should read zero when no pressure is applied; and the mercury should fall freely when the pressure is reduced.

THE OSCILLOMETRIC TECHNIQUE

This technique was first demonstrated by Marey in 1876,[89] and it was shown subsequently that when the oscillations of pressure in a sphygmomanometer cuff are recorded during gradual deflation, the point of maximal oscillation corresponds to the mean intra-arterial pressure.[92] The oscillations begin approximately at SP and continue below DP, so that both can be estimated only indirectly, according to some empirically derived algorithm. One advantage of the method is that placement of the cuff is not critical, because a transducer is not used. Other potential advantages are that it is less susceptible to external noise (but not to low-frequency mechanical vibration), and the cuff can be removed and replaced by the patient, for example, to take a shower. The main disadvantage is that such recorders do not work well during physical activity, when there may be considerable movement artifact.

The oscillometric technique has been used successfully in ambulatory (am) BP monitors (such as the U.S. Spacelab recorders) and home monitors. Note that different brands of oscillometric recorders use different algorithms, and there is no generic oscillometric technique. However, comparisons of several different commercial models with intra-arterial and Korotkoff sound measurements have shown generally good agreement.[20,26]

Devices Used for BP Measurement

MERCURY AND ANEROID SPHYGMOMANOMETERS

Many studies of BP in the workplace require screening of subjects, and for this purpose mercury sphygmomanometers remain the gold standard. Aneroid devices commonly are used as a substitute, but they are not as accurate: in one survey, 30% of aneroid dials had errors greater than 4 mmHg.[25] The reliability of clinic pressure for estimating true BP can be improved by increasing the number of readings taken per visit and the number of visits, and by eliminating sources of error, such as digit preference.

ELECTRONIC SELF-MONITORS

In the past few years automatic electronic devices have become increasingly popular. Early versions were mostly inaccurate,[118,151] but currently available ones are often satisfactory.[48,59] Unfortunately, only a few have been subjected to proper validation tests such as the AAMI and BHS protocols.[106] The advantages of electronic monitors have begun to be appreciated by epidemiologists, who have always been greatly concerned about the accuracy of clinical BP measurement.[30] Cooper, et al. have asserted that ease of use and relative insensitivity to who is taking the reading can outweigh any inherent inaccuracy compared to the traditional sphygmomanometer method.[30] Electronic devices are now available that take BP from the upper arm, wrist, or finger. While more distal sites may be more convenient, measurement of BP from the arm (brachial artery) always has been the standard method, and is likely to remain so for the foreseeable future. Neither wrist nor finger monitors can be recommended for worksite studies.

The standard type of monitor for home use is an oscillometric device that records pressure from the brachial artery. Oscillometric monitors are easy to use, since cuff placement is not as critical as with devices that use a Korotkoff sound microphone. One of the limitations of earlier models of electronic monitors was that they required the subject to write down the readings, which is not only inconvenient for worksite studies, but also allows the potential for misreporting.[96] Some devices have a printer attached, which at least avoids observer bias. Others have a memory that can store several hundred readings, from which the data can be downloaded (for example, into the physician's computer, as in the Omron IC).

24-HOUR AMBULATORY MONITORS

First developed more than 30 years ago, amBP monitoring is only now beginning to find acceptance as a clinically useful technique, but it is widely used in research studies, particularly when BP in the natural environment is of interest. Recent technological advances have led to the introduction of monitors that are small, relatively quiet, and take up to 100 readings over 24 hours, while subjects go about their normal activities. They are reasonably accurate while the subject is at rest, but less so during physical activity.

When last systematically surveyed (in 1995) there were 43 different devices on the market. Only 18 had been validated according to the AAMI or BHS criteria, and of these only 9 satisfied the criteria for accuracy.[107] Ambulatory monitors can, in theory, provide information about the three main measures of BP—the average level, the diurnal variation, and short-term variability. Because the currently available monitors take readings intermittently rather than continually and are unreliable during exercise, they give a crude estimate of the short-term variability.

Determining Which Measures Are Clinically Important

In clinical practice, a patient's BP typically is characterized by a single value of the SP and DP, to denote the average or true BP level. Such readings normally are taken in a clinic setting, but there is extensive evidence that in hypertensive patients clinic pressures are consistently higher than the average 24-hour pressures recorded with ambulatory monitors,[80] and in some cases may be within the normal range, leading to a diagnosis of white coat hypertension. Given that there is a discrepancy between the clinic and ambulatory pressures, it is reasonable to suppose that the prediction of risk will be different. Cross-sectional studies have shown that amBP predicts the extent of CV damage better than clinic pressures,[37] and there are now several prospective studies showing that amBP is a better predictor of risk than clinic pressure.

The diurnal rhythm of BP is pronounced, with a decrease of 10–20 mmHg during sleep and a prompt increase on waking and getting up in the morning. The highest BP levels usually occur between 6 AM and noon, which is also the time at which the prevalence of many CV morbid events tends to be highest.[116] The pattern of BP during the day is, to a large extent, dependent on the pattern of activity, with pressures tending to be higher during the hours of work and lower while at home.[29] In hypertensive patients, the diurnal BP profile is reset at a higher level of pressure, with preservation of the normal pattern in the majority. The short-term BP variability is increased when expressed in absolute terms (mmHg), but the percentage changes are no different. Thus, hypertension can be regarded as a disturbance of the **set point** or **tonic level** of BP with normal short-term regulation. The normal diurnal rhythm of BP is disturbed in some individuals, with loss of the normal nocturnal fall of pressure. This disturbance has been observed in a variety of medical conditions, including renal disease and diabetes, but also occurs as a normal variant, particularly among African-Americans. Subjects whose pressure remains high at night ("nondippers") may have more target-organ damage than those who show the normal pattern ("dippers"), and there is evidence that women nondippers are at greater risk of CV morbidity than dippers,[152] but these findings are not sufficiently well established to be applied to routine clinical practice.

Even less information is available for defining the clinical significance of short-term BP variability, although it may be a risk factor for CV morbidity.

Practical and Technical Issues for Workplace Measurement

The choice of which technique should be used for measuring BP in worksite studies is dictated largely by the study design. Some of the advantages and limitations of the different types of monitors are shown in Table 1. The conventional sphygmomanometer is still the preferred method for screening large numbers of subjects, although electronic monitors are beginning to be used. The disadvantage of the sphygmomanometer is that it gives a restricted view of what happens to BP in different situations; thus, readings may or may not be representative of the subject's true BP.

Electronic (home) monitors are advantageous because they can monitor BP changes over long periods of time. To date, for unknown reasons, they have been little used in research on occupational stress. At this author's facility, electronic monitors were employed to evaluate BP changes associated with the approach of major work deadlines; subjects took their BP daily at the same time of day for many weeks.

Ambulatory monitoring can be performed at the worksite, and is normally done for 24 hours to provide a profile covering work and leisure hours. In most

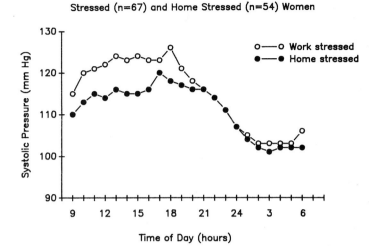

FIGURE 1.   Comparison of the blood pressure profiles recorded over 24 hours in two groups of employed women: "work stressed" and "home stressed." (From James GD, Moucha OP, Pickering TG: The normal hourly variation of blood pressure in women: Average patterns and the effects of work stress. J Hum Hypertens 5:505–509, 1991; with permission.)

people, BP is higher at work than at home (Fig. 1); diaries can help determine to what extent this is due to physical activity as opposed to mental stress. It is possible to determine to what extent the effects of work carry over to the evening hours, for example.

There are some special considerations related to worksite measurement:

1. **Effects of posture**. For routine clinical measurement it usually is recommended that the patient be sitting.[113] However, ambulatory monitoring studies of subjects at work may include measurements in the standing position. The BP changes associated with standing are usually modest—little change in systolic pressure and a slight increase in diastolic. However, analyses based on diary entries comparing sitting and standing BP have shown much bigger changes.[49] The most likely explanation is that these differences are due to the activities associated with the different postures, rather than to the postures themselves.

2. **Effects of physical activity**. During dynamic exercise there is an increase of SP but not DP, while isometric exercise increases both. Both types of activity may occur during work, but BP measurement becomes technically difficult even with ambulatory monitors, which may register artifactual readings. Monitoring people with sedentary jobs is more reliable.

3. **Effects of noise and vibration**. The oscillometric method of BP measurement, incorporated by most ambulatory monitors, is relatively immune to the effects of noise, but is affected by mechanical vibration, e.g., driving a taxi.

4. **The use of diaries**. When ambulatory monitoring is used to evaluate BP changes in the workplace, subjects should keep diaries describing their location, postures, moods, and activities, with entries made at the time of each BP reading. This documentation enables correlations to be made between work-related activities and BP.[133] A compromise on quantity of information is advisable, however, since very elaborate diaries tend to result in poor compliance.

JOB STRAIN

The Job Strain Model has been used mainly to study the effects of job strain on the development of CHD, but it also provides a good example of the use of workplace BP monitoring to study the effects of occupational stress on BP.[128] In the Cornell Worksite BP Study, men in high-strain jobs were found to have higher amBP than men in less stressful jobs.[131] Interestingly, this elevation of pressure was seen not only during working hours, but also while at home and during sleep. Furthermore, the association between job strain and BP could not be accounted for by any of the following factors known to influence BP: sodium intake, body mass, race, alcohol intake, education level, smoking, and level of physical activity.

Two other interactive effects were observed: (1) the highest BPs were observed in subjects who were in high-strain jobs and drank regularly; (2) the effects of job strain on BP were much greater in older than in younger subjects.

In a recent analysis of 3-year followup data from the worksite study, a cross-sectional association between job strain and amBP was found to closely parallel the association observed at baseline.[129] Furthermore, longitudinal analyses indicated that after controlling for baseline BP, the followup systolic and diastolic amBPs at work of those classified as having high-strain jobs at both baseline and followup were significantly greater than the BPs of those classified as having low-strain jobs at both baseline and followup. Though not statistically significant, those who switched from low-strain to high-strain jobs showed an increase in amBP, while those who switched from high strain to low strain showed a decrease. These findings have received support from other ambulatory monitoring studies.[85,146,150]

Exposure to job strain also is associated with increased left ventricular mass (LVM),[128] which is consistent with an earlier finding that LVM correlates more closely with the BP measured at work than at other times.[38]

SHIFT WORK

Studies of shift workers also have shown a close linkage between activity and BP. Several studies using ambulatory monitoring have found that BP is highest during the working hours in people who work different shifts, whatever the shift. Furthermore, when the shift ichanges, BP rhythm immediately follows the work shift.[8,28,143] Yamasaki, et al. monitored 24-hour BP in 105 nurses who worked different shifts: day, evening, or night.[157] Awake and sleep times were evaluated from subjects' diaries. The work-time BPs were similar, but the sleep-time pressures were higher in the evening and in nightshift workers, probably because quality of sleep for nightshift workers was not as good as for dayshift workers.

AMBULATORY ELECTROCARDIOGRAPHIC MONITORING: STRESS-MEDIATED CLINICALLY RELEVANT ENDPOINTS
by Karen Belkić, MD, PhD

The impressive body of data linking high-strain jobs and other adverse occupational conditions to increased amBP during work has provided empirical corroboration for a mechanistic link between the work environment and risk of CVD.[129] Perhaps most striking is the association between salutogenic changes in the levels of psychological demands and decision latitude on the job and lowered amBP measured at work. Compared to the findings concerning amBP and the work environment, ambulatory electrocardiographic (ECG) endpoints that are clinically relevant and affected by stress mechanisms and/or other factors in the workplace have been, for the most part, less systematically investigated.

Heart Rate Variability

DEFINITION AND MAJOR PHYSIOLOGIC DETERMINANTS

Heart rate variability (HRV) reflects the beat-to-beat oscillations in the sinus rate. The major determinant of the fluctuations between consecutive heart beats is the respiratory cycle; hence, the term respiratory sinus arrhythmia. Intrapleural pressure changes during the respiratory cycle affect venous pressures; these, in turn, activate reflex mechanisms leading to variations in beat-to-beat intervals. Chemoreceptor feedback also affects sinus rhythm.[76] These phasic, respiratory-related changes in the R-R interval are controlled by parasympathetically-mediated acetylcholine secretion. In contrast, the sympathetic nervous system is mainly responsible for the tonic control of heart rate.[14,64,76]

MEASUREMENT TECHNIQUES

HRV can be assessed in the **time domain**. An estimate of the overall HRV can be obtained by taking the standard deviation (SD) of all the normal sinus (N-N) intervals (SDNN). The long-term components of HRV can be estimated by mean SD of the averages of N-N intervals in all 5-minute segments, while the short-term components can be estimated by several techniques. The root-mean-square successive difference is preferred.[144] Time domain measurement is detailed elsewhere.[74,144]

Measurements in the **frequency domain** (power spectral analysis) quantitate the relative contribution of various frequency bands to total variance. Respiratory sinus arrhythmia has a frequency of about 0.15–0.4 Hz; this component, measured by spectral analysis, is termed the high frequency (HF) component. At baseline, it shows a significant relation to vagal tone.[42] Oscillations in heart rate of a somewhat longer periodicity (0.04–0.15 Hz); the low frequency [LF] component) have been ascribed to sympathetic outflow, possibly together with some parasympathetic modulation. The LF/HF ratio has been said by some investigators to represent sympathetic/parasympathetic balance, such that the greater this ratio, the higher the sympathetic influence and the more parasympathetic tone withdrawn.[144] However, Eckberg and others have called into question some of the latter premises.[42] Particularly controversial is how well the 0.1 Hz RR rhythm reflects sympathovagal balance. Caution must be exercised in relating these spectral parameters to the influence of the limbs of the autonomic nervous system (ANS).

The advantages and disadvantages of the various methods used for power spectral analysis, e.g., autoregression or the nonparametric Fast Fourier Transform, are thoroughly discussed elsewhere.[15,119] There is a growing appreciation for the role of nonlinear, parametric transforms to substantially improve the signal/noise ratio.[9,57,86,124] However, the eventual advantages of these latter techniques have yet to be demonstrated in biomedical investigations.[144] Overall, there is no consensus on optimal approach. However, particularly for autoregression, specific parameters such as choice of order can affect the results. Thus, comparisons among studies require attention to methodologic consistency.[15]

Regardless of the analytic method chosen, meticulous standards concerning ECG equipment, proper choice of sampling rate, and exclusion of artifact and nonsinus beats must be met.[15,144] Manual editing of the R-R data is recommended "to a very high standard, ensuring correct identification and classification of every QRS complex."[144] HRV cannot be measured in patients with large numbers of ectopics, atrial fibrillation, or sinus node dysfunction.[17] Although there are no formal recommendations, a high percentage (> 95%) of sinus-beats is optimal for reliable HRV analysis. Details on the equipment and other technical requirements for HRV analysis can be found elsewhere.[15,144]

Baseline short-term (5-minute) measures of HRV are stable and reproducible; these should be made using frequency domain methods.[144] Time domain methods are not considered appropriate for psychophysiologic studies.[15] Long-term recordings can be made using time domain analysis (e.g., standard deviation of the normal R-R interval) over a 24-hour period; power spectral analysis also can be performed. In the latter, an ultra-low frequency component (< 0.03 Hz) also appears, and there is a lack of stationarity over lengthy periods. Berntson and colleagues suggest analyzing short epochs at "strategic points" in a 24-hour recording when using frequency domain methods.[15] It is critical to distinguish interpretations of short versus long recordings.[76,144]

Factors Affecting HRV: Covariates and Confounders

Age has a major effect on HRV. O'Brien and colleagues report that the standard deviation of the R-R intervals declines with age, both at rest and during activities such as deep breathing, Valsalva maneuvers, and standing.[108] Normally there is an increased power of the LF component with postural changes such as upright tilt, but this response is attenuated among the elderly.[110] The increased heart rate level associated with physical activity is accompanied by a decrease in HRV.[83] Conversely, respiratory sinus arrhythmia can be pronounced in trained athletes at rest, and is considered a sign of physical fitness.[76]

There also may be gender differences in HRV parameters, although they probably are of lesser importance than age differences.[62] The interaction between HRV and age seems to vary according to gender.[138] Ramaekers and colleagues found that below age 40, men had significantly greater LF power and LF/HF ratio, as well as 24-hour SDNN.[122] Stein and colleagues reported that among younger men all 24-hour time domain indexes of HRV, except those that reflect vagal modulation of heart rate, were significantly higher than among similarly aged women.[138]

Changes in respiratory patterns affect HRV.[15] Relaxation training that included deep breathing exercises was found to be associated with increased time-domain measures of HRV.[147] In contrast, abnormal respiration, for example as seen in sleep apnea, is associated with untoward alterations in HRV.[76] Irregular breathing patterns can diminish the reliability of HRV measures.[99]

Kageyama and colleagues reported that after adjusting for age, the power of the HF component during supine rest with normal breathing among 282 healthy, white-collar, Japanese male workers was significantly decreased among those who were mildly to moderately obese (BMI 21–36).[67] On that basis, the authors concluded that obesity should be considered as a covariate when possible relationships between cardiac parasympathetic activity and other environmental factors are examined.

Among healthy subjects there usually is circadian variation in HRV, with greater power in the LF component during the day and in the HF component at night. The HF component normally increases during nonREM sleep. The nadir of HRV (largest LF, smallest HF power) is in the early morning hours, which is the time of highest incidence of transient myocardial ischemia, MI, and sudden cardiac death.[110,144] These circadian changes are attenuated or lost after acute MI and in advanced hypertension. Menstrual phase–related changes in HRV have been reported, with LF significantly greater, HF lower, and LF/HF greater during the luteal compared to the follicular phase.[125]

Myocardial dysfunction has been consistently associated with a reduction in time domain measures of HRV, while both HF and low LF components may be lost in advanced heart failure.[110,144] Absolute power of both LF and HF also is lost in autonomic neuropathy. Medications affecting the ANS also influence HRV.

Clinical Significance

Depressed HRV has been found to powerfully predict post-MI mortality and the occurrence of life-threatening ventricular tachyarrhythmias, independently of other post-infarction predictive factors such as left ventricular ejection fraction (LVEF) and the presence of late potentials.[144] The predictive strength of the HRV index (a time domain parameter based on the width of the distribution of N-N intervals, obtained from 24-hour Holter recordings) measured 5–10 days after infarction was found to be equal to or even greater than LVEF among 385 patients who were followed for at least 5 months post-MI. For arrhythmic complications, the sensitivity of the HRV index was 75% and specificity 76%. In comparison, a LVEF < 40% showed a sensitivity of 42% and specificity of 75% for this outcome.[109]

HRV also appears to predict incident CHD. Liao and colleagues performed a population-based case-cohort study in which there were 137 patients with incident CHD and 2252 healthy patients after 3 years.[84] The HF power taken from a baseline supine, resting recording was a significant predictor of CHD, after adjusting for age, race, gender, and other cardiac risk factors (lowest quartile compared with upper three quartiles adjusted relative risk 1.72; 95% CI, 1.17–2.51). Low frequency power, HF/LF ratio, and standard deviation of RR were not significant predictors.

Time and frequency domain analyses of HRV also have been used to investigate autonomic changes associated with various stages of essential hypertension.[86] This information may help indicate mechanisms mediating risk for cardiac events among hypertensives. SNS activation, consistent with the defense reaction, appears to be predominant in the early stages of hypertension.[47,65] Possibly supporting this formulation, the power of the low frequency HRV has been reported to be elevated among patients with mild-moderate hypertension.[115] In contrast, among 40 hypertensive patients with diastolic BP consistently over 95 mmHg compared to age-matched normotensive patients, there was significantly less power of the HF component, together with a greater LF component.[50] Hypertensive patients with left ventricular hypertrophy, but without evidence of coronary artery disease, were found to show not only a 24-hour decrease in time domain–measured HRV, but also a lack of nocturnal rise in occurrence of N-N interval differences > 50 msec.[27] Reviewing these and other studies, Lombardi and Fiorentini conclude that "a reduction in heart rate variability and in particular a marked attenuation of the circadian variation of spectral indices of sympathetic and vagal modifications of heart period seem to characterize the most advanced phases of the disease."[86]

HRV and Environmental Stressors

A large body of laboratory investigation among healthy subjects demonstrates an association between mental workload and attenuation or disappearance of respiratory sinus arrhythmia.[21,53,69,83,87,105,123,124,126] Kalsbeek ascribed the complete suppression of respiratory sinus arrhythmia to performance at peak capacity with "no reserve capacity left unoccupied."[69] This contention is corroborated by field studies among pilots, who during the time of landing exhibit a total loss of HRV. Among pilots learning to handle a new type of aircraft, there was a prolonged duration of attenuated HRV during the approach period, prior to touch down.[64]

Exposure to certain physical factors may be associated with stress-mediated and/or autonomic neuropathic alterations in HRV. Male tool operators with vibration white finger disease have been found to have a significantly lower power of the respiratory sinus arrhythmia components compared to healthy controls.[3] Corroborative results concerning vibration exposure and HRV have been reported.[51,52] Occupational exposure to lead has been associated with a dose-related decrease in HRV during deep breathing among 172 male workers.[145]

Assessment of HRV also provides insight into the acute and chronic effects of fatiguing work conditions, as these may relate to untoward CV outcomes. Kageyama and colleagues found that among 223 male, white-collar workers in greater Tokyo, working more than 60 hours of overtime per month was associated with short-term HRV changes while standing at rest.[68] The authors interpreted these findings to be consistent with decreased vagal and increased SNS activity.

Long work hours that include a night shift appear to be associated with profound alterations in the circadian pattern of HRV, with a nearly complete loss of HF surge over 24 hours, reminiscent of the patterns described for post-MI and advanced hypertensive patients. Kobayashi and colleagues examined these effects among 12 healthy nurses who demonstrated normal circadian HRV patterns when working the day shift only.[75] When, after having worked the full day shift, these same nurses went on to work the midnight to 8:30 AM shift, the LF/HF ratio remained at or even above usual daytime levels for all but 3 of the 24 hours. Matsuzaki and coworkers in their study of seven male factory workers reported a significant decrease in power of the HF component with day sleep after night shiftwork compared to night sleep after day work.[91] These findings are particularly intriguing in light of the possible relation between night shiftwork and CVD.

The clinical relevance of HRV renders it a potentially useful endpoint for assessing workplace interventions aimed at promoting CV health. The above-described study of Kobayashi, et al. illustrates this point.[75] These authors also examined the circadian pattern of LF/HF power when, prior to working the night shift, the nurses worked a half- rather than full-day schedule and thereby had a chance to sleep for an average of 4 hours in the late afternoon and early evening, prior to going to work. A distinct drop in LF/HF lasting about 7 hours was observed during this period, although these values were still not as low as during a normal night sleep after day shiftwork. These findings are coherent with the statement of Kristal-Boneh and colleagues that "spectral analysis of HRV may be used to predict optimal worktime under a combination of enhanced mental load and other stressors."[76] More widespread examination of HRV, as a psychophysiologic parameter with importance to cardiovascular well-being, is warranted in various work environments.

Myocardial Ischemia

The definition and physiologic determinants of myocardial ischemia, as well as a review of empirical data linking stress mechanisms and other workplace exposures to myocardial ischemia are presented in Chapter 5. Here, the focus is on ambulatory measurement techniques and the clinical significance of myocardial ischemia detected during Holter monitoring.

Measurement Techniques, Reliability, and Validity

Among patients with documented or a high likelihood of coronary disease, ambulatory recording of ST segment depression of 1 mm or more, lasting for at least 1 minute, has been demonstrated to be a reliable and valid marker of myocardial ischemia. This finding is based on simultaneous investigation using radionuclide or echocardiographic evaluation of ventricular function as well as positron emission tomographic assessment of myocardial perfusion.[4]

Verification of automatically-detected ST segment changes should be made by review of the analog ECG waveform,[81,90] with confirmation of a horizontal or downsloping configuration. At least 1 minute—according to some authors, 5 or 10 minutes—should separate individual episodes of ST segment depression.[112,120,142] Among patients with variant angina, transient elevation of the ST segment can be detected using ambulatory monitoring.[24,79]

Most ambulatory monitoring systems use two bipolar leads, and sites can be chosen to detect likely maximum ischemia based on exercise testing or coronary angiography data.[142] The use of three leads increases the chance of detecting extant ischemia.[77] The diagnostic accuracy of ST analysis may be improved by excluding ST segment depression associated with: an increase in R wave amplitude; PQ and ST segments that run a parallel course; and an abrupt onset and offset of ST segment deviation.[11,154] The coexistent finding on ambulatory monitoring of frank T wave inversion may indicate that horizontal or downsloping ST segment depression is of ischemic origin, since this feature significantly distinguished a large series of women with CAD from healthy controls.[11] Interestingly, cohort data by Daviglus, et al. indicate that incident minor ST-T abnormalities on resting ECG independently predict CV mortality among men.[32]

Many authors exclude patients from analysis who have artifactual postural ST deviation; this can be done by review of an initial recording in supine, sitting, standing, and left and right lateral decubitus positions.[120,142] Patients taking digitalis medications or with left bundle branch block, pre-excitation, or uncorrected hypokalemia also usually are not included in analysis of ST segment deviation.[7,35] LeClercq and Coumel and Sheffield, et al. offer detailed discussion of the technical aspects of ambulatory monitoring of ST changes, including standards of instrumentation.[81,135]

Clinical Significance

A correlation is found among coronary patients between the total duration and number of episodes of ischemic ST segment changes during daily activities and ischemic changes during exercise testing. However, the correlation is of limited magnitude, indicating that each of these tests can provide useful diagnostic information in these patients.[136,142] While there is still some controversy about the precise predictive value of ischemia detected on ambulatory monitoring versus on exercise, it is generally concluded that transient ischemia during daily life independently has an adverse prognostic significance among various subsets of patients with IHD.[18,31,36,41,60,63,73,121,148] At least 75% of myocardial ischemia detected on Holter monitoring is asymptomatic,[4] and the prognostic significance of this finding is not diminished if unaccompanied by symptoms.[5,34,140]

The QT Interval

Definition and Standard Measurement Techniques

Left stellate ganglion sympathetic outflow leading to temporal dispersion of ventricular repolarization is manifested on the ECG by a prolonged QT interval.

This is associated with a lowered threshold for ventricular fibrillation and vulnerability to life-threatening ventricular tachycardia.

There are numerous formulations and criteria for defining a long QT interval; dilemmas in this regard have been ongoing for decades.[33,70] The QT corrected for heart rate by Bazett's formula, or the QTc (QT/square root of the R-R interval in seconds) is most frequently used, with a pathologically long QTc being > 0.44–0.46.[88,104] The QT interval ideally should be measured on a 12-lead ECG from the earliest onset of the QRS to the end of the T wave, where it merges with the baseline. An eventual subsequent, discrete U wave should not be included. Leads II, V3, and V4 or V5 are usually the most helpful in distinguishing T and U waves. At least three consecutive QT intervals should be measured and averaged to increase precision.[100,101] Measurement of the QT interval is difficult or impossible with flat T waves. The above-cited criteria are not valid for QRS ≥ 0.12 sec. Further, the correction of QT for heart rate should not be applied in the tachycardic range, especially for heart rate over 125/min.[88] Hypocalcemia, as well as quinidine and several other antiarrhythmics, prolong the QT interval. Women appear to have longer QTc than men, according to normative, age-stratified data among Caucasians.[88]

CLINICAL SIGNIFICANCE

Patients with the hereditary long QT syndrome are known to be at risk for polymorphic ventricular tachycardia, syncope, and sudden cardiac death.[102] Resting QTc is normal in 5–10% of gene carriers for this disorder.[134] Furthermore, the long QT syndrome can occur sporadically without evidence of inheritance.[43] In apparently healthy, population-based samples, approximately 6–8% of men and 3% of women were found to have a QTc > 0.44 on resting ECG.[10,132]

In a population-based cohort study among 1583 men and 1508 women aged 40–65 at baseline, at 15-year followup among the men there was a significantly increased risk of CVD and IHD mortality associated with a QTc > 0.44 (RR 1.8 and 2.1, respectively) after adjusting for age and standard cardiac risk factors.[132] There was no significant relation among the women, however.

Dynamic assessment of QTc using ambulatory monitoring reveals that among post-MI patients the mean 24-hour QTc was significantly greater in those with, compared to those without, subacute or late-occurring life-threatening ventricular arrhythmias. The patients with these arrhythmias also had significantly more peaks of QTc > 0.500.[56] Among 6693 consecutive patients undergoing Holter monitoring, those with a mean QTc > 0.44 over 24 hours had a risk ratio of 2.3 (CI 1.3–4.5) for sudden cardiac death at 2-year followup.[1]

Sympathetic outflow associated with emotional stress, sensory stimuli, and/or physical activity can precipitate ventricular arrhythmias in persons with the long QT syndrome.[82,103,155] Antimony exposure is associated with QT interval prolongation, and an epidemic of sudden death has been described in relation to occupational exposure to antimony trisulfide.[23] Among healthy subjects with normal resting QTc, both the cold pressor and the glare pressor tests elicit significant prolongation of the QTc.[13,153] Recently, validated automatic monitoring techniques suggest that the QTc feasibly could be assessed during work activity.[56]

Bradyarrhythmias and Ventricular Tachyarrhythmias

Notwithstanding medications and structural abnormalities affecting the cardiac conducting system, intense, unopposed vagal outflow can result in various degrees of sinus bradycardia. In extreme, rare cases, Stokes-Adams attacks or even sudden death[97] can occur from vagally mediated sinus node arrest and asystole. Hyper-vagotonia in the carotid sinus syndrome and vaso-vagal syncope are seen.[156] It is es-timated that about 8% of the population responds to novel or conditional stimuli with extreme vagotonia. Case reports reveal that repeated intense emotional stimuli can trigger multiple Stokes-Adams attacks in extreme vago-dominant individuals.[127] Ambulatory ECG recording is well suited to detect symptomatic or asymptomatic bradyarrhythmias of various degrees of severity in relation to working activity.

While ventricular tachyarrhythmias are responsible for the vast majority of sudden arrhythmic deaths, the evidence is conflicting as to the value of any of the various forms of ventricular ectopy for independently predicting the occurrence of cardiac events, particularly among those without underlying heart disease.[16,17,71,139] It is increasingly recognized that examination of the interaction among relevant para-meters can yield more diagnostically important, predictive information.[55,78,139] For example, Hoberg and colleagues observed that silent myocardial ischemia–related complex ventricular arrhythmias can be triggered by physical activity among a large percentage of patients with clinically stable CAD.[54] These authors propose that "silent myocardial ischemia may be the missing link between the increased risk of cardiac arrest and the lack of premonitory symptoms" during physical exercise. A significant positive association has been found during ambulatory monitoring among women with CHD between the extent of ST segment depression and degree of complexity of ventricular arrhythmias, with a mean 2.2-mm horizontal depression in lead CMV5, when episodes of ventricular tachycardia were recorded.[11] These em-pirical findings are concordant with clinical-physiologic data demonstrating that myocardial ischemia can act as a promoting substrate for electrical instability of the ventricle.

Dilaveris and colleagues have reported that diminished HRV preceded ST seg-ment depression and was significantly related to the magnitude and duration of my-ocardial ischemia.[40] Seen in this light, the observations concerning abrupt and total loss of respiratory sinus arrhythmia with work performance at peak capacity acquire a potential clinical relevance. Integrative examination of the interaction among these relevant parameters can be performed in relation to the work environment, using ambulatory ECG monitoring. Because of the intimate interrelation between many of these ECG endpoints and hemodynamic changes, a more complete view of the ef-fects of the occupational milieu on CV well-being would be gained if ECG and BP monitoring were assessed in concert.

POINT ESTIMATES OF BLOOD PRESSURE AT THE WORKSITE   *by Peter Schnall, MD, and Karen Belkić, MD, PhD*

There are several major reasons why blood pressure (BP) should be measured at the workplace:

1. **Public health**. Surveillance of the workplace to determine the prevalence of hypertension or elevated BP is important from a public health perspective, espe-cially in light of the evidence that workplace factors play a significant role in the eti-ology of essential hypertension. Worksite screenings are the only way to identify those groups of individuals with normal clinic BP and elevated worktime BP—the "false negatives"—who are at a high risk for a hypertension-related morbid event.

2. **Improved clinical diagnosis**. Collecting worksite estimates of BP should result in improved diagnosis and treatment of patients. The level of an individual's

worktime BP is important for diagnosis, as a predictor of subsequent illness, and for evaluation of clinical treatment.

3. **Studies of etiology**. To the extent that psychosocial workforce factors play an important etiologic role in the genesis of hypertension, *where* one measures BP matters, because these factors are not static and may or may not be present at any moment. All BP measures are influenced by some set of psychosocial factors. For example, BP in the clinic is subject to the "white coat" effect. BP at home can be affected by home stressors and likely carry-over from work. Sleep BP may be influenced by dreaming (REM sleep), which is associated with elevation of BP and disinhibition of CV control mechanisms.[19] Factors such as work-related stressors, physical activity, and posture are important in workplace BP assessment.

A significant association also has been found between left ventricular mass index and exposure to job strain.[130] Left ventricular enlargement is correlated more highly with average BP at work than at other locations.[6,38,39] These authors propose that the observed associations between job strain, left ventricular hypertrophy, and hypertension suggest a pathophysiologic process that may explain the reported association between job strain and CHD mortality. Measurement of BP at the workplace represents the critical node for further elucidating these inter-relations.

4. **Reliability and validity**. Workplace amBPs are more reliable and have greater validity than casual clinic BPs, and this also may be true for point estimates of worktime BP.

5. **Reduced cost**. It is usually less expensive to collect BP at the workplace than to send individuals to a medical center.

Basal Blood Pressures

The concept of casual BP is derived from the work of Smirk in the 1940s.[137] His idea was that the clinic BP had two independent components—the basal and the supplemental. Basal BPs were those obtained in a seated subject in a comfortable environment after a 30-minute rest by a single observer. The difference between this BP and the initial BP (the casual BP) was the supplemental BP. Smirk found that basal BPs and supplemental readings did not correlate. It was proposed that the basal BP represented the structural or fixed elements of an individual's hypertension, while the supplemental pressure was the elevation attributable to the effects of physical and mental activity.

The fact that casual BP did not correlate with basal BP in Smirk's research requires explication. It is plausible that the psychosocial, mental, and physical factors associated with a visit to the doctor's office reflect a small percentage of actual exposures impacting on an individual's basal tonic BP. In contrast, picture a universe of exposures that influence BP (the frequency and intensity of these exposures determine the ultimate impact on BP). Work stressors, since they occur more frequently (longer hours of the days, more days of the year, more years of a life) and with greater intensity than does the stress of a visit to the doctor's office play a major role in elevating an individual's BP.[129]

The possibility of obtaining a basal BP uninfluenced by psychosocial factors seems unlikely. There is a real question whether 30 minutes or more (rarely achieved in practice) of rest in a comfortable environment is a true reflection of basal BP. Even under such conditions humans are not free of psychosocial influences. In fact, we often have observed increases in BP in patients at rest (anxious subjects may worry increasingly as they "rest"). Even among those persons who manage to fully relax and shut out nearly all psychosocial stimuli, this approximation of basal BP may not be reflective of clinically relevant BP status.

The very concept of basal BP—a BP free of all psychosocial and other stimuli providing a best estimate of tonic true BP—is not compatible with our current notions of the etiology of essential hypertension of neurogenic origin. We now believe that in most cases of essential hypertension, psychosocial factors, especially at work, play an important role in elevation of BP. Basal BP eventually reflects these influences. This process leads to three identifiable stages: (1) When individuals first are exposed to putative causes such as workplace stressors, BPs are elevated at work and basal BP is normal. (2) Chronic exposure to these stressors leads to elevated workplace BPs as well as basal BPs.[46,47] At this stage the psychosocial factors likely are correlated with both measures of BP (structural changes in the cardiovascular system are occurring). (3) In end-stage hypertension, self-sustaining structural processes in the vascular system may lead to disjuncture between reported psychosocial factors and BP (both workplace and basal) since the individual may no longer be exposed to the psychosocial factors (e.g., promotion, retirement) and the BP process is now autonomous.

These stages are consistent with the presumed mechanisms of neurogenic hypertension—an initial reversible stage with predominant elevation of systolic BP as the defense response is elicited. With repeated exposure, structural changes occur in the heart and vasculature.[46,47]

Problems with Clinic Measures

In the clinic setting there are a number of psychosocial stimuli present that can affect BP. For some individuals the presumably unpleasant experience of the clinic setting can produce an elevation. This may be a unique response (i.e., totally unrelated to the usual universe of BPs during daily life). It has been called the "white coat" phenomenon and is characterized by normal ambulatory BP and high clinic casual BP. Most studies of individuals who display this unique response appear to show they are at relatively low risk for morbid events compared to those with sustained hypertension.[117a] However, Julius, et al. argue to the contrary, on the basis of point measurements at home versus clinic.[66] They found an increased prevalence of cardiovascular metabolic syndrome (SNS driven) among young adults with white coat hypertension, and postulate that white coat hypertension is mediated by over-activity of the SNS.

According to Pickering: "True blood pressure may be regarded as the average level over a prolonged period of time, which is generally thought to be the most important determinant of target organ damage."[117] The interest in and subsequent research with amBP monitoring arose out of the observation that the typical casual clinic BP is highly variable and does not reliably reflect BP during daily life. A body of evidence that workplace amBP is a better predictor of morbidity and mortality has emerged. BPs obtained with an ambulatory monitor are more reliable and valid than other assessments of BP (see pages 191–196).

Combining information from both clinic BPs and amBPs allows identification of four groups—two in which the clinic and ambulatory measures agree and two crossover groups:

• Individuals with normal amBPs and elevated BPs are the **false positives** (i.e., those with white coat hypertension) if one accepts amBP as the definitive measure of BP.

• Individuals with normal clinic BP but elevated amBP are the **false negatives**. This group is potentially at risk of an untoward event since amBPs are increased, yet these individuals remain undiagnosed. It has been found, for example, that among individuals in stressful professions (e.g., journalists, professional drivers) selected to have normal clinic BP, worktime DBP averaged to nearly 90 mmHg, and some individuals had sustained increases in work BP that failed to decrease below 150/100 during the entire recording period.[149] Obtaining estimates of BP at the workplace in such individuals is extremely important from a clinical perspective, and alone is justification for worksite BP screenings.

Problems with Ambulatory Measures

First, logistics at the workplace frequently are complicated. Participants wearing a monitor require time to don the equipment, experience frequent interruptions of work—albeit of short duration—when BP is measured and a diary filled out, and need time to remove the monitor at the end of the work period. For some work activities these interruptions may have serious consequences for job performance and productivity, especially when large numbers of participants are involved.

Second, costs are high for several reasons. Equipment, including the monitors themselves and the necessary computers, are expensive. Moreover, amBP measurement is a technologically sophisticated and labor-intensive process requiring highly trained personnel to collect and process data. Trained technicians hook the subject up to the equipment; insure its proper working; explain its use to the wearer, including the completion of an accompanying diary (for location and activity codes); and enter and code the obtained data into a computer.

Point Estimates as an Alternative to AmBP Monitoring

What is needed is a point estimate of BP that approximates a typical amBP reading in the same subject (Table 2). We can imagine a subject wearing an amBP monitor at work and wanting to obtain several readings during the same period, which approximate those that the machine is obtaining when it records BP every 15 minutes or so during the working day.

No current protocol exists for obtaining point estimates of BP at the workplace. Below we outline a new BP protocol for obtaining point estimates of BP while a

TABLE 2. Point Estimates of Workplace Blood Pressure

Advantages	Disadvantages
Cost effective and feasible as means of screening an entire workplace to determine prevalence of hypertension. Less expensive than amBP monitoring.	Fewer samples and therefore lower reliability compared to amBP. However, individual point estimates are likely more reliable than an individual amBP reading (individual machine readings are imprecise).
Comprehensive database development for a variety of public health and research purposes.	Logistics of workplace screenings may be difficult.
Enhanced reliability and validity in comparison to clinic BPs. As compared to office-obtained casual BPs, they better reflect real work life—not contaminated by spurious, clinic-related stimuli. Workplace-obtained, casual BPs correlate well with workplace amBP in contrast to casual clinic BPs and are better correlated with workplace psychosocial risk factors such as job strain.	
Can inform treatment decisions. Identify those subjects who are false positive or false negative on casual clinic BP.	

subject is actually working (contrast with the current American Heart Association protocol for casual clinic BP recording, 1998[2]).

Protocol for Obtaining a Point Estimate of Worktime BP

Part 1. Checklist. Use prior to obtaining point measurements at the workplace—before the workday on which BP is to be measured:

1. Obtain informed consent
2. Obtain arm circumference
3. Provide instructions regarding clothing (e.g., loose shirts, accessible arms)
4. Collect medication and medical history (and other relevant data)
5. Use simplest accurate equipment—a carefully calibrated Anaeroid device (not a mercury column)

Part 2. Protocol for obtaining two sets of point estimates. Conducted while individuals are working.

1. Trained observer can measure (not necessarily health professional)
2. Avoid "clinic atmosphere"—no white coats; don't act like a clinician.
3. Aim for informal interactions and neutral conversations—avoid conversations that are of personal relevance to the participant; do not discuss controversial issues until after BP collection.
4. Obtain two sets of point estimates in one workday while subject is at usual work activity.

> **First BP estimate** should be obtained near start time at beginning of shift (workday) This helps maximize number of workers examined during each day if part of a large population screening.
> - Record time(s) of BP measurements
> - Record subject's body position
> - BPs to be determined with worker in same position as at work (e.g., standing if stands at work)
>
> **Second BP estimate** should occur later in same workday or at same time on second day.

5. Equipment: calibrated aneroid sphygmomanometer (determine proper cuff size)
6. Conducting actual point estimate measurements

> **First set**
> - Taken at workstation, shortest possible interruption of work process
> - Three readings for each point estimate
> - 1 minute between readings
>
> **Second set**
> - Repeat above. *This is probably the best single estimate because subject is desensitized.*

7. Average first and second readings for best estimate; discard third
8. Subject feedback

> Give BP results only after second set of estimates obtained

Part 3. Protocol for obtaining related data. Needed to complement point estimate of BP at the workplace.

1. Diary

> Obtain diary data if possible (elective)
> Include observations about job and individual (requires separate protocol and training)
> Work environment (see Chapters 6 and 8)—record usual and atypical for the day of estimate

Assess job characteristics (see Chapters 6 and 8)—including subjective evaluation of work by subject (home life as well, if desired)
2. Medical history, demographics, and other potential confounders
   Potential confounders include alcohol, body-mass index, age, race, gender, family history of hypertension, medications (antihypertensives and oral contraceptives as well as other medications that may potentially affect BP), smoking, caffeine, body position, and physical activity.
3. Data analysis (depends on purpose of measurement)
4. Some unresolved questions
   Start time of BP Screening—possibilities include at beginning of shift or at fixed intervals during shift
   Heart rate abnormalities
   • Bradycardia (extreme)—bear in mind the need to more slowly deflate the BP cuff in the presence of extreme bradycardia that may occur, for example, in well-trained athletes and those with clinical conduction abnormalities.
   • Tachycardia

REFERENCES

1. Algra A, Tijssen JGP, Roelandt JRTC, et al: QT interval variables from 24-hour electrocardiography and two-year risk of sudden death. Br Heart J 70:43–48, 1993.
2. American Heart Association: Blood pressure testing and measurement (http://www.americanheart.org/Heart_and Stroke_A_Z_Guide/bpest.htm), American Heart Association, 1998.
3. Araki S, Murata K, Yokoyama K: Assessment of central, peripheral, and autonomic nervous system functions in vibrating tool operators: Neuroelectrophysiologic studies. Environ Research 62:272–282, 1993.
4. Armstrong PW: Stable ischemic syndromes. In Topol EJ (ed): Textbook of Cardiovascular Medicine. Philadelphia, Lippincott-Raven, 1998, pp 333–364.
5. Assey ME: The recognition and treatment of silent myocardial ischemia. In Hurst JW, Logue RB, Rackley CE, et al (eds): The Heart. New York, McGraw-Hill, 1990, pp 1079–1086.
6. Baba S, Nakamoto Y, Ueshima H, et al: Variations of blood pressures under regularly recurring stress in daily life and its relation to left ventricular hypertrophy in urban hypertensive men. J Hypertens 6:S695–S696, 1988.
7. Banai S, Moriel M, Benhorin J, et al: Changes in myocardial ischemic threshold during daily activities. Am J Cardiol 66:1403–1406, 1990.
8. Baumgart P, Walger P, Fuchs G, et al: 24-hour blood pressure is not dependent on endogenous circadian rhythm. J Hypertens 7:331–334, 1989.
9. Belkic D: New spectral estimations for ICR and NMR. Nobel Institute, Manne Siegbahn Laboratory Newsletter No. 2, 1997.
10. Belkic K: Neural mechanisms and risk of sudden cardiac death. An epidemiologic approach. Belgrade, University of Belgrade, Center for Multidisciplinary Studies, 1989.
11. Belkic K: Psychosocial triggers of myocardial ischemia in women. Research Report to the Swedish Medical Research Council, 1995.
12. Belkic K: Neurocardiologic mechanisms of heart disease risk in professional drivers. Project Report to the Swedish Work Environment Fund, 1996.
13. Belkic KL, Mickovic L, Milic B, Savic S: Blood pressure and electrocardiographic changes elicited by the glare pressor test. Arch Environ Health 42:37–43, 1987.
14. Benditt DG: Syncope. In Topol EJ (ed): Textbook of Cardiovascular Medicine. Philadelphia, Lippincott-Raven, 1998, pp 1807–1831.
15. Berntson GG, Bigger JT Jr, Eckberg DL, et al: Heart rate variability: Origins, methods, and interpretive caveats. Psychophysiology 34:623–648, 1997.
16. Bjerregard P, Sorensen KE, Molgaard H: Predictive value of ventricular premature beats for subsequent ischaemic heart disease in apparently healthy subjects. Eur Heart J 12:597–601, 1991.
17. Blake LM, Goldschlager N: Risk stratification of potential sudden death victims after myocardial infarction. Prim Cardiol 21:8–15, 1995.
18. Bonaduce D, Petretta M, Lanzillo T, et al: Prevalence and prognostic significance of silent myocardial ischaemia detected by exercise test and continuous ECG monitoring after acute myocardial infarction. Eur Heart J 12:186–193, 1991.
19. Bond WC, Bohs C, Ebey J Jr, Wolf S: Rhythmic heart rate variability (sinus arrhythmia) related to stages of sleep. Conditional Reflex 8:98–107, 1973.
20. Borrow KM, Newburger JW: Noninvasive estimation of central aortic pressure using the oscillometric method for analyzing systemic artery pulsatile blood flow: Comparative study of indirect systolic, diastolic, and mean brachial artery pressure with simultaneous direct ascending aortic pressure measurements. Am Heart J 103:879–886, 1982.

21. Boyce PPR: Sinus arrhythmia as a measure of mental load. Ergonomics 17:177–183, 1974.
22. Breit SN, O'Rourke MF: Comparison of direct and indirect arterial pressure measurements in hospitalized patients. Aust NZ Med J 4:485–491, 1974.
23. Brieger H, Semisch CS, Stasneg J, et al: Industrial antimony poisoning. Ind Med Surg 23:521–523, 1954.
24. Bugiardini R, Borghi A, Sassone B, et al: Prognostic significance of silent myocardial ischemia in variant angina pectoris. Am J Cardiol 68:1581–1586, 1991.
25. Burke MJ, Towers HM, O'Malley K, et al: Sphygmomanometers in hospital and family practice: Problems and recommendations. Br Med J (Clin Res Ed) 285:469–471, 1982.
26. Cates EM, Schlussel YR, James GD, Pickering TG: A validiation study of the Spacelabs 90207 ambulatory blood pressure monitor. J Ambul Monitor 3:149–154, 1990.
27. Chakko S, Mulingtapang RF, Huikuri HV, et al: Alterations in heart rate variability and its circadian rhythm in hypertensive patients with left ventricular hypertrophy free of coronary artery disease. Am Heart J 126:1364–1372, 1993.
28. Chau N, Mallion J, de Gaudemaris R, et al: 24-hour ambulatory blood pressure in shift workers. Circulation 80:341–347, 1989.
29. Clark LA, Denby L, Pregibon D, et al: A quantitative analysis of the effects of activity and time of day on the diurnal variations of blood pressure. J Chronic Dis 40:671–681, 1987.
30. Cooper R, Puras A, Tracy J, et al: Evaluation of an electronic blood pressure device for epidemiological studies. Blood Press Monitor 2:35–40, 1997.
31. Currie P, Ashby D, Saltissi S: Prognostic significance of transient myocardial ischemia on ambulatory monitoring after acute myocardial infarction. Am J Cardiol 71:773–777, 1993.
32. Daviglus ML, Liao Y, Greenland P, et al: Association of nonspecific minor ST-T abnormalities with cardiovascular mortality. The Chicago Western Electric Study. JAMA 281:530–536, 1999.
33. de Bruyne MC, Hoes AW, Kors JA, et al: Prolonged QT interval: A tricky diagnosis? Am J Cardiol 80:1200–1304, 1997.
34. Deedewania PC: Asymptomatic ischemia during predischarge Holter monitoring predicts poor prognosis in the postinfarction period. Am J Cardiol 71:859–861, 1993.
35. Deedewania PC, Carbajal EV: Exercise test predictors of ambulatory silent ischemia during daily life in stable angina pectoris. Am J Cardiol 66:1151–1156, 1990.
36. Deedwania PC, Nelson JR: Pathophysiology of silent myocardial ischemia during daily life. Hemodynamic evaluation of simultaneous electrocardiographic and blood pressure monitoring. Circulation 82:1296–1304, 1990.
37. Devereaux RB, Pickering TG: Ambulatory blood pressure in assessing the cardiac impact and prognosis of hypertension. In O'Brien ET, O'Malley K (eds): Handbook of Hypertension. Amsterdam, Elsevier Science Publishers B.V., 1991, pp 261–286.
38. Devereux RB, Pickering TG, Harshfield GA, et al: Left ventricular hypertrophy in patients with hypertension: Importance of blood pressure response to regularly recurring stress. Circulation 68:476–479, 1983.
39. Devereux RB, Roman MJ: Hypertensive cardiac hyptertrophy: Pathophysiological and clinical characteristics. In Laragh JH, Brenner BM (eds): Hypertension: Pathophysiology, Diagnosis, and Management. New York, Raven Press, Ltd., 1995, pp 409–432.
40. Dilaveris PE, Zervopoulos GA, Psomadaki KD, et al: Assessment of time domain and spectral components of heart rate variability immediately before ischemic ST segment depression episodes. PACE 19:1337–1345, 1996.
41. Echevarria P, Saucedo A, Molinero E, et al: Angiographic, exercise, and Holter monitoring variables in patients with stable angina: 5-year followup. J Amb Monitor 8:279–288, 1995.
42. Eckberg DW: Sympathovagal balance: A critical appraisal. Circulation 96:3224–3232, 1997.
43. Eggeling T, Hoeher M, Osterhues H-H, et al: Significance of noninvasive diagnostic techniques in patients with long QT syndrome. Am J Cardiol 70:1421–1426, 1992.
44. Eilertsen E, Humerfelt S: The observer variation in the measurement of arterial blood pressure. Acta Med Scand 184:145–157, 1968.
45. Fauci AS, Braunwald E, Isselbacher KJ, et al: Harrison's Principles of Internal Medicine. New York, McGraw-Hill, Inc., 1998.
46. Folkow B: Psychosocial and central nervous influence in primary hypertension. Criculation 76:10–19, 1987.
47. Folkow B: Autonomic nervous system in hypertension. In Swales JD (ed): Textbook of Hypertension. London, Blackwell Scientific Publications, 1994, pp 427–438.
48. Foster C, McKinlay S, Cruickshank JM, Coats AJS: Accuracy of the Omron HEM 706 portable monitor for home measurement of blood pressure. J Hum Hypertens 8:661–664, 1994.
49. Gellman M, Spitzer S, Ironson G, et al: Posture, place, and mood effects on ambulatory blood pressure. Psychophysiology 27:544–551, 1990.
50. Guzetti S, Piccaluga E, Casati R, et al: Sympathetic predominance in essential hypertension: A study employing spectral analysis of heart rate variability. J Hypertens 6:711–717, 1988.
51. Harada N, Yoshida I, Kimura K: Heart rate variability and dopamine beta hydroxylase in workers exposed to vibration. Int Arch Occup Environ Health 61:369–373, 1989.
52. Heinonen E, Farkklia M, Forsstrom J, et al: Autonomic neuropathy and vibration exposure in forestry workers. Br J Ind Med 44:412–416, 1987.
53. Hitchen M, Brodie DA, Harness JB: Cardiac responses to demanding mental load. Ergonomics 23:379–385, 1980.
54. Hoberg E, Schuller G, Kunze B, et al: Silent myocardial ischemia as a link between lack of premonitory symptoms and risk of cardiac arrest during physical stress. Am J Cardiol 65:583–589, 1990.
55. Hohnloser SH, Klingenheben T, Zabel M, Gang Li Y: Heart rate variability used as an arrhythmia risk stratifier after myocardial infarction. PACE 20:2594–2601, 1997.

56. Homs E, Marti V, Guindo J, et al: Automatic measurement of correct QT interval in Holter recordings: Comparison of its dynamic behavior in patients after myocardial infarction with and without life-threatening arrhythmias. Am Heart J 134:181–187, 1997.
57. Huikuri HV: Heart rate dynamics and vulnerability to ventricular tachyarrhythmias. Ann Med 29:321–325, 1997.
58. James GD, Moucha OP, Pickering TG: The normal hourly variation of blood pressure in women: Average patterns and the effect of work stress. J Hum Hypertens 5:505–509, 1991.
59. Jamieson MJ, Webster J, Witte K, et al: An evaluation of the A&D UA-751 semi-automatic cuff-oscillometric sphygmomanometer. J Hypertens 8:377–381, 1990.
60. Janosi A, Hankoczy J, Vertes A, et al: Preoperative silent myocardial ischemia has it prognostic significance? Cardiology 78:95–98, 1991.
61. Jennison EA, Parker JE: Recognition and evaluation of occupational and environmental health problems. In Rom WN (ed): Environmental and Occupational Medicine. Philadelphia, Lippincott-Raven Publishers, 1998, pp 11–18.
62. Jensen-Urstad K, Storck N, Bouvier F, et al: Heart rate variability in healthy subjects is related to age and gender. Acta Physiol Scand 160:235–241, 1997.
63. Jereczek M, Andresen D, Schroder J, et al: Prognostic value of ischemia during Holter monitoring and exercise testing after acute myocardial infarction. Am J Cardiol 72:8–13, 1993.
64. Jorna PGAM: Heart rate and workload variations in actual and simulated flight. Ergonomics 36:1043–1054, 1993.
65. Julius S: The defense reaction—A common denominator of coronary risk and blood pressure in neurogenic hypertension? Clin Exper Hypertension 17:375–386, 1995.
66. Julius S, Mejia A, Jones K, et al: "White coat" versus "sustained" borderline hypertension in Tecumseh, Michigan. Hypertension 16:617–623, 1990.
67. Kageyama T, Nishikido N, Honda Y, et al: Effects of obesity, current smoking status, and alcohol consumption on heart rate variability in male white-collar workers. Int Arch Occup Environ Health 69:447–454, 1997.
68. Kageyama T, Nishikido N, Kobayashi T, et al: Long commuting time, extensive overtime, and sympathodominant state assessed in terms of short-term heart rate variability among male white-collar workers in the Tokyo megapolis. Ind Health 36:209–217, 1998.
69. Kalsbeek JWH: Do you believe in sinus arrhythmia? Ergonomics 16:99–104, 1973.
70. Kautzner J, Malik M: QT interval dispersion and its clinical utility. PACE 20:2625–2640, 1997.
71. Kennedy HL, Whitlock JA, Sprague MK, et al: Long-term follow-up of asymptomatic healthy subjects with frequent and complex ventricular ectopy. N Engl J Med 312:193–197, 1985.
72. King GE: Influence of rate of cuff inflation and deflation on observed blood pressure by sphygmomanometry. Am Heart J 65:303–306, 1963.
73. Kishida H, Saito T: Cardiac events in patients with silent myocardial ischemia. Japan Heart J 33:1–13, 1992.
74. Kleiger RE, Stein PK, Bosner MS, Rottman JN: Time domain measurements of heart rate variability. Cardiol Clin 10:487–498, 1992.
75. Kobayashi F, Furui H, Akamatsu Y, et al: Changes in psychophysiological functions during night shift in nurses: Influences of changing from a full-day to a half-day work shift before night duty. Int Arch Occup Environ Health 69:83–90, 1997.
76. Kristal-Boneh E, Raifel M, Froom P, Ribak J: Heart rate variability in health and disease. Scand J Work Environ Health 21:85–95, 1995.
77. Krucoff M: Identification of high-risk patients with silent myocardial ischemia after percutaneous transluminal coronary angioplasty by multilead monitoring. Am J Cardiol 61:29F–34F, 1988.
78. La Rovere MT, Schwartz PJ: Baroreflex sensitivity as a cardiac and arrhythmia mortality risk stratifier. PACE 20:2602–2613, 1997.
79. Lanza GA, Pedrotti P, Pasceri V, et al: Autonomic changes associated with spontaneous coronary spasm in patients with variant angina. J Am Coll Cardiol 28:1249–1256, 1996.
80. Lauer MS, Anderson KM, Levy D: Influence of contemporary versus 30-year blood pressure levels on left ventricular mass and geometry: The Framingham Heart Study. J Am Coll Cardiol 18:1287–1294, 1991.
81. LeClercq JF, Coumel P: Ambulatory electrocardiographic monitoring. In MacFarlane PW, Veitch Lawrie TDF (eds): Comprehensive Electrocardiography. New York, Pergamon Press, 1989, pp 1063–1106.
82. LeClercq JF, Maisonblanche P, Cauchemez B, et al: Troubles du rhythme ventriculaires polymorphes familiaux incessants avec anomalies de la repolalisation ventriculaire: forme frontiere du syndrome du QT long congenital? (Polymorphic familial incessant ventricular arrhythmias with abnormalities of ventricular repolarisation: an intermediate form of the long QT syndrome?) Arch Mal Coeur 77:1013–1019, 1984.
83. Lee DH, Park KS: Multivariate analysis of mental and physical load components in sinus arrhythmia scores. Ergonomics 33:35–47, 1990.
84. Liao D, Cal J, Rosamond WD, et al: Cardiac autonomic function and incident coronary heart disease: A population-based case-cohort study. Am J Epidemiol 145:696–706, 1997.
85. Light KC, Turner JR, Hinderliter AL: Job strain and ambulatory work blood pressure in healthy young men and women. Hypertension 20:214–218, 1992.
86. Lombardi F, Fiorentini C: Hypertension, left ventricular hypertrophy, and heart rate variability. In Zanchetti, et al (eds): Hypertension and the Heart. New York, Plenum Press, 1997, pp 181–187.
87. Luczak H, Laurig W: An analysis of heart rate variability. Ergonomics 16:85–97, 1973.
88. MacFarlane PW, Veitch Lawrie TD: Comprehensive Electrocardiology. New York, Pergamon Press, 1989.
89. Marey EJ: Pression et vitesse du sang. Paris, Physiologie Experimentale. Pratique des hautes etudes de M. Marey, 1876.
90. Mark JB: Atlas of Cardiovascular Monitoring. New York, Churchill Livingstone, 1998.
91. Matsuzaki I, Nishimura A, Morita N, et al: Autonomic nervous activity changes due to shift-work: An evaluation by spectral components of heart rate variability. J Occup Health 38:80–81, 1996.

92. Mauck GW, Smith CR, Geddes LA, Bourland JD: The meaning of the point of maximum oscillations in cuff pressure in the indirect measurement of blood pressure. Part II. J Biomech Eng 102:28–33, 1980.
93. Maxwell MH, Waks AV, Schroth PC, et al: Error in blood pressure measurement due to incorrect cuff size in obese patients. Lancet 2:33–35, 1982.
94. McCubbin JA, Wilson JF, Bruehl S, Brady M, Clark K, Kort E: Gender effects on blood pressures obtained during an on-campus screening. Psychosom Med 53:90–100, 1991.
95. McNamee R, Binks K, Jones S, et al: Shiftwork and mortality from ischemic heart disease. Occ Env Med 53:367–373, 1996.
96. Mengden T, Hernandez-Medina RM, Beltran B, et al: Reliability of reporting self-measured blood pressure values by hypertensive patients. Am J Hypertens 11:1413–1417, 1998.
97. Milstein S, Buetikofer J, Lesser J, et al: Cardiac asystole: A manifestation of neurally mediated hypotension-bradycardia. J Am Coll Cardiol 14:1626–1632, 1989.
98. Mitchell PL, Parlin RW, Blackburn H: Effect of vertical displacement of the arm on indirect blood-pressure measurement. N Eng J Med 271:72–74, 1964.
99. Miyake S: Factors influencing mental workload indexes. Sangyo Ika Daigaku Zasshi 19:313–325, 1997.
100. Morganroth J: Relations of QTc prolongation on the electrocardiogram to torsades de pointes: Definitions and mechanisms. Am J Cardiol 72:10B–13B, 1993.
101. Moss AJ: Measurement of the QT interval and the risk associated with QTc interval prolongation: A review. Am J Cardiol 72:23B–25B, 1993.
102. Moss AJ: The long QT syndrome revisited: Current understanding and implications for treatment. PACE 20:2879–2881, 1997.
103. Moss AJ, Clinical significance of ventricular arrhythmias in patients with and without coronary artery disease. In Sonnenblick EH, Lesch M (eds): Sudden Cardiac Death. New York, Grune & Stratton, 1981, pp 125–144.
104. Moss AJ, Robinson J: Clinical features of the idiopathic long QT syndrome. Circulation 85 Suppl I:I140–I144, 1992.
105. Mulder G, Van Der Meulen M: Mental load and the measurement of heart rate variability. Ergonomics 16:69–83, 1973.
106. O'Brien E, Atkins N: A comparison of the British Hypertension Society and Association for the Advancement of Medical Instrumentation protocols for validating blood pressure measuring devices: Can the two be reconciled? J Hypertension 12:1089–1094, 1994.
107. O'Brien E, Atkins N, Staessen J: State of the market. A review of ambulatory blood pressure monitoring devices. Hypertension 26:835–842, 1995.
108. O'Brien IAD, O'Hare P, Corrall RJM: Heart rate variability in healthy subjects: Effect of age and the derivation of normal ranges for tests of autonomic function. Br Heart J 55:348–354, 1986.
109. Odemuyiwa O, Malik M, Farrell T, et al: Comparison of the predictive characteristics of heart rate variability index and left ventricular ejection fraction for all-cause mortality, arrhythmic events and sudden death after acute myocardial infarction. Am J Cardiol 68:434–439, 1991.
110. Ori Z, Monir G, Weiss J, Sayhouni X, Singer DH: Heart rate variability: Frequency domain analysis. Cardiology Clinics 10:499–537, 1992.
111. Padfield PL, Jyothinagaram SG, Watson DM, et al: Problems in the measurement of blood pressure. J Hum Hypertens 4 Suppl 2:3–7, 1990.
112. Panza JA, Quyyumi AA, Diodati JG, et al: Long-term variation in myocardial ischemia during daily life in patients with stable coronary artery disease: Its relation to changes in the ischemic threshold. J Am Coll Cardiol 19:500–506, 1992.
113. Perloff D, Grim C, Flack J, et al: Human blood pressure determination by sphygmomanometry. Circulation 88:2460–2470, 1993.
114. Petrie JC, O'Brien E, Littler WA, De Swiet M: British Hypertension Society Recommendations on Blood Pressure Measurement. Brit Med J 293:611–615, 1986.
115. Picirillo G, Bucca C, Durante M, et al: Heart rate and blood pressure variabilities in salt-sensitive hypertension. Hypertension 28:952–994, 1996.
116. Pickering TG: Diurnal rhythms and other sources of blood pressure variability in normal and hypertensive subjects. In Laragh JH, Brenner BM (eds): Hypertension: Pathophysiology, Diagnosis, and Management. New York, Raven Press, 1990, pp 1397–1405.
117. Pickering TG: Ambulatory Monitoring and Blood Pressure Variability. London, Science Press, 1991.
117a. Pickering TG: White-coat hypertension. Curr Opin Nephrol Hypertens 5(2):192–198, 1996.
118. Pickering TG, Cvetkovski B, James GD: An evaluation of electronic recorders for self-monitoring of blood pressure. J Hypertens 4 Suppl 5:S328–S330, 1986.
119. Porat B: A Course in Digital Signal Processing. New York, John Wiley & Sons, Inc., 1997.
120. Quyyumi AA, Panza JA, Diadati JG, et al: Relation between left ventricular function at rest and with exercise and silent myocardial ischemia. J Am Coll Cardiol 19:962–967, 1992.
121. Raby KE, Barry J, Treasure CB, et al: Usefulness of Holter monitoring for detecting myocardial ischemia in patients with a nondiagnostic exercise treadmill test. Am J Cardiol 72:889–893, 1993.
122. Ramaekers D, Ector H, Aubert AE, et al: Heart rate variability and heart rate in healthy volunteers. Is the female autonomic nervous system cardioprotective? Eur Heart J 19:1334–1341, 1998.
123. Rohmert W, Laurig W, Philipp U, Luczak H: Heart rate variability and work-load measurement. Ergonomics 16:33–44, 1973.
124. Sammer G: Heart period variability and respiratory changes associated with physical and mental load: Non-linear analysis. Ergonomics 41:746–755, 1998.
125. Sato N, Miyake S, Akatsu J, Kumashiro M: Power spectral analysis of heart rate variability in healthy young women during the normal menstrual cycle. Psychosom Med 57:331–335, 1995.

126. Sayers BM: Analysis of heart rate variability. Ergonomics 16:17–32, 1973.
127. Schlesinger Z, Barzilay J, Stryjer D, Almog CH: Life-threatening "vagal reaction" to emotional stimuli. Israel J Med Sci 13:59–61, 1977.
128. Schnall PL, Devereux RB, Pickering TG, Schwartz JE: The relationship between "job strain," workplace diastolic blood pressure, and left ventricular mass index: A correction [letter; comment]. JAMA 267:1209, 1992.
129. Schnall PL, Landsbergis PA, Schwartz J, et al: A longitudinal study of job strain and ambulatory blood pressure: Results from a 3-year followup. Psychosom Med 60:697–706, 1998.
130. Schnall PL, Pieper C, Schwartz JE, et al: The relationship between job strain, workplace diastolic blood pressure, and left ventricular mass index. Results of a case-control study [published erratum appears in JAMA 1992 Mar 4:367(9):1209]. JAMA 263:1929–1935, 1990.
131. Schnall PL, Schwartz JE, Landsbergis PA, et al: Relation between job strain, alcohol, and ambulatory blood pressure. Hypertension 19:488–494, 1992.
132. Schouten EG, Dekker JM, Meppelink P, et al: QT interval prolongation predicts cardiovascular mortality in an apparently healthy population. Circulation 84:1516–1523, 1991.
133. Schwartz JE, Pickering TG: Work-related stress and blood pressure: Current theoretical models and considerations from a behavioral medicine perspective. J Occup Health Psychol 1:287–310, 1996.
134. Sgarbossa EB, Wagner G: Electrocardiography. In Topol EJ (ed): Textbook of Cardiovascular Medicine. Philadelphia, Lippincott-Raven Publishers, 1998, pp 1545–1589.
135. Sheffield LT, Berson A, Bragg-Remschel D, et al: Recommendations for standards of instrumentation and practice in the use of ambulatory electrocardiography. Circulation 71:626A–636A, 1985.
136. Shell WE, Dobson D: Dissociation of exercise tolerance and total myocardial ischemic burden in chronic stable angina pectoris. Am J Cardiol 66:42–48, 1990.
137. Smirk FH: Casual and basal blood pressures. IV. Their relationship to the supplemental pressure with a note on statistical implications. Brit Heart J 6:174–182, 1944.
138. Stein PK, Kleiger RE, Rottman JN: Differing effects of age on heart rate variability in men and women. Am J Cardiol 80:302–305, 1997.
139. Steinbach K, Nurnberg M: Present and future role of ambulatory Holter monitoring for arrhythmia risk stratification. PACE 20:2587–2593, 1997.
140. Stern S, Gavish A, Zin D: Clinical outcome in silent myocardial ischemia. Am J Cardiol 61:16F–18F, 1988.
141. Stokols D, Pelletier KR, Fielding JE: Integration of medical care and worksite health promotion. JAMA 273:1136–1142, 1995.
142. Stone PH, Chaitman BR, McMahon RP, et al: Asymptomatic cardiac ischemic pilot (ACIP) study. Relationship between exercise-induced and ambulatory ischemia in patients with stable coronary disease. Circulation 94:1537–1544, 1996.
143. Sundberg S, Kohvakka A, Gordin A: Rapid reversal of circadian blood pressure rhythm in shift workers. J Hypertens 6:393–396, 1988.
144. Task Force of the European Society of Cardiology and the North American Society of Pacing and Electrophysiology: Heart rate variability standards of measurement, physiological interpretation, and clinical use. Eur Heart J 17:354–381, 1996.
145. Teruya K, Sakurai H, Omae K, et al: Effect of lead on cardiac parasympathetic function. Int Arch Occup Environ Health 62:549–553, 1991.
146. Theorell T, de Faire U, Johnson J, et al: Job strain and ambulatory blood pressure profiles. Scand J Work Environ Health 17:380–385, 1991.
147. Toivanen H, Lansimies E, Jokela V, Hanninen O: Impact of regular relaxation training on the cardiac autonomic nervous system of hospital cleaners and bank employees. Scand J Work Environ Health 19:319–325, 1993.
148. Tzivoni D, Stern S: Prognostic significance and therapeutic implications of silent myocardial ischaemia. Eur Heart J 11:288–293, 1990.
149. Ugljesic M, Belkic K, Boskovic S, et al: Porast arterijskog krvnog pritiska tokom rada i profil rizika kod stresogenih profesija: novinari i vozaci gradskog saobracja (Increased arterial blood pressure during work and risk profile among high-stress occupations: journalists and city mass transit drivers). Kardiologija 13:150–154, 1992.
150. van Egeren LF: The relationship between job strain and blood pressure at work, at home, and during sleep. Psychosom Med 54:337–343, 1992.
151. van Egmond J, Lenders JW, Weernink E, Thien T: Accuracy and reproducibility of 30 devices for self-measurement of arterial blood pressure. Am J Hypertens 6:873–879, 1993.
152. Verdicchia P, Porellati C, Schillaci G, et al: Ambulatory blood pressure: An independent predictor of prognosis in essential hypertension [published erratum appears in Hypertension 1995 Mar; 25(3):462]. Hypertension 24:793–801, 1994.
153. Victor R, Mainardi JA, Shapiro D: Effects of biofeedback and voluntary control procedures on heart rate and perception of pain during the cold pressor test. Psychosom Med 40:216–225, 1978.
154. Voller H, Andresen D, Bruggemann T, et al: Transient ST segment depression during Holter monitoring: How to avoid false positive findings. Am Heart J 124:622–629, 1992.
155. Wellens HJJ, Vermeulan A, Durrer D: Ventricular fibrillation occurring on arousal from sleep by auditory stimuli. Circulation 46:661–665, 1972.
156. Wolbrette DL, Naccarelli GV: Bradycardias sinus nodal dysfunction and AV conduction disturbances. In Topol EJ (ed): Textbook of Cardiovascular Medicine. Philadelphia, Lippincott-Raven, 1998, pp 1637–1660.
157. Yamasaki F, Schwartz JE, Gerber LM, et al: Impact of shift work and race/ethnicity on the diurnal rhythm of blood pressure and catecholamines. Hypertension 32:417–432, 1998.

CARDIOVASCULAR EVALUATION OF THE WORKER AND WORKPLACE: A PRACTICAL GUIDE FOR CLINICIANS

by Karen Belkić, MD, PhD, Peter Schnall, MD, and Mirjana Uglješić, MD

While the empirical evidence presented in Chapter 2 strongly suggests that psychosocial, ergonomic, and physical workplace stressors make an important contribution to risk of CVD, the workplace has yet to become an integral consideration for clinical cardiology. In recent textbooks and/or millennium reviews in cardiology, hypertension, and internal medicine,[8,13,14,25,43,47,51] the work environment is only minimally discussed with respect to CVD; most often this area is ignored entirely. Consequently, there are very few guidelines (with the exception of those related to physical activity levels) to help clinicians make informed recommendations concerning occupational factors as these pertain to individual patients with various degrees of CVD severity. The challenge remains, as articulated over a decade ago by Giorgio Maisano,[28] to offer the cardiac patient a style of life and of work that protects both his or her health and right to be productive.

THE OCCUPATIONAL HISTORY AS IT RELATES TO THE CARDIOVASCULAR SYSTEM

Maisano insisted that in order to achieve the aforementioned goal, understanding of the job and the work environment, in addition to a functional evaluation of the patient, is absolutely essential.[28] This recommendation would be more feasible if it applied to medical disciplines such as pulmonology, hepatology, nephrology, or hematology, for which assessment of exposure to specific (albeit numerous) chemical agents should suffice. However, given the large panoply of diverse workplace factors potentially affecting the CV system and, especially, the seeming difficulty of evaluating psychosocial stressors, the clinician might well be disinclined to even attempt such an endeavor.

The following text outlines a fairly streamlined, systematic, and comprehensive approach (Table 1) to taking an occupational history as it relates to the CV system. This approach facilitates the inclusion of a single, concise paragraph as an obligatory part of the standard clinical history. An example of such a paragraph is presented. This information provides other colleagues with insight not only into the fixed characteristics of a given occupation, but also about modifiable work conditions which could most acutely affect CV well-being.

The first step (see A) is to indicate the current occupation, and determine whether it falls into the high-risk category.[6] Be as specific as possible; for example,

TABLE 1. Clinical Evaluation of Objective Occupational Stressors Relevant to the Cardiovascular System: Present and Past History

Step A: Type of Occupation. High Risk Category?	Step B: Job Characteristics	Step C: Specific Work Conditions	Step D: Exacerbating (New) Conditions	Step E: Larger Questions
Strong Evidence Professional drivers* Air traffic controllers Sea pilots Smelter workers Workers in the explosives industry Chimney sweeps *Possible High Risk* Lumbermen Police officers Journalists Clerical/sales workers Waste incinerator workers Certain industrial and physical worker categories: (metal processing, paper board workers, sawyers, cement workers, fine mechanics)	*Disaster Potential* Danger of serious accidents (hazardous tasks)* Serious (even fatal) consequences of error or lapse of attention (threat-avoidant vigilant work)** Threat of physical violence from other people** *Underload* Monotonous work* Sits out work time with nothing to do Doesn't learn anything new* *High Psychological Demand* Rapid flow of new information** Receives and transmits important job-related information to other people** Many things going on simultaneously/ must divide attention** Must focus attention on devices** Complicated decision making and/or tasks Supervises work of others *Low Control/Physical Constraints* Strict time schedule** Paced work No chance for creativity* No influence over work conditions* Works in a confined space/fixed body position** Heavily supervised *Socially Isolated*	Long work hours* Night work/other unphysiologic schedule* Few/no rest breaks** Physical exposures: noise*, cold*, heat*, vibration*, heavy lifting Cardiotoxins (e.g., carbon monoxide, carbon disulfide, cadmium, mercury, lead, hydro- and fluorocarbons)* Working two or more jobs Conflicting demands on time and space* Interpersonal conflicts (especially with supervisor)	More overtime work than usual New deadlines Recent involvement in or witnessing serious work accident, or other threatening situation* New interpersonal conflicts	Looming possibility of layoff or permanent unemployment Need to change occupation or workplace Minority/refugee/immigrant: discrimination and/or status incongruity Restructuring within the work organization Additive burden from major nonwork stressors

* Factors present in the sample history, ** Factors strongly present in the sample history

rather than merely noting that the patient is a nurse, indicate where (intensive care unit? well-baby clinic?). Ascertain the number of years in the current job, and obtain a list of all jobs held with approximate dates of employment and relevant details of past work conditions. Pay attention to worsening of cardionoxious working conditions over time. There are, for example, consistent tendencies, albeit of borderline statistical significance, indicating that worsening job decision latitude over time is associated with increased risk of MI.[46]

Next (see B), define the underlying work characteristics. These include many factors that are relatively fixed features of a given job. Modification of these features, if possible, often requires major organizational change. As the clinician becomes more familiar with the occupations of his or her patients, this step can become shorter. Many of the job attributes will be obvious, so that the number of queries posed will be reduced. The clinician should be particularly concerned with jobs exhibiting low control or decision latitude, given the importance of the axis with respect to cardiac risk (see Chapters 2 and 3). When low control is combined with high psychological demand and/or low support, the resulting job strain and isostrain represent a major psychosocial burden that can threaten CV health.

Step C outlines cardionoxious physical, psychosocial, and ergonomic factors that may vary to some extent within an occupation, and may be more amenable to change. The exacerbating conditions listed in Step D could represent trigger mechanisms for acute cardiac events. Finally, in Step E, the larger questions (often cardionoxious) affecting the working individual are considered, such as threat of unemployment; work reorganization requiring change of occupational activity; and minority, refugee, or immigrant status that may result in discrimination and/or status incongruity. Some of these elements are part of the low-reward dimension of the Effort-Reward Model. Note also any nonwork stressors, keeping in mind the additive burden. The latter may be of particular importance to women workers.

This qualitative approach, which we and our colleagues have used successfully in the clinical setting, is based on the Occupational Stress Index[6]; it also incorporates much of the full Job Content Questionnaire,[20] as well as elements from the Effort-Reward Model[41] and the Position Analysis Questionnaire (elements from the latter being associated with cardiovascular disability).[32] Alternatively, much of this information can be acquired using these and other available instruments with a computer-based system, thus streamlining data collection. This type of approach provides the clinician with more time to explore factors that appear to be of critical importance. Whenever possible, information should be obtained using these and other standardized methods and sources (as outlined in Chapter 6). Carefully review any data available from the company and/or the trade union. Insights gained from observational analysis of the worksite are invaluable, and we strongly encourage direct observation, if at all possible. Jennison and Parker note the particular value of open-ended discussion with workers on the job.[18]

Here is a **sample paragraph**, derived from this five-step approach, that could be included in a clinical history:

> The patient has worked for 10 years (prior to this he was a mechanic for 2 years), as an urban bus driver (sole occupational activity) mainly on congested inner-city routes with high threat of violence (has been physically assaulted three times, most recently 2 months ago with superficial lacerations to the right hand) and without a conductor or any ancillary workers in his vehicle. He predominantly works the split shift, starting at 6 AM and driving until 10 AM, then from 2 PM until 6 PM and he does not have time to

go home for the 4 intervening hours. His schedule is very strict; due to heavy traffic he usually is several minutes behind and therefore rarely has any rest breaks. He usually works Monday through Friday; however, at least once and often twice per month he voluntarily works an extra 4 to 8 hours on the weekends, including late night shifts, at the request of the dispatcher. The vehicle which he drives has a major breakdown at least once per month, and there are frequent minor mechanical problems. He has to raise his voice to be heard due to the combinations of vehicular and traffic noise; shock absorption is poor; he feels vibration and fumes inside the cabin; it becomes drafty with temperatures well below 18°C in the winter. His is isolated. There is no air-conditioning. Interpersonal relations within his team are good. He has had no driving accidents. There are no known upcoming changes in organization or work status.

Overall, this patient can be considered to have a cardionoxious job. The patient works in a high-CVD-risk occupation, with a high disaster potential. He is exposed to many elements of high demand and low control, leading to job strain. Numerous additional cardiodeleterious conditions include: long work hours, an unphysiologic work schedule, rare rest breaks, and physical and chemical noxins. The significant negatives include no moonlighting, lack of interpersonal conflicts and driving accidents, and apparently stable macro-work environment.

OCCUPATIONAL CARDIOLOGIC SCREENING AND EVALUATION

After completing an occupational history, if a global assessment is made that the patient's job is potentially cardionoxious, an occupational cardiologic screening and evaluation should follow. A large and ever-expanding array of diagnostic modalities can be applied to the workplace (see Chapter 7). These possibilities present the clinician with a practical dilemma: "For whom and when?" The clinician could aptly bemoan, particularly in the current climate of managed care and cost containment, that it is utterly impossible to nonselectively use these tests in all patients exposed to work conditions potentially harmful to the CV system. The astute clinician is well aware that new, *proactive* paradigms are needed. The very changes underway in the medical system argue for such an approach. Drew and Coye elaborate on this possibility with regard to occupational health and managed care in the 21st century: "It . . . becomes prudent to encourage preventive medicine (wellness) in order to reduce expensive (acute illness, chronic disease state) demand . . ."[11] They encourage health screenings and healthy lifestyle choices. Furthermore, there are increasing efforts to coordinate care and avoid duplications.[11]

In Table 2 we attempt to address these issues by proposing an integrated and *graded* approach to occupational cardiologic workup, based on the degree of acquired CVD severity. We also distinguish between what could be considered the minimal workup needed and those assessments that are either strongly recommended or advised only if feasible. These guidelines have been formulated after taking into consideration existing empirical data on risk stratification and the likelihood of each proposed diagnostic step yielding new, relevant information for clinical decision-making, as it relates to the workplace. (Clinico-physiologic rationale for these guidelines can be found in Chapters 5 and 7.)

We have assumed for this discussion that the clinician is based at a site outside the workplace. Insofar as the clinician has access to the workplace, blood pressure (BP) should be measured at work in *all* patients, including those with normal casual clinic

TABLE 2. Proposed Occupational Cardiology Workup for Patients with Cardionoxious Jobs

Screening Evaluation		Findings: ACVD Severity	Next Diagnostic Steps*		
Minimum	Strongly Recommended		Minimum	Strongly Recommended	Recommended If Feasible
Medical history	Worksite BP measurement	Normal-normotensive	Continued surveillance†	Worksite BP measurement	Ambulatory BP monitoring (during work)
Physical exam (BP × 2)	5-minute resting ECG (measure heart rate variability)	Lone borderline HTN	Worksite BP measurement	Ambulatory BP monitoring (during work) Echocardiogram (LV mass)	Holter monitoring (during work) Exercise testing Laboratory testing of work stressors**
Resting 12-lead ECG		Borderline HTN + other signs of CV metabolic syndrome or Frank primary HTN	Ambulatory BP monitoring (during work) Echocardiogram (LV mass)	Exercise testing Holter monitoring (during work)	Laboratory testing of work stressors**
Cardiac risk factors Smoking Obesity Sedentary Family history Blood pressure HDL/LDL cholesterol Fasting blood glucose Triglycerides Behavior patterns (e.g., hostility)		HTN + increased LV mass	The above plus: Exercise testing Holter monitoring (during work)		Laboratory testing of work stressors**
Alcohol (for hypertension) Atherogenic diet		Myocardial ischemia and/or previous cardiac events	Clinical cardiology consultation (see Chapter 9)		

* With increasing number of cardiac risk factors, and/or low heart rate variability, upgrade workup

** See text for description

† At least yearly, as per American Heart Association

BP = blood pressure, HTN = hypertension, LV = left ventricular, ACVD = acquired cardiovascular disorders

BP. The limited reliability and diagnostic validity of casual clinic BPs is becoming increasingly recognized. Most importantly, BP measurement at the workplace offers the possibility of detection of at-risk patients whose casual clinic BP remains normal.

Here are a few examples of the logic used to generate these guidelines: Since the cardiovascular metabolic syndrome frequently is associated with an increased left ventricular mass (LVM), echocardiography is indicated for those patients with borderline hypertension together with other evidence of this syndrome. The close relation between amBPs during work and large LVM as well as risk of cardiovascular morbidity should be borne in mind. Patients with increased LVM are at heightened risk for myocardial ischemia. Thus, work-related ST segment depression should be evaluated by Holter monitoring in these patients. Given the septadian data on increased Monday morning risk of cardiac events, recordings should be performed on Mondays or the first day after a nonwork period, if possible.

Laboratory CV testing of workplace stressors can be considered, at present, an ancillary diagnostic modality. In clinical cardiologic practice, laboratory simulation of work activity has been limited primarily to assessing cardiovascular responses to various combination of static and dynamic workplace physical activity, e.g., shoveling, heavy lifting, other upper extremity activity.[10,15,21,23,24,42] Laboratory testing of physiological responses to other physical stressors that affect the cardiovascular system, such as noise, cold, heat, cardionoxious chemicals, glare, and vibration, has been performed in the research setting.[4,7,12,22,27,30,35,50] In principle, testing of this type could be applied routinely in clinical practice—for example, to evaluate the patient's CV reactions to each of the physical noxious agents to which he or she is exposed at work. This type of approach is already well established in other occupational medical disciplines, notably pulmonary medicine.

In the laboratory, it has been consistently reported that "personally relevant mental stress" is a potent stimulus of myocardial ischemia in coronary patients.[17,36,38,39] Discussions about painful or otherwise emotionally-charged events experienced by the cardiac patient are found to elicit heart rate and galvanic skin responses, as well as signs of cardiac electrical instability.[26,48] For 22 young, healthy, male, mainly blue collar workers, discussion in the laboratory during a 10-minute semi-structured interview about intensely stressful workplace events was a more powerful stimulus of pressor reactions (+12.4 / +15.1) than any of five standard mental stress tests.[2] In another report, discussion in the laboratory of a threatening work situation triggered bouts of ventricular tachycardia in a post-MI patient.[45] The only other topic that provoked these arrhythmias was the MI experience itself.

These findings could be used as the basis for laboratory clinical testing in specific relation to the workplace. It may be feasible, in the future, to routinely register CV responses during a semi-structured interview focusing on painful, difficult, and/or dangerous aspects of a patient's work. This approach might be particularly helpful for patients in high-strain jobs or emotionally-intensive work, for those obliged to maintain a high level of vigilance to avert potentially disastrous consequences, and for those exposed to other major psychosocial hazards.

As a general principle, the greater the exposure to potential cardionoxins from the workplace, the more intensive the workup should be, especially if multiple standard cardiac risk factors are present. The independent prognostic significance of low heart rate variability for various patient strata also suggests that the workup be upgraded with this finding. The clinician should be particularly cognizant of the potential association between work stressors and modifiable risk factors such as smoking, obesity, and sedentary leisure time (see Chapter 2).

Screening evaluation or further workup may reveal CV abnormalities other than the acquired CV disorders, which merit clinical attention. Any relation to workplace exposures should be evaluated; e.g., cobalt-, arsenic- or other toxic cardiomyopathy; antimony exposure and prolonged QT interval; nephrotoxin-induced secondary (renal) hypertension.

MODIFICATION OF THE CARDIONOXIOUS WORK ENVIRONMENT: WHY WE CAN'T WAIT

The impact of workplace intervention on CV well-being is the subject of intense investigation (see Chapter 13). Some experts have contended that without data from controlled workplace intervention trials, it is premature to recommend workplace modifications. Muir states that while such recommendations may "seem pragmatically to make good sense, evidence is lacking from intervention studies that introducing these changes will reduce the likelihood of CHD events."[31]

There is, however, an emerging body of observational data suggesting that changes in psychosocial working conditions (as well as lack of such) may have an important impact on clinical CV outcomes among hypertensive and young MI patients. Schnall and colleagues demonstrated among hypertensive men followed over 3 years that change from exposure to nonexposure to job strain (N = 10) was associated with a mean fall in unmedicated ambulatory workplace BP levels of –11.3/–5.8 mmHg, after adjusting for age, body mass index, alcohol, and smoking status.[40] Those hypertensive patients who continued to work at high-strain jobs for the 3 years showed persistently high BP levels. Among 79 men who had survived a first MI before the age of 45, return to work at a high-strain job was a significant, independent predictor of mortality related to ischemic heart disease (IHD) after 5 years of followup, in a study by Theorell and coworkers.[44] The predictive strength of return to high-strain work was of comparable magnitude to degree of angiographically assessed coronary atheromatosis, and more powerful than left ventricular ejection fraction. This finding remained robust after adjustment for standard cardiac risk factors.

Among professional drivers a significant relation has been found between number of years on the job and development of hypertension.[3,5,34] Furthermore, in a small cohort study with 4-year followup of male workers up to the age of 40 at intake, Uglješić and colleagues reported that 66 professional drivers who continued in that occupation had a mean increase in casual BP of +10.9/+9.6; this was approximately twice the BP rise found among 31 examined building trade workers.[49] In contrast, the drivers had only a mean increase of 1.7 kg body weight over followup, while the building workers gained 2.2 kg.

In our opinion, the above-cited data coupled with clinical experience argues that *ethically* we cannot wait for the definitive results of intervention trials to begin to address what the clinician can do to promote cardiovascular well-being in a cardionoxious workplace. Table 3 presents a suggested approach, based on the degree of acquired CVD severity. For workers who are still healthy or have lone borderline hypertension, the recommendations are more or less educational, and linked to public health efforts to improve the workplace. However, even among these workers, overtime work should be strongly discouraged, given the evidence implicating long work hours and CVD and suggesting that the total burden of cardionoxious work increases in relation to duration of exposure.

Since borderline hypertension is an early pathologic state, which may revert to normotension or progress to frank primary hypertension,[1,9,19] based on the data of Schnall, et al.[40] it seems justified to recommend that the patient lower his or her job

TABLE 3. Clinician Options for Promoting Cardiovascular Well-Being
in a Cardionoxious Workplace

Degrees of Acquired CV Disorder Severity	Suggested Approach
Normotensive–healthy	Educate and promote empowerment/bolster social support
	Encourage positive changes at work
	Facilitate longitudinal study and workplace intervention trials
	Strongly discourage overtime work
	Promote salutogenic use of break time (exercise, positive social interaction, relaxation)
Lone borderline hypertension	*The above plus:*
	Advise patient to lower job strain profile, if at all possible
	Retain a high index of suspicion that this may be a "sentinel event"
	Help initiate workplace intervention trials whenever feasible
Borderline hypertension + CV metabolic syndrome or Frank primary hypertension (especially if LVH)	*The above plus:*
	Use ambulatory BP monitoring to find and then recommend work schedule or conditions with minimum BP
	Strongly discourage split and night shiftwork; noise, heat, or vibration exposure; heavy lifting
	Eliminate overtime work and exposure to pressogenic chemicals (e.g., lead)
Silent myocardial ischemia	*The above plus:*
	Use Holter monitoring to find and then recommend work schedule or conditions with minimum ischemia
	Minimize job strain and exposure to heat and cold
	Eliminate early AM, night, and split shifts, and heavy lifting
Post-acute cardiac events	Maximal efforts by clinician to realize all of the above (see Chapter 9)

CV = cardiovascular, LVH = left ventricular hypertrophy

strain profile, if at all possible (of course, without creating other major life perturbations). The clinician should retain an index of suspicion that borderline hypertension or more severe manifestations of acquired CVD in the face of a cardionoxious workplace may represent an occupational sentinel event, defined as: "a disease, disability or untimely death which is occupationally related and whose occurrence may: (1) provide the impetus for epidemiologic or industrial hygiene studies; or (2) serve as a warning signal that materials substitution, engineering control, personal protection, or medical care may be required."[29]

In addition to the standard clinical measures and cardiac risk factor interventions that comprise usual care for patients with more advanced degrees of acquired cardiovascular disorders, individualized workplace modifications could represent another therapeutic modality. Here, the clinician could play a unique role in integratively evaluating the results of ambulatory monitoring to find work schedules or conditions that are the least deleterious to the cardiovascular system. Some individual reports of the success of this type of approach have been published.

Kavanagh and Matosevic present several cases of coronary patients in whom exercise testing was normal, but for whom situations involving mental overload combined with exposure to physical stressors evoked hemodynamic signs of marked sympathetic arousal, leading to several millimeters of ST segment depression.[21] Specific modifications in the patient's work environment were consequently instituted, with favorable clinical results as well as preservation of the patients' employment status. Thus, it has been recommended that the prevalence and severity of ischemic, arrhythmic, and hemodynamic abnormalities be assessed during actual work, with a detailed diary kept so that the influence of specific occupational activity on CV parameters can be followed.[21,23,24,42]

Belkić and colleagues presented a case report of an obese, hyperlipidemic, borderline hypertensive city bus driver—a current smoker with a very strong family history of IHD—admitted to the coronary care unit for chest pain.[6] His occupational history was similar, though somewhat less severe, than the one presented on page 215. In conjunction with standard risk factor and pharmacologic measures, the clinician suggestion that the patient change from a split-shift to the afternoon shift (which the patient preferred) was implemented. At 4-month followup, the patient had quit smoking, lost 14 kg, and lipid and BP levels were diminished. It was concluded that "this case demonstrates that modifiable workplace and standard cardiac risk factors can be closely interrelated . . . When the clinician can recognize this and intervene in both of these spheres, there is a much better chance for successful prevention in high-risk patients."[6]

The above-cited cases illustrate another important principle with regard to the role of the clinician in suggesting workplace modifications. Namely, that the suggestions be made with careful consideration of the wishes of the patient. It is important to keep in mind that these patients are, more often than not, in their most productive years and highly motivated for work. Depriving them of their occupational activity can have devastating consequences for themselves and their families.[16,23,28,33] Thus, iatrogenically compromising employability should be avoided and respect for confidentiality scrupulously maintained—particularly when there are looming possibilities of lay-offs within the work organization. With the consent and, optimally, the participation of the patient, "medical practitioners or their designates" should try to work with employers to create a more salutogenic work environment for cardiac patients.[37] If queried, patients themselves may give realistic, insightful ideas into how this might be accomplished. Ambulatory monitoring then offers the possibility of objectively examining whether and how specific modifications in work conditions actually provide some benefit to the patient.

REFERENCES

1. Australian National Blood Pressure Study: The Australian therapeutic trial in mild hypertension. Lancet 1:1261–1267, 1980.
2. Belkic K: Methodology for detecting individuals at high risk for developing the acquired cardiovascular disorders. Master's Thesis, Center for Multidisciplinary Studies, Belgrade, University of Belgrade, 1984.
3. Belkic K, Gluhak M, Ugljesic M, et al: Ucestalost abnormalnosti arterijskog krvnog pritiska i elektrokardiograma kod vozaca gradskog saobracajnog preduzeca Beograd (Prevalence of high blood pressure and electrocardiologic abnormalities among Belgrade mass transit drivers). Revija Rada 20:50–60, 1990.
4. Belkic K, Ercegovac D, Savic C, et al: EEG arousal and cardiovascular reactivity in professional drivers: The glare pressor test. Eur Heart J 13:304–309, 1992.
5. Belkic K, Pavlovic S, Djordjevic M, et al: Determinants of cardiac risk in professional drivers. Kardiologija 13:145–149, 1992.
6. Belkic K, Savic C, Theorell T, Cizinsky S: Work Stressors and Cardiovascular Risk: Assessment for Clinical Practice, Part I. Stockholm, National Institute for Psychosocial Factors and Health. Section for Stress Research, Karolinska Institute, WHO Psychosocial Center, 1995.
7. Borsky I, Hubacova L, Hatiar K, et al: Combined effect of physical strain, noise and hot environmental conditions on man. Arch Complex Environ Studies 5:75–83, 1993.
8. Braunwald E: Cardiovascular medicine at the turn of the millennium: Triumphs, concerns, and opportunities. New Engl J Med 337:1360–1369, 1997.
9. de Faire U, Lindvall K, Nilsson B: Noninvasive ambulatory 24th blood pressures and basal blood pressures predict development of sustained hypertenion from borderline state. Am J Hypertens 6:149–155, 1993.
10. DeBusk RF: Determination of cardiac impairment and disability. J Am Coll Cardiol 14:1043–1044, 1989.
11. Drew DC, Coye MJ: Occupational health and managed care into the 21st century. In Rom WN (ed): Environmental and Occupational Medicine. Philadelphia, Lippincott-Raven Publisher, 1998, pp 79–85.
12. Egan CE, Espie BH, McGrann S, et al: Acute effects of vibration on peripheral blood flow in healthy subjects. Occup Environ Med 53:663–669, 1996.

13. Fauci AS, Braunwald E, Isselbacher KJ, et al: Harrison's Principles of Internal Medicine. New York, McGraw-Hill, Inc., 1998.
14. Goldman L, Braunwald E: Primary Cardiology. Philadelphia, WB Saunders Co., 1998.
15. Haskell WL, Brachfeld N, Bruce RA, et al: Determination of occupational working capacity in patients with ischemic heart disease. J Am Coll Cardiol 14:1016–1042, 1989.
16. Hellerstein HK: Work evaluation. In Wenger NK, Hellerstein HK (eds): Rehabilitation of the Coronary Patient. New York, Churchill Livingstone, 1992, pp 523–542.
17. Ironson G, Taylor CB, Boltwood M, et al: Effects of anger on left ventricular ejection fraction in coronary artery disease. Am J Cardiol 70:281–285, 1992.
18. Jennison EA, Parker JE: Recognition and evaluation of occupational and environmental health problems. In Rom WN (ed): Environmental and Occupational Medicine. Philadelphia, Lippincott-Raven Publishers, 1998, pp 11–18.
19. Julius S, Shork MA: Borderline hypertension—A critical review. J Chronic Dis 23:723–754, 1971.
20. Karasek RA, Gordon G, Pietroskovsky C, et al: Job Content Instrument: Questionnaire and User's Guide. Los Angeles/Lowell MA, University of Southern California/University of Massachuesetts, 1985.
21. Kavanagh T, Matosevic V: Assessment of work capacity in patients with ischaemic heart disease: Methods and practices. Eur Heart J 9 Suppl L:67–73, 1988.
22. Kjelberg A, Wikstrom BO: Whole-body vibration: Exposure time and acute effects—A review. Ergonomics 28:535–544, 1985.
23. Knapp D, Gutman MC, Tristani F, Sheldahl L, Wilke N: Returning the patient to work. In Pollock ML, Schmidt DH (eds): Heart Disease and Rehabilitation. New York, John Wiley & Sons, 1986, pp 647–677.
24. Landes I, Rod JL: Return to work evaluation after coronary events. Special emphasis on simulated work activity. Sport Medicine 13:365–375, 1992.
25. Laragh JH, Brenner BM: Hypertension Pathophysiology, Diagnosis, and Management. NY, Raven Press, 1995.
26. Lown B: Role of higher nervous activity in sudden cardiac death. Jpn Circ J 54:581–602, 1990.
27. Lundstrom R, Landstrom U, Kjelberg A: Combined effects of low-frequency noise and whole body vibrations on wakefulness, annoyance and performance. Arch Complex Environ Studies 2:1–7, 1990.
28. Maisano G: Summary and conclusions towards guidelines for return to work after myocardial infarction and myocardial revascularization. Eur Heart J 9 Suppl L:120–122, 1988.
29. Markowitz SB: The role of surveillance in occupational health. In Rom WN (ed): Environmental and Occupational Medicine. Philadelphia, Lippincott-Raven Publishers, 1998, pp 19–29.
30. Matoba T, Mizobuchi H, Ito T, et al: Further observation of the digital plethysmography in response to auditory stimuli and its clinical applications angiology. Angiology 32:62–72, 1981.
31. Muir J: Personality and psychological environment. In Lawrence M, Neil A, Fowler G, Mant D (eds): Prevention of Cardiovascular Disease: An Evidence-Based Approach. Oxford, Oxford University Press, 1996, pp 93–104.
32. Murphy LR: Job dimensions associated with severe disability due to CVD. J Clin Epidemiol 44:155–166, 1991.
33. Picard MH, Dennis C, Schwartz RG, et al: Cost-benefit analysis of early return to work after uncomplicated acute myocardial infarction. Am J Cardiol 63:1308–1314, 1989.
34. Ragland DR, Greiner BA, Holman BL, Fisher JM: Hypertension and years of driving in transit vehicle operators. Scand J Soc Med 25:271–279, 1997.
35. Razmjou S: Mental workload in heat: Toward a framework for analyses of stress states. Aviat Space Environ Med 67:530–538, 1996.
36. Rozanski A, Bairey N, Krantz DS, et al: Mental stress and the induction of silent myocardial ischemia in patients with coronary artery disease. N Engl J Med 318:1005–1012, 1988.
37. Russell RO, Abi-Mansour P, Wenger NK: Return to work after coronary bypass surgery and percutaneous transluminal angioplasty: Issues and potential solutions. Cardiology 73:306–322, 1986.
38. Schiffer F, Hartley LH, Schulman CL, Abelmann WH: The quiz electrocardiogram. Am J Cardiol 37:41–47, 1976.
39. Schiffer F, Hartley LH, Schulman CL, Abelmann WH: Evidence for emotionally-induced coronary arterial spasm in patients with angina pectoris. Br Heart J 44:62–66, 1980.
40. Schnall PL, Landsbergis PA, Schwartz J, et al: A longitudinal study of job strain and ambulatory blood pressure: Results from a 3-year follow-up. Psychosom Med 60:697–706, 1998.
41. Siegrist J: Adverse health effects of high-effort/low-reward conditions. J Occup Health Psychol 1:27–41, 1996.
42. Stoltz I, Erdelyi A: Practical aspects of identifying and correcting worksite stress in a post-infarction patients returning to work. Eur Heart J Suppl L:82–83, 1988.
43. Swales D: Textbook of Hypertension. London, Blackwell Scientific, 1994.
44. Theorell T, Perski A, Orth-Gomer K, et al: The effects of the strain of returning to work on the risk of death after a first myocardial infarction before age of 45. Int J Cardiol 30:61–67, 1991.
45. Theorell T: Medical and physiological aspects of job interventions. In Cooper CL, Robertson IT (eds): International Review of Industrial and Organizational Psychology, Vol. 8. New York, John Wiley, 1993, pp 173–192.
46. Theorell T, Tsutsumi A, Hallqvist J, et al: SHEEP Study Group. Decision latitude, job strain, and myocardial infarction. Am J Public Health 88:382–388, 1998.
47. Topol EJ: Textbook of Cardiovascular Medicine. Philadelphia, Lippincott-Raven, 1998.
48. Tsouna-Hadjis ED, Mitsibounas DN, Kallergis GE, Sideris DA: Autonomic nervous system responses to personal stressful events in patients with acute myocardial infarction. Psychoth Psychosom 97:31–36, 1998.
49. Ugljesic M, Belkic K, Simeunovic-Mickovic L, Vukajlovic M: Realization of a preventive plan for cardiovascular disease prevention among professional drivers: a high risk group. Srp Arh Lek 120 Suppl 1:49–51, 1992.
50. Verdun di Cantogno L, Dallerba R, Teagno PS, et al: Urban traffic noise, cardiocirculatory and coronary risk factors. Acta Otolaryng Suppl 339:55–63, 1976.
51. Willerson JT, Cohn JN: Cardiovascular Medicine. New York, Churchill Livingstone, 1995.

CLINICAL ISSUES: RETURN TO WORK AND PUBLIC SAFETY *by Regis de Gaudemaris, MD*

Cardiovascular disease (CVD) commonly occurs before the age of retirement, and some of those who suffer a heart attack are still in normal, full-time employment. By virtue of their age, such subjects are highly experienced and are often in positions of responsibility. Indirect costs associated with sick leave can be high. Thus, exactly when a patient can go back to work is an important issue for employers and for the worker. By way of reference, in England in 1983 the prevalence of coronary heart disease (CHD) among industrial workers was 10.4 cases for every 1000 individuals,[19] and the disease was responsible for 13% of all health-related early retirements.

Advances in cardiovascular therapy (e.g., fibrinolysis, coronary angioplasty, coronary bypass surgery, pacemaker technology, automatic implantable cardioverter-defibrillators, and drugs) mean that the cardiovascular function of many patients is restored to such an extent that returning to work is possible.[9] However, CVD can entail a whole range of medical problems: the need for physical rehabilitation; how to assess residual functional capacity; the short- and medium-term prognosis for the disease; the risk of a heart attack putting at risk either the life of the patient and/or their colleagues; being sure that the treatment administered will not interfere with the subject's ability to perform his or her job. Even with ideal medical treatment, many subjects should not go back to work for a variety of psychological or social reasons, all of which have to be taken into account. Work can only be resumed with the cooperation of several parties, i.e., the patient's personal physician, cardiologist, and employer (job modifications may be required of the latter). Therefore, in technical terms, the decision whether or not to go back to work involves not only weighing medical considerations but also the patient's psychosocial profile and factors associated with his or her particular job.

MEDICAL ASSESSMENT AND PSYCHOSOCIAL PROFILE

Studies on going back to work have shown that a number of different elements are involved:

1. The exact nature of the original cardiovascular event that led to the patient stopping work. The most common reason is **coronary artery disease** (CAD) which can range from myocardial infarction (MI) to angina treated with coronary artery bypass, angioplasty, or just drugs. In CAD, whatever its particular form, certain clinical issues always dominate: whether or not the patient still experiences angina during exercise; whether there is a risk of arrhythmia; and the level of left ventricular function, if this is likely to limit the capacity for physical exertion. It is important to note that, for patients with no residual angina, neither their cardiovascular status (whether there is any infarction or not) nor the nature of the treatment (whether it involves only drugs or also a coronary artery bypass) is important when it comes to deciding on return to work. The possibility of silent myocardial ischemia also should be considered, given its prognostic importance; and systematic maximal exercise test and/or ECG Holter monitoring should be recommended in at-risk patients, especially those with diabetes. Although patients tend to go back sooner following coronary angioplasty than after bypass surgery, figures show that long-term employment prospects are the same.[10]

Unmanaged high blood pressure (BP) can make returning to work difficult, partly because of symptoms (e.g., headaches, dizziness, feeling unwell) that interfere with the patient's ability to perform the job, but more importantly because the very fact of working tends to exacerbate high BP. Static and dynamic effort can induce significant increases in BP load, and psychological factors can disrupt key balance mechanisms, thereby perturbing the patient's BP level, not only during working hours but also throughout the rest of the circadian cycle.

Feelings of **malaise** and **cardiac syncope** are strong indicators of a risk of relapse and all the associated consequences vis-à-vis the working environment. Different conclusions have been arrived at concerning physical examinations and function tests,[13,14] but sending a patient back to work should not even be contemplated until an overall evaluation has been performed and a stable treatment strategy has been definitively established.

Improvements in the drugs available for treating heart failure (ACE inhibitors, specific beta-blockers) and in rehabilitation techniques have significantly increased the number of patients able to resume their professional lives. The main clinical consideration in this case is how well the heart problem that originally gave rise to the heart failure is being managed.

2. The extent of loss of function. Going back to work always entails some extra physical effort corresponding to routine actions (e.g., commuting and moving around in the workplace) and, beyond that, specific forms of exertion associated with the job. During a standard cardiologic examination, a patient's **functional capacity** can be assessed in an exercise stress test (for hypertension and CAD) or an exercise stress test with measurement of oxygen consumption (for heart failure). Although not part of the usual cardiologic examination, some of the physical as well as psychological workplace noxins can be simulated in the laboratory while monitoring cardiovascular response[12] (see Chapter 8).

Functional capacity can be increased by cardiac rehabilitation, so consider sending patients to a physical therapy center before they return to work. These centers offer programs geared towards preparing patients for a variety of different types of working conditions—for example, by carrying progressively heavier loads or practicing increasingly more demanding arm manipulations.[12]

Once the patient is working again, the physical stress involved in the job can be estimated using a Holter ambulatory ECG monitor or a heart rate integrator in conjunction with specific, validated indices.[6] In many workplaces, it is also possible to measure ambulatory BP. In addition to gauging the dynamic-aerobic demands of work, ambulatory monitoring (ideally Holter and BP monitoring together) is of great utility for assessing the impact of other work stressors (e.g., physical, chemical, psychosocial, ergometric)—especially their additive burden—on clinically relevant cardiovascular parameters. With the help of such techniques, physicians can review their decision to allow the patient to go back to work.

3. Prognosis and the risk factors associated with the heart disorder. A return to work is only worthwhile if it is to be for a significant period of time. Thus it is important to weigh the probability that a subject will be able to continue his or her professional life through the medium and perhaps the long term. This **prognostic assessment** must include: the likelihood of the condition deteriorating; any job-related risk factors (e.g., stress, heavy physical demands); any other risk factors (smoking, blood cholesterol levels, BP); patient compliance level.

4. Personal factors involved in deciding whether or not to go back to work. **Psychological and social factors** are more important than medical considerations when it comes to deciding whether or not to go back to work.[4] To do so means that the patient will have to stick to the agreed upon plan, especially if job reassignment or professional retraining is necessary. Many studies have used multivariate analysis to identify the key factors that determine or modify whether and when patients return to work.[5] These factors can be broken down into a number of different groups:

- The probability of going back is inversely proportional to the length of time away from work, whatever the prognosis of the cardiovascular event.
- The psychological representation of the cardiovascular event that caused the patient to stop working becomes particularly significant when the episode of malaise or unconsciousness occurred in the workplace (in front of others), or if the patient was treated surgically and is suffering complications of sternotomy (i.e., if the healing of the operative wound is causing pain).
- The worker's age and level of retirement coverage are closely linked: the older the patient (i.e., the closer to retirement age), the more they will be eligible for anticipated redundancy provisions and the more likely they will be to stop work before the statutory retirement age.
- The motivation to go back to work corresponds to the patient's daily interest in getting up and undertaking the job. Patients are less likely to go back to monotonous, routine work that makes no demands on their personal talents or skills.
- The patient's level of education or training and their suitability for retraining is an important factor. When necessary, reassignment tends to mean changing to a less physical job, but one which might be more mentally or psychologically demanding (e.g., in information technology). Such a change is not always consistent with the patient's original training and skills.

5. The physician's motivation. Physicians often are reluctant to send their patients back to work, even in the face of a nonischemic exercise test, based on their concern about prognosis.[18]

THE JOB AND THE WORK ENVIRONMENT

All the relevant information normally can be obtained in the course of an in-depth interview with the patient, but in some cases a visit to the patient's workplace also may be necessary. It is essential to work together with the employer's health and safety department. The interview should cover any aspects of the patient's job which could affect the return to work and should highlight any working conditions that might exacerbate the patient's condition.

Job Aspects to Consider

Different jobs combine, to different extents, physical activity (static and dynamic work) with psychosensory stress. The most common argument against an early return to work is that the job involves heavy and/or sustained physical work (either static or dynamic). However, a job that involves a moderate level of physical effort probably protects against the recurrence of CAD more effectively than completely sedentary work. In the context of coronary insufficiency, it is also necessary to identify factors that might exacerbate any residual coronary ischemia, e.g., work at high altitudes or extreme temperatures (either hot or cold), or the possibility that the patient may be exposed to carbon monoxide (particularly if the patient is continuing to smoke). It is especially important to identify patients in high-risk jobs—jobs in which the operative, in the event of sudden cardiac incapacitation (cardiac syncope, serious arrhythmia), could be at risk or could risk other lives.

Potentially Harmful Work Practices

Shift work can exacerbate heart disease (hypertension and cardiac or coronary insufficiency) by upsetting the circadian rhythms that regulate BP and heart rate. Working the night shift or getting up for the early morning shift (4–5 AM) coincides with the time when the cardiovascular system is normally at rest (with catecholamines at their lowest levels). Moreover, if the daily routine is constantly changing, it is difficult to schedule medications to cover the 24-hour period effectively.

Long work hours are of interest, for they are a cardionoxious factor that could be prevented.

Work-related psychological stress, as defined by Karasek or Siegrist can exacerbate high BP and CHD. If the support system in the workplace is poor, the therapeutic equilibrium can be thrown off, and new symptoms may develop.[23] Even when no direct link can be proven, patients sometimes blame such stress for their condition, and this should be taken into account when there is a strong possibility that the patient will refuse to go back to work. In most return-to-work studies, the psychosocial quality of the work environment has not been assessed in relation to prognostic criteria.[1,3,7,9,11,16,20] Furthermore, studies examining prognosis often have not had sufficient followup periods. However, in a clinical prospective study of a group of men up to the age of 45 who were followed for 5 years, the prognostic significance of returning to high-strain work after MI was comparable to the degree of angiographically assessed coronary atherosclerosis, and of greater importance than the left ventricular ejection fraction.[21] On the basis of these data, together with numerous cohort studies showing an excess risk of CHD morbidity and mortality among workers exposed to job strain or other untoward psychosocial work conditions, Theorell and Karasek have questioned whether heart attack patients should return to stressful jobs.[21]

Deciding About a Return to Work

It is only possible to send a patient back to work if he or she wants to go. Problems arise when it is necessary, because of diminished functional capacities, to modify working conditions or completely change to another job. The final decision on whether the patient should go back to work is up to the cardiologist, optimally, together with the occupational health specialist.[17] Every country (every state in the U.S.) has its own regulations. In Europe, especially in France and Germany where occupational health is mainly dealt with by specialists, return to work is most easily organized with full participation of the company, because it is familiar with all the relevant working conditions and the possibilities for reassignment within the company. The approach is necessarily more complicated in countries where occupational health is less tightly regulated and mainly concerns safety issues.

It is useful to let patients with less severe cardiovascular problems who wish to go back to work at any price return for a predefined period of up to 6 months. Ensure that the resources are available to check that they are responding well. This followup may include a physical examination, an ECG during working hours, and an assessment of cardiovascular risk factors.

PUBLIC SAFETY ISSUES

A job is considered high risk if the worker involved puts lives at risk in the event of experiencing a sudden loss of ability to carry out the job duties. Such abrupt deterioration can take the form of a profound malaise, syncope, or even sudden death. From a cardiologic point of view, a sudden loss of consciousness is usually due to arrhythmia exacerbating a pre-existing cardiac problem. Although ventricular arrhythmia traditionally has been considered the main danger, certain kinds of supraventricular arrhythmia which have hitherto been thought of as relatively benign as well as bradyarrhythmias also can cause syncope or sudden death. Accurately gauging the risk of syncope is difficult, and it is not always possible to predict its appearance, even when a comprehensive cardiologic examination is performed.

The Type of Job

Most of the jobs presenting public safety problems are those that involve operating vehicles, e.g., trucks, public transport vehicles, machines used in the construction industry, cars, airplanes, and trains. However, other jobs, such as operating cranes and handling dangerous industrial processes, also are implicated. Additionally, although perhaps not directly associated with the job, driving a car—essential to many people for getting to the workplace—can affect public safety.

Risk assessment for driving a car remains complicated, but figures have been extensively studied for professional drivers on the road: U.S. and Canadian studies indicate that less than 0.1% of all accidents can be attributed to a health problem, and only 10–25% of these are associated with a cardiac event. In a study of the London Public Transport system, only six accidents over a 20-year period were found to have happened as a result of the driver suffering a coronary heart problem; during that time, 6.8 million miles were covered, corresponding to 334,000 driver-hours.[19] It is reasonable to conclude that asymptomatic drivers who match the current criteria laid down by cardiologic experts[2,24] can go back to their jobs without significantly endangering themselves, their passengers, or other drivers.

Commercial airplane accidents associated with health problems also are rare. Although one-third of pilots have developed some kind of transient incapacitation (mainly gastrointestinal) while flying,[8] in each case there was enough time for the copilot to take over. In Europe, the estimate for fatal commercial airplane accidents is 1 for every 10^7 flying hours, and of these only 1% can be attributed to health problems. Epstein and colleagues state: "A review of the International Air Transport Association of 36,000 pilots at risk over 10 years found 26 cardiovascular or neurological medical events that could have jeopardized safety if they occurred at a critical time (i.e., takeoff or approach)."[8] No figures are available for other high-risk jobs.

The Risk of Losing Consciousness

Assessing any individual's risk of syncope relies on a diagnostic approach based on the guidelines recently issued by the American College of Physicians.[13,14] These take into account the patient's clinical history and the results of a variety of examinations, e.g., electrocardiography, electrophysiology, Holter monitoring or telemetry, loop monitoring, and tilt testing.

The decision whether or not to go back to a high-risk job depends on the exact nature of the cardiac disorder and the likelihood of its inducing serious arrhythmia. In practice, the main factors to be taken into account are: the probability that the patient's arrhythmia might reappear following treatment; the probability that any such arrhythmia might lead to the patient losing control of any machinery or procedure for which he or she is responsible; and the probability that any such loss of control might lead to an accident. With respect to car driving, a mathematical model for calculating this risk has been developed.[2] This calculation takes into account the vehicle type, the number of hours of driving per year, the risk of syncope or sudden death within the year, and the chance that loss of control might endanger other road users.

Following an assessment of the various risks, the medical/scientific statement of the American Heart Association estimates the risk of an accident occurring as very low, but emphasizes that it is the chance of arrhythmia which should be taken most seriously in making the decision as to whether or not to send a patient back to a high-risk job.[8] Although every case should be treated on its own merits, taking into account the particularities of the work and especially the period within the workday during which there is a genuine danger, the following typical circumstances can be considered for reference.

- Those for whom the possibility of going back to a high risk job is completely excluded: patients with Class III or IV heart failure; those who are waiting for cardiac transplantation; those who have recently had an MI coupled with serious loss of ventricular function, with ventricular arrhythmia, or with reduced variability of their heart rate; or those who have already experienced cardiac arrest and been revived.
- Patients who should be able to go back to work without any problem: if asymptomatic, those with sinus bradycardia or tachycardia, paroxysmal supraventricular tachycardia, and first or second-degree type 1 atrioventricular block.
- For all other kinds of arrhythmia (ventricular dysrhythmia, atrioventricular node re-entry, Wolff-Parkinson-White syndrome, neurally mediated syncopal syndromes): a cardiologist's opinion should be sought for diagnosis, treatment strategy, and decisions about return to work.

Cardiac Pacemakers and Cardiovascular Pharmacological Agents

Carrying a pacemaker does not automatically exclude working in a high-risk job, but special care should be taken if the work involves intense magnetic fields (e.g., electrolysis technicians and electricians). The decision whether or not to send patients with implanted defibrillators back to work does not depend on the presence of the device, but rather on the reason the device was implanted in the first place. A European study of 46 queried pacemaker cardiologists, regarding driving advice, actual practices, and outcomes among patients with automatic implanted cardioverterdefibrillators, showed that over half the patients advised not to drive by their physicians had done so within 6 months of implantation, and no arrhythmia-related fatal accidents were reported.[15]

Out of all the drugs that may be prescribed, particular caution should be attached to β-blockers and antiarrhythmic agents. The former can induce diminution of mental alertness, somnolence, or depression, possibilities to consider when prescribing. Class I and III antiarrhythmic drugs should not be used in cases of benign arrhythmia because, as is widely recognized amongst cardiologists, they can themselves induce more pronounced arrhythmia (proarrhythmic effect). In all cases of arrhythmia, continuous ECG monitoring should be undertaken to check that the drugs are working before the patient is allowed to return to work.

Ethical Considerations

Despite the fact that many patients may derive great benefit from radical treatment (e.g., correction of coronary insufficiency or heart failure, surgery or other techniques designed to ablate conduction pathways, or implantation of a pacemaker), they may still be barred from resuming their work because of specific regulations related to insurance policies, driving license suspension, or other professional restrictions. The physician responsible for treating the heart disorder is subject to all the rules of medical confidentiality, but adhering to them may raise ethical problems if a patient is intent on ignoring the risk entailed in going back to work, especially if the patient refuses to consent to fully informing the physician who will be responsible for allowing resumption of a high-risk job. The attending physician is open to censure if he or she fails to maintain medical confidentiality, but a personal sense of responsibility may demand that confidentiality be breached.

This type of ethical problem most often arises with the drivers of heavy vehicles, for whom professional and social lives often are one and the same, and who often are reluctant to abandon their work. Moreover, the regulations stipulating the physical examination criteria that must be fulfilled to keep the special driver's licenses required for heavy goods and public service vehicles are not always relevant to patients with cardiac problems. The regulations do not address the shortcomings of physicians nor the work conditions (e.g., lone driving, long working hours, stress associated with delivery deadlines, heavy physical work involved in unloading, drastic temperature changes).

Therefore, the best approach is to conduct a series of interviews—possibly including the patient's family or a qualified psychologist—to try and make the patient see reason. This is the only possible option, because there is nothing to stop the patient from finding a job in another transportation company where it is not known that he has a heart problem.

REFERENCES

1. Almeida D, Bradford JM, Wenger NK, et al: Return to work after coronary bypass surgery. Circulation 68 (Suppl II):II205–II213, 1983.
2. Brennan FJ: Assessment of the cardiac patient for fitness to drive: Update. Can J Cardiol 12:1164–1170, 1996.
3. Cay EL, Vetter N, Philip A, Dugard D: Return to work after heart attack. J Psychosom Res 17:213–243, 1973.
4. Cay EL, Walker DD: Psychological factors and return to work. Eur Heart J 9:L74–81, 1988.
5. DeBusk RF, Davidson DM: The work evaluation of the cardiac patient. J Occ Med 22:715–721, 1980.
6. De Gaudemaris R, Frimat P, Chamoux A: Mesure de la pression arterielle et de la frequence cardiaque en activite professionnelle. Collection explorations fonctionnelles humaines (Measuring blood pressure and heart rate at work. Human Function Tests Collection). Editions Medicales Internationales. 94234 Cachan cedex France, 1998.
7. Dennis C, Houston-Miller N, Schwartz RG, et al: Early return to work after uncomplicated myocardial infarction. JAMA 260:214–220, 1988.
8. Epstein AE, Miles WM, Benditt DG, et al: Personal and public safety issues related to arrhythmias that may affect consciousness: Implications of regulations and physician recommendations. A medical/scientific statement from the American Heart Association and the North American Society for Pacing and Electrophysiology. Circulation 94:1147–1166, 1996.
9. Fitzgerald ST, Becker DM, Celentano DD, et al: Return to work after percutaneous transluminal coronary angioplasty. Am J Cardiol 64:1108–1112, 1989.
10. Hlatky MA, Boothroyd D, Horine S, et al: Employment after coronary angioplasty or coronary bypass surgery in patients employed at the time of revascularization. Ann Intern Med 129:543–547, 1998.
11. Johnson WD, Kayser KL, Pedraza PM, Shore RT: Employment patterns of males before and after myocardial revascularization surgery: A study of 2229 consecutive male patients followed for as long as 10 years. Circulation 65:1086–1093, 1982.

12. Landes J, Rod JL: Return to work evaluation after coronary events. Special emphasis on simulated work activity. Sport Med 13:365–375, 1992.

13. Linzer M, Yang EH, Mark Estes III NA, et al: Diagnosing syncope: Part 1. Value of history, physical examination, and electrocardiography. Ann Int Med 126:989–996, 1997a.

14. Linzer M, Yang EH, Mark Estes III NA, et al: Diagnosing syncope: Unexplained syncope. Ann Int Med 127:76–86, 1997b.

15. Luderitz B, Jung W: Driving a motor vehicle after implantation of a cardioverter-defibrillator in malignant heart rhythm disorders. Criteria for the medical assessment of driving fitness in Europe. Dtsch Med Wochenschr 212:119–123, 1996.

16. Mark DB, Lam LC, Lee KL, et al: Identification of patients with coronary disease at high risk for loss of employment. A prospective validation study. Circulation 86:1485–1494, 1992.

17. Monpere C, Francois G, Rondeau du Noyer C, Van JP: Return to work after rehabilitation in coronary bypass patients. Role of the occupational medicine specialist during rehabilitation. Eur Heart J 9:L48–53, 1988.

18. Pilote L, Thomas RJ, Dennis C, et al: Return to work after uncomplicated myocardial infarction: A trial of practice guidelines in the community. Ann Intern Med 117:383–389, 1992.

19. Scott AR: Employment of workers with cardiac diseases. J Soc Occup Med 35:99–102, 1985.

20. Smith R, O'Rourke DF: Return to work after a first myocardial infarction. Test of multiple hypotheses. JAMA 259:1673–1677, 1988.

21. Theorell T, Karasek R: Should heart attack patients return to stressful jobs? Stress Med 11:219–220, 1995.

22. Theorell T, Karasek R: Should heart attack patients return to stressful jobs? Stress Med 11:219–220, 1987.

23. Theorell T, Perski A, Orth-Gomer K, et al: The effects of the strain of returning to work on the risk of death after a first myocardial infarction before age of 45. Int J Cardiol 30:61–67, 1991.

24. U.S. Department of Transportation FHA: Conference on Cardiac Disorders and Commercial Drivers. Publication No. FHWA-MC-88-040. Bethesda, MD, 1987.

SCREENING AND MANAGEMENT OF THE WORKPLACE FOR CVD RISK

INDIVIDUAL STRESS MANAGEMENT: EFFECTIVE OR NOT?
by Kenneth M. Nowack, PhD

Individual stress-management interventions are defined as techniques designed to help employees modify their appraisal of stressful situations or deal more effectively with symptoms of stress. Diversity of stress techniques, use of varying health outcome measures, and methodological limitations make it difficult to reach firm conclusions about the efficacy of stress-management interventions. Current research suggests that individual stress-management interventions generally are effective in reducing negative individual health outcomes, but do not consistently affect job/organization-relevant outcomes such as absenteeism, turnover, productivity, and job satisfaction.

Concern with the effects of occupational stress on productivity, absenteeism, and health-related problems have increased dramatically during the past decade.[88] Although causal relations between job stressors and outcomes have not been conclusively demonstrated, associations between specific types of job stressors (e.g., job strain), individual (e.g., physiologic) and organizational (e.g., job satisfaction) outcomes have been observed consistently.[71,84] These outcomes, regardless of the antecedents, inevitably generate high organizational medical care expenditures, litigation, and operational costs. Organizations have been making efforts to implement individual stress-management interventions to reduce the cost associated with these negative consequences.

According to Ivancevich, Matteson, Freedman, and Phillips, worksite stress-management interventions refer to any cooperative action initiated by an organization for reducing the presence of work-related stressors, or for helping individuals to reduce and/or cope with the negative consequences of these stressors.[43] The goals of these interventions are to reduce specific occupational stressors,[53] modify individual's cognitive appraisal of stressful events,[64] or help individuals cope more effectively. Stress-management interventions traditionally implemented in the worksite can be categorized by the type of exposure the intervention is designed to reduce or eliminate, including: environmental (e.g., chemical and biologic stressors), physical and ergonomic (e.g., noise, rotating shiftwork, equipment); and psychosocial. Psychosocial interventions are aimed at various points in the stress process and can be classified as **organizational change** (*primary interventions*), **stress reduction** (*secondary interventions*), or **stress treatment**, such as employee assistance programs (*tertiary interventions*).

Organizational change interventions focus on identifying worksite stressors, either through comprehensive assessments and modifications[46] or participatory processes during which employees identify stressors and develop solutions.[57] Participatory processes typically include enhanced employee involvement in decision-making, job redesign, participatory action research, autonomous work teams, re-engineering, team building, and 360-degree feedback.

The first type of stress reduction intervention focuses on developing **individual strategies** for alleviating stress-related symptoms. It is the most common type in the workplace. Some examples include progressive muscle relaxation, visualization, biofeedback, meditation, and exercise. The second type of stress reduction intervention is assumed to occur through increased confidence and **interpersonal coping skills**. Examples include assertiveness training, conflict management, communication skills, and leadership development. The third type of stress reduction intervention is assumed to occur through increased **intrapersonal awareness** and insight of cognitive and affective reactions to job stressors. Examples include cognitive restructuring, stress inoculation training, and cognitive-behavioral skills training.

Evidence of the success of occupational stress management interventions generally is confusing and imprecise in light of the considerable heterogeneity of published studies. Interpretation of the occupational stress management literature is difficult because of numerous methodological and conceptual issues, including the use of diverse measures of stressors, moderator variables, strains, and health outcomes; short-term evaluation periods; and a preponderance of self-report measures often confounded with negative affectivity.[42,71,76] Despite these issues, the practicality and effectiveness of worksite stress-management interventions generally support individual, but not organizational, impact.[9,19,46,71,109] Overall, it appears that individual stress management interventions may have a positive effect, but if employees return to an unchanged work environment and its intrinsic stressors, those beneficial effects are likely to be eroded. Published studies suggest that the differential effectiveness of worksite stress-management interventions may depend entirely on the unique individual and organizational outcomes targeted.[9,84,109] A comprehensive review of the occupational stress-management literature allows a summary of the effectiveness of individual-oriented techniques on diverse health and organizational outcomes:

1. Subject matter experts in the occupational stress management field rated **relaxation** as the most practical and least expensive intervention, and the easiest to implement. With respect to effectiveness, exercise and muscle relaxation were considered to be the most effective interventions to alter somatic symptoms and psychological outcomes, whereas stress inoculation and assertiveness training were rated least effective.[9]

2. Stress-management interventions that include a **combination of training techniques** (e.g., muscle relaxation and cognitive-behavioral skills training) seemed to produce the most consistent and significant results across diverse health-outcome measures. The combination of relaxation and cognitive strategies appears to be the most effective type of individually oriented worksite stress-management intervention.[71,72]

3. As the main intervention technique, **biofeedback** appeared to be used least frequently of all interventions, and its effects on most health-outcome and job/organizational measures appeared unremarkable.[71]

4. Recent research examining the impact of **lifestyle and health programs** (e.g., exercise) shows consistently positive effects on psychological outcomes (e.g., depression), but the benefits may not be sustained. Ivancevich, et al. suggest that,

after a short time, 70% of individuals fail to maintain long-term commitment to exercise habits and are likely to revert to their previous lifestyle.[43]

5. In assessing the efficacy of stress-management interventions on *specific* outcomes, relaxation appears to consistently produce significant effects on some physiologic outcomes (e.g., blood pressure) and little change on other outcomes. **Cognitive-behavioral skills** training was the single intervention technique most frequently cited in stress management studies and produced the most consistent effects on psychologic outcomes, particularly anxiety. For somatic complaints, a combination of stress-management techniques appears most effective, and for job/organizational outcomes, job redesign, participatory action research, autonomous work teams, and organizational change interventions appear to be the most effective.[71,72,77,84]

6. None of the **individual stress-management interventions** were consistently effective in producing effects on job/organization-relevant outcomes such as absenteeism, turnover, accidents, health care costs, productivity, or job satisfaction. Murphy found that of individual stress-management strategies, cognitive techniques produced changes in job/organizational measures in 75% of the studies he reviewed.[71] However, in most of these studies cognitive techniques were associated primarily with subjective (e.g., job satisfaction) and not objective endpoints (e.g., absenteeism, productivity).

7. Recent findings suggest that **participatory organizational change** efforts (e.g., job redesign, participatory action research, and autonomous work teams) may be particularly effective in reducing or eliminating specific occupational stressors (e.g., job strain), and as a result, affecting both diverse individual and organizational outcome measures (e.g., productivity, blood pressure).[46,109]

Researchers have assessed the effectiveness of various stress-management interventions practiced in the workplace. Current research suggests that the effects of any one type of individual or organizational outcome typically depend on the specific stress-management technique used. Researchers and practitioners should continue to design and evaluate more comprehensive stress-management programs that attempt to change stressful aspects of the work environment as well as help individual employees learn to manage stress through improved coping. To maximize the effectiveness of occupational stress-management interventions, practitioners should attempt to integrate current findings on individual and organizational change, including readiness to change models,[87] relapse prevention,[66] transfer of training,[4] job redesign,[37] and participatory action research.[46]

HYPERTENSION: COULD LOWERING JOB STRAIN BE A THERAPEUTIC MODALITY?   *by Peter Schnall, MD*

There is a well-established link between hypertension (elevated BP) and increased risk for stroke and heart disease. Indeed, recognition of rapidly rising rates of stroke and heart attack following World War II led to intensive efforts by private organizations like the American Heart Association and agencies of the U.S. government to modify known risk factors for CVD. This led, in turn, to the conduct of a number of clinical trials[2,16] that demonstrated the effectiveness of treating hypertension with medications to lower BP with consequent reduction in stroke and CVD morbidity and mortality. It is now well-established medical practice to place individuals on medication for hypertension if clinic-ascertained BPs exceed 140/90 mmHg.[25]

Unfortunately, the primary cause(s) of hypertension and CVD—which recent evidence suggests is, in part, a product of the organization and nature of work—remains neglected as potential arenas for intervention and primary prevention. In the U.S., the focus is on medical treatment of individuals with elevated BP. Given the widespread availability of effective pharmacologic and nonpharmacologic treatment for hypertension, the reader may appropriately ask, "Why should we bother with interventions aimed at preventing/reducing work-related stress and/or changing the workplace?" The following pages address this question.

Evidence that Elevations in BP Increase Risk of Stroke and Heart Disease

Evidence from epidemiological studies shows that an increase of 5 mmHg in BP has a considerable impact on stroke and heart attack rates in the general population. A meta-analysis of nine prospective studies[16] conducted among women and men concluded that a persistent elevation of 5 mmHg of diastolic BP increases the risk of strokes by 34% and the risk of coronary heart disease by 21%.[63] Furthermore, the association between daytime ambulatory BP and these endpoints is stronger than that of casual BP.[85,86]

Evidence that Treatment of Hypertension Leads to Reduction in Risk

During the past three decades, considerable evidence for the benefit of treating hypertension has been documented through a series of clinical trials beginning with the Veterans Administration Cooperative Study Group on Antihypertensive Agents in 1967.[111] Two forms of treatment for hypertension are widely available and in common use. For individuals with mild levels of BP elevation (BP ≤ 140/90 mmHg), nonpharmacologic interventions such as salt restriction, weight loss, and relaxation techniques are preferred. In the event of a nonresponse or further increase in BP despite these treatments, medications intended to lower BP are prescribed. Treatment of hypertension with antihypertensive medication generally results in BP reductions proportionate to the amount and number of medications.[1]

LIMITATION OF MEDICAL TREATMENT OF HYPERTENSION

Three serious limitations are associated with hypertension medications: issues of efficacy, side effects, and high cost. First, with respect to efficacy, there is the observation that lowering BP in clinical studies (e.g., a 10 mmHg decrease in diastolic BP from 100 mmHg to 90 mmHg) does not lower future morbidity and mortality to the same level as exists in an untreated population with BPs of 90 mmHg.[2] In addition, antihypertensive drugs are even less effective in preventing CVD than in preventing stroke.[2] Second, the greater the drug intervention, the greater the side effects experienced by the patient. These side effects not only can have a substantial, negative impact on an individual's quality of life, but can cause morbidity and mortality as well.[1,94] Third, chronic treatment is associated with substantial cost.

These limitations argue for nonpharmacologic interventions. However, while such nonpharmacologic interventions as weight loss, relaxation therapy, and salt restriction frequently are effective, they often are less so than medications and usually do not return BP to normal in individuals with sustained elevations of BP.[25] The problems with intervening exclusively on these "proximate" causes of disease and the need for a social-ecologic-public health approach are discussed on pages 245–252.

Evidence that Job Strain Is Linked to Hypertension

Several threads of evidence now link the workplace to hypertension and ultimately to CVD. Specifically, during the past two decades many studies have linked job strain to increases in ambulatory BP (amBP) and to CVD (see Chapter 2). The largest study of job strain and hypertension that uses AmBP monitoring in a longitudinal design has been the ongoing Cornell Worksite AmBP Study, which is designed to investigate the hypothesis that exposure to job strain is causally related to increases in mean AmBP.[98]

The sample consists of 285 healthy male employees, aged 30–60 at initial recruitment (Time 1), at eight New York City worksites; 195 were restudied 3 years after their initial participation (Time 2), and 194 were restudied 6 years later (Time 3). Mean systolic (S) and diastolic (D) AmBP at work, home, and during sleep were computed from 24-hour recordings and diary entries specifying location. The relationship of job strain to AmBP was examined cross-sectionally at each round of data collection. In addition, to take advantage of our information on job strain status at each assessment and to evaluate the impact of changes in exposure, a job strain change variable was constructed with four categories: those defined as having no job strain at either Time 1 or Time 2 (N = 138), those reporting job strain at both times (N = 15), and two groups that changed job strain status. We repeated this analysis comparing Times 1 and 3 as well as Times 2 and 3.[95] Multiple regression analysis was used to examine the cross-sectional associations of AmBP with job strain, as well as to predict 3-year and 6-year change in AmBP (from Time 1 to Time 2, Time 2 to Time 3, and Time 1 to Time 3) with job strain change, controlling for age, body mass, race/ethnicity, smoking status, alcohol consumption, education, sodium, and physical exertion level of the job.

Among the findings from the Cornell Worksite AmBP study is the observation in all three cross-sectional analyses (Times 1, 2, 3) of consistent significant effects of job strain on AmBP.[95] Subjects with job strain had work SAmBP/DAmBP that was 5–7/3–5 mmHg higher than subjects without job strain. Moreover, those men facing chronic job strain—working in high-strain jobs at two points in time—had work SAmBP/DAmBP on average 10–12/6–8 mmHg higher than those with no job strain at both times. The two crossover groups had intermediate levels of BP. Effect sizes for chronic 3-year exposure to job strain were larger than the estimated effect of aging 25 years or gaining 50 pounds in weight. In longitudinal analyses, subjects who changed from exposure to job strain to no exposure 3 years later had a decrease in SAmBP/DAmBP of about 5/3 mmHg.[95]

These findings lead to the following conclusions: (1) The relationship between job strain and AmBP has been replicated on three separate occasions, enhancing the validity of the initial observation first reported in 1992.[95,97] (2) Repeated exposure to job strain is associated with the highest levels of AmBPs. (3) Changes in job strain status predict change in AmBP over 3- and 6-year periods. (4) Job strain emerges in this research project as a consistent and substantial risk factor for hypertension in men.

Most importantly, these findings for men have been replicated in recent studies conducted among women. Four out of six studies of job strain that used AmBP found an effect.[12,52,106,110] There is evidence in the study by Laflamme and colleagues that the effect of exposure to job strain on AmBP is persistent beyond working hours, as university-educated women exposed to high job strain had an average of 6 mmHg (p = .012) higher SAmBP than nonexposed women over a 24-hour working day.[52] In addition, as in the Cornell Worksite AmBP study, repeated exposure to job strain showed a substantially greater effect on AmBPs than exposure at only one point in time.[52]

Evidence that Changing Job Characteristics Leads to Lower BP

The question arises whether or not *preventing* exposure to job strain (including taking action to remove job strain for those already exposed) might not lead to lower BPs for working men and women, and to the prevention of stroke and CVD. The Cornell study sheds some light on this issue of the impact of changing job characteristic on AmBP. The authors reported that:

Those with job strain at Time 1 but not at Time 2 had a significant decrease in AmBP at work and home after controlling for other risk factors. Based on a comparison of regression coefficients, the effect of no longer being exposed to job strain at Time 2 on change in work and home SAmBP is comparable in magnitude, but opposite in direction, to the effect of aging 15 years or gaining more than 40 pounds. The decrease of 5/3 mmHg in work and home AmBP is larger than the observed treatment effect on BPs (2–4 mmHg systolic, 2–3 mmHg diastolic) of a weight-reduction intervention in four clinical trials. Moreover, the fall in work AmBP in this group is largest (–11.3 mmHg SAmBP and –5.8 mmHg DAmBP) among those subjects who entered the study as cases (i.e., subjects with elevated casual BPs at recruitment, N = 10). This finding suggests that the removal of job strain, especially for those with elevated BP, can result in a substantial reduction in AmBP. The amount of decrease in AmBP when job strain is removed is proportional to the initial height of AmBP—the greater the entry AmBP, the greater the fall.[97]

The following case is illustrative of the potential impact of changes in job characteristics on AmBP. One of the employees in the Cornell study went from reporting having job strain at Time 1 to not having job strain at Time 2, accompanied by a dramatic fall in his AmBP. His interview on the NBC Nightly News on November 23, 1998 provides anecdotal support that positive changes in his worklife led to lowered job strain.

Reporter: *This participant from the Cornell Study was one of those middle-level managers for a liquor manufacturer. He had very high blood pressure, until he got a promotion.*

Participant: *I had accomplished a couple of key things that gave me a track record, which made me feel good, and I feel much more in control of what I'm doing.*

In addition to the evidence from the Cornell Worksite BP study, two recent intervention studies have examined the impact of worksite changes on casual measures of BP. Kawakami, et al. implemented a stress reduction program among blue-collar workers that included organizational changes.[48] This was intended to alleviate symptoms of depression due, in part, to overwork. Machine work was streamlined, production steps were reduced, and on-the-job training to enhance skills was introduced, thereby reducing job strain. While the study design was not optimized to detect workplace BP changes, nonetheless there was observed a decrease in casual systolic and diastolic BP of 4.4 mmHg and 2.5 mmHg, respectively, that approached statistical significance. A study of urban bus drivers by Rydstedt and colleagues found that an intervention intended to improve traffic conditions, thereby decreased route time and perceived workload among drivers, led to significantly fewer job hassles and lower systolic BP in the intervention group.[93] These studies provide evidence of the feasibility of worksite interventions intended to reduce worksite stressors and lower BP.

The Best Intervention for Elevated BP

A 5 mmHg decrease in BP brought about by nonpharmacologic means (such as weight loss) may result in lower risk of heart disease than a comparable fall in BP due to antihypertensive drug treatment. The effect of no longer being exposed to job strain in the Cornell AmBP Worksite Study was comparable in magnitude to losing more than 40 pounds. However, the effort needed for large numbers of working people to successfully achieve this goal is daunting indeed! These findings support the potential benefit of a public health approach. Workplace interventions to reduce or prevent job stress (e.g., increased job control to reduce job strain) should receive priority as an important preventive and therapeutic modality for individual workers and, probably most importantly, for groups of workers. Nonpharmacological interventions (such as weight reduction) to lower BP are recommended for individuals with mild elevations of BP, while treatment with medications is reserved for those who have developed sustained hypertension.

There are a number of possible worksite interventions to reduce psychosocial stressors, such as job strain, associated with increased BP. It is feasible to intervene at the worksite on each or all of the key dimensions that constitute iso-strain (demands, control, and support).

First, workload demands can be limited by, for example, attenuation of time pressure and more realistic deadlines and caseloads. As conflict is an important component of the Karasek demand scale, clarifying roles and diminishing conflicting instructions may result in lowered perceived demands by an employee. Note that when people report working hard, they often are referring to excessive work hours; thus, interventions to limit the length of the work week, and work day as well as increase work breaks may reduce reports of psychological demand.

Second, decision latitude can be increased—for example, through training to increase skills, or by providing workers with enhanced authority over their work.

Third, social support can be increased in a number of ways, including improved supervisory techniques and group activities. Most importantly, efforts to promote collective work activities should be maximized. A consequence of enhanced collectivity is usually an increased sense of empowerment, which impacts favorably on decision latitude.

In addition, while other identified work stressors have not been examined here, a number of work related psychosocial variables, such as effort-reward imbalance, are amenable to change (see Chapter 2).

Discussion and Conclusions

Readers of this article may reasonably point to a great need for additional evidence that reducing job strain leads to lowered BP, and assert that an intervention trial should be conducted. This author concurs that a high priority should be given to further validating the role of job strain and other psychosocial stressors in causing hypertension and CVD and in determining that changes in these risk factors result in improved health and cardiovascular status (see Chapter 13 for a further discussion of interventions).

However, while intervention studies are highly desirable in establishing causal relationships, from a public health perspective they are not believed absolutely essential before acting to reduce an exposure believed harmful to the public (e.g., cigarettes and lung cancer).[92] This is especially true if the benefits from an intervention greatly outweigh any possible harm. Assessments of harm must include the potential negative impact on both the individual and the workplace, with the latter including an assessment of the *social costs* of workplace change as well as the economic impact on the company. In addition, much of the economic costs of work-induced CVD have been transferred from business to society (an externality of costs), as illnesses become particularly burdensome after employees retire from work. These costs need to be included in any cost-benefit analysis.

The lack of definitive evidence regarding the benefits of reducing job strain on hypertension should not deter individuals, especially clinicians, in a position to effect changes at the workplace from doing so, for the following reasons:

• Reducing work stress (e.g., job strain) may lower BP and reduce risk for heart attack.

• Lowering work stress has a number of potentially salutary effects on employees (e.g., improved mental status).

• Work reorganization may prove cost effective as a means of controlling CVD. The costs of interventions that enhance decision latitude, reduce demands, and increase social support should prove less expensive and more effective in the long run as a means of reducing cardiovascular risk than current medical and drug treatments or other interventions (e.g., weight loss for BP control).

• Employers gain twofold from work reorganization, first through a healthier work force and second because reducing work stress frequently leads to greater job productivity and job satisfaction for employees.

• Most importantly, it is unethical to withhold an effective intervention.

The recent exciting discovery that work stress (e.g., job strain) is an important risk factor for hypertension and CVD and, most importantly, that a reduction of job strain is associated with a substantial reduction in BP opens the door to possible interventions at the workplace aimed at reducing work stress and thereby lowering BP or preventing its increase. The critical question becomes—Do we have enough evidence to justify initiating these interventions? We need not wait for definitive evidence of the causal role of job strain. Both the employee and the employer stand to gain from interventions. The reduction of work stress promises wide-ranging benefits to individuals in the form of better CVD health, improved mental status, greater job satisfaction, and more energy for the rest of their lives. For companies the initial economic costs will be offset in the long run by reduced medical costs and a healthier, more productive workforce. A win-win situation, if there ever was one.

THE CLINICIAN'S ROLE   *by Samuel Melamed, PhD, and Paul Froom, MD*

Evidence from well-designed, methodologically rigorous studies points to the effectiveness of worksite-based intervention targeted to modify risk behaviors, reducing physiological CV risk factors.[39,61,71,83,114] However, evidence that such interventions subsequently lower CV morbidity and mortality is limited, based on relatively old studies, and contradictory.[6,51,91]

Worksites have become increasingly attractive points for such interventions for a number or reasons: (1) many adults who would not otherwise seek out risk reduction service through traditional healthcare outlets can be reached repeatedly and at relatively low cost; (2) the convenience of preventive services offered at the worksite, even on work time, may increase participation rate; (3) environmental factors (e.g., cafeteria food choices and no-smoking policies) and social support of coworkers are likely to increase the effectiveness of worksite health promotion and disease prevention programs; and (4) employers assume that such programs offset their cost in reduced medical expenditures.[83]

The conduction of worksite CV risk management interventions is supported by senior management and decision makers for a variety of reasons, including enhanced moral and company image, productivity improvement, and yield for health and medical care cost containment. Clinicians (e.g., company physicians and nurses, medical consultants, occupational health physicians and nurses) often are consulted and may be advocates for the disease prevention effectiveness of such programs. Furthermore, ample evidence suggests that program effects are more likely to be maintained if the worksite continues to support and reinforce employee risk reductions. Thus, continuous input from clinicians is warranted to motivate senior management to institute CV risk management interventions and health promotion programs as an integral part of the fabric and culture of the organization. In addition, clinicians may take an active role in conducting various parts of the worksite intervention, and in the ongoing evaluation of their effectiveness.

Types of Worksite Interventions

Worksite interventions that are designed to reduce CV risk can be roughly classified as primary, secondary, or tertiary in nature, each having different aims. The aim of primary interventions is to reduce the risk factors or to change the nature of the job stressors; the aim of secondary interventions is to alter the ways individuals respond to risks or job stressors; and the aim of tertiary interventions is to heal those who have been traumatized.[41] These interventions may be categorized as health promotion programs; stress management; or alterations of the sources of stress, through job design or organizational change.

HEALTH PROMOTION PROGRAMS

These interventions target both healthy workers (as a way of primary prevention) and employees at risk (secondary prevention). The initial step of such programs frequently is obtaining self reports of risky behaviors through various Health Risk Appraisal (HRA) questionnaires.[3] HRAs often are combined with biometric measures of blood pressure (BP), serum cholesterol (and other lipids), obesity, or aerobic fitness. After participation in the screening, employees typically are given personalized feedback by mail: by forwarding the results to the employee's healthcare provider with consent of the employee; by computerized feedback from the HRAs; and/or by individualized risk reduction counseling.[83]

Experienced practitioners realized over the years that feedback given to employees on the basis of HRAs and medical screening results did not motivate employees to reduce their health risks.[3] Thus, health promotion and disease prevention programs introduced interventions based on theories and models of behavior change and behavior modification techniques to assist employees to make lifestyle changes, gain control of CV risk factors, and maintain those benefits over time.

The majority of health promotion programs target single risk factor reduction or health-promoting behaviors, such as weight control, smoking cessation, nutrition and cholesterol reduction, and fitness exercise. Furthermore, many "workplace" health promotion programs really have nothing to do with the workplace even when located there. They are a form of secondary medical intervention aimed at individuals with risk factors for some disease (e.g., hypertension). In recent years, however, an increasing number of larger companies have developed and implemented multi-component programs that address multiple CV risk factors. Such programs can meet different needs of different employees. Programs that address multiple risk factors have a greater opportunity of attracting the participation of "high-risk" employees, due to numerous points of access. Furthermore, after employees have successfully managed one risk factor, they may be more motivated and more confident to try to change other behaviors.[39,83]

Multi-component CV risk management interventions vary in scope and intensity. Many include assessment of major risk factors for CVD, with personalized feedback provided to each employee. High-risk employees are referred to their physicians. Opportunities to learn and practice new skills are provided through self-help material and workshops and seminars on nutrition, weight control, and other health-promoting behaviors. Some of the programs incorporate modifications in organizational policy or the physical work environment to facilitate employee behavioral change. Modifications include policies restricting or banning smoking on the work premises, eliminating cigarette vending machines, providing onsite exercise facilities, offering cafeteria food that is lower in fat and calories, and providing financial incentives for risk behavior reduction.

The focus of multi-component programs can be on the entire employee population or on the subset of employees who exhibit elevated risk factors. Several programs use intensive individualized activities that focus on specific factors. It is increasingly clear that programs successful in reducing CV risk include extensive and sustained personal and behavioral counseling by physicians, nurses, and dietitians for high-risk employees. Such personal followup is maintained through the duration of the intervention trials.[39,83] This finding implies that company physicians and nurses could play crucial roles in CV risk management by instituting periodical HRAs along with long-term medical followup and counseling of high-risk employees. Interventions that are designed for high-risk employees can stand alone. However, many experts maintain that designing health promotion activities for other workers and creating a supportive environment can facilitate and contribute to the endurance of intervention effects among high-risk employees.

STRESS-MANAGEMENT INTERVENTIONS

Stress management strategies may be part of comprehensive health promotion programs, but often are conducted by themselves. They are defined as techniques designed to help employees modify their appraisal of stressful situations (secondary prevention) and/or to deal more effectively with symptoms of stress (tertiary intervention). Typically, stress management interventions are prescriptive and person-oriented, such as progressive muscle relaxation, biofeedback, meditation, and cognitive behavioral skill training.[71] Such programs show positive trends in reducing cholesterol levels and lowering BP in normotensives as well as in hypertensive workers. Related outcomes of these programs include desired changes in catecholamine levels (adrenaline and nonadrenaline), plasma rennin, cardiac function, and pulse rate.[71]

ORGANIZATIONAL PREVENTION STRATEGIES

There is a long-standing call to broaden the scope of work-based CV risk prevention programs to include organizational prevention strategies,[20,47,56] and also to include the often-neglected target groups of blue-collar and rank-and-file employees.[20]

Organizational prevention strategies are conceived to be a primary prevention[41,88] and represent preferred approaches to contain the adverse effect of job stress because they focus on reducing or eliminating the sources of the problem (generally referred to as job stressors) in the work environment.[41] The envisaged benefits of organizational prevention strategies are based on the compelling evidence for the association between job stress (including job strain) and risky behaviors such as smoking and lack of physical exercise,[34,40,45,69] elevated ambulatory BP levels,[68,96,97] serum lipid levels,[100,101] and CV disease morbidity and mortality.[96]

A variety of organizational strategies have been developed over the years and are now available for creating healthy organizations and altering the sources of stress at work.[18,47,73,74,88] These strategies include, for example, job redesign, job enrichment, participative management, implementing self regulating teams, Total Quality Management (TQM), and participatory action research. It should be noted, however, that in referring to organizational change, techniques that are potentially salutogenic are not distinguished from those that increase job strain, e.g., lean production. TQM has elements of both, as demonstrated clearly in a recent article on lean production by Landsbergis, Cahill, and Schnall.[54]

Tertiary intervention programs usually are in the form of employee assistance programs (EAPs).[10,13] In practice, tertiary intervention programs are more common in the workplace than primary intervention programs, with secondary intervention programs intermediate in frequency.[73] EAPs are job-based strategies designed to help troubled employees and their families identify problems and resolve them through confidential, short-term, in-house or external counseling (referrals are made for more specialized services and for followup services). EAPs also may offer supervisory training, education and prevention programs, and health promotion activities.

Because of their access to organizations, EAPs have significant potential for reducing stress-related problems. However, for this potential to be realized, EAPs need to incorporate a primary (as well as secondary) intervention component and begin to provide feedback to organizations about stressful work environment factors. Feedback from an EAP in the form of summary statistics (which protect worker confidentiality) permits organizations to pinpoint high-stress departments or areas to establish a starting point for more in-depth intervention efforts.[41]

The outcomes selected to assess the effectiveness of the EAPs are derived from the EAP objectives and usually include the percentage of employees who take up the service, changes in job satisfaction, mental and physical well-being, individual turnover, absenteeism, and job performance. Rigorous and methodologically sound studies to evaluate EAP effectiveness are lacking.

Organizational prevention methods (including EAPs) were designed primarily to attain organizational objectives as well as to improve workers mental and physical well being. To date, only a few studies investigate the impact of these prevention methods on reducing CV risk factors or lowering CV morbidity and mortality. Orth-Gomer, et al. demonstrated that an organizational intervention was associated with an improved lipid profile.[81] Barrios, et al. showed that an "inner quality management" program resulted in increases in contentment, job satisfaction, and communication, and decreases in physical symptoms of stress and of BP levels in hypertensive individuals.[5] Finally, Landsbergis, et al. showed that increase in job decision latitude was associated with smoking cessation.[55]

Evaluation studies are needed to examine the effectiveness of organizational prevention strategies, alone or in combination with traditional health promotion

TABLE 1.   Outcomes of Worksite Interventions

Direct Outcomes	Indirect Outcomes
Blood pressure (clinic & ambulatory)	*Costs Reduction*
Serum cholesterol	Health care costs reduced
Body mass index & weight control	Disability costs reduced
Body fat	Workers' compensation costs reduced
Aerobic fitness	Insurance costs reduced
Smoking cessation	*Individual Outcomes*
Heart rate variability	Satisfaction with the intervention
ST changes	Employee morale
Carotid atherosclerosis	Reduction of physical exhaustion and burnout
Metabolic/neuroendocrine parameters	Injury rate
Self-reported symptoms	*Organizational Outcomes*
Overall Health Outcomes	Performance/productivity
Cardiovascular morbidity	Organizational effectiveness
Cardiovascular mortality	Absenteeism, turnover
Total mortality	Improved safety (fewer accidents)

programs, in reducing CV disease risk. There is some evidence that introduction of organizational prevention strategies, such as EAPs, facilitates the adoption of health promotion programs by the workers.[11] Various professionals associated with the occupational health care setting—physicians, nurses, social workers, psychologists, technicians, and physiotherapists—can play a pivotal role in evaluating the outcomes of organizational prevention strategies.

Outcomes of Worksite Intervention Programs

Worksite CV risk reduction programs that increase employees awareness, encourage health-promoting activities, and teach new skills are likely to yield a variety of outcomes that may go beyond reduction of CV risk factors and/or risk for CVD (Table 1). Reviews of the literature suggest that a program must be sustained for a minimum of 1 year to bring about risk reductions among employees. Risk reduction may be maintained for 5 years or more after the program is ended.[39,83] The expected long-term health outcomes of CV risk reduction—reduced morbidity and mortality—has been demonstrated to date only in one study.[51] More long-term followup studies are needed to determine whether such endpoints are achieved.

Senior management/decision makers who might invest in worksite health promotion programs for a clear business purpose expect the favorable changes in employees' health to result in cost reduction outcomes. Other individual and organizational outcomes also are possible. Those most frequently measured are satisfaction with the program and fullfilment of individuals' needs. These outcomes are important since they relate to whether workers will persist in the current program and join future programs. Additional benefits to employees are increased morale and reduction of physical exhaustion, burnout, and injuries. Financial benefits to the company include increased productivity and organizational effectiveness, reduced absenteeism and turnover, and improved safety.

Evaluation of Worksite Intervention Programs

Evaluation of worksite intervention programs is needed to provide scientific evidence that they are successful in achieving their objectives (Table 2). To conduct a high-quality evaluation, the method should be determined to advance—at the stage of designing the intervention program—so that the needed data is collected from the

TABLE 2.   Evaluation Criteria for Worksite Interventions

I. Outcome evaluation Short- and long-term effectiveness in changing/ modifying risk factors for CVD and/or facilitating health promoting behaviors Impact on overall health outcomes Attaining indirect outcomes II. Participation rates % completing an initial risk assessment and screening % completing a minimal proportion of the program	III. Attrition from the sample (e.g., nonresponse to post intervention assessment) IV. Cost outcomes Cost effectiveness Cost savings Cost-benefit analysis

outset. Goetzel provided an excellent description of different types of intervention designs.[32]

The most immediate role that the clinician may play is in the evaluation of the direct medical outcomes. Clinicians should be aware, however, of other facets for evaluating intervention programs (see Table 2), and consider this information when arriving at conclusions concerning program effectiveness. This information is needed if one wishes to explore additional benefits of the intervention programs, to ensure validity of inference made concerning their effectiveness, and to examine various aspects of cost outcomes.

OUTCOME EVALUATION

Basic program effectiveness assessment examines whether or not direct outcomes were attained. Using a proper experimental design, one can test if there was a favorable post-intervention change in biometric measures, risky behaviors, and/or health-promoting behaviors compared to pre-intervention baseline levels; and whether these changes exceeded those that occurred in the comparison groups. The recommended length of followup to detect intervention effect is at least 1 year, although length of followup does not seem to be associated with the strength of study results.[39] Preferably, followup assessment should be performed during the same season as the baseline assessment (12 or 24 months following the baseline study) to avoid the problem of a seasonal effect on the results.

A secular trend for improved health behavior in the general population also needs to be taken into account.[6] An excellent example of the need for a comparison group in the face of secular trends can be found in the study by Johanning, Landsbergis, Geissler, and Karazmann.[44] In this study of the effectiveness of a worksite CV health promotion program among mass transit operators, equal benefits were seen in both intervention and control groups.

Multiple followup assessments are warranted to demonstrate the extent to which early intervention effects are maintained over time. Longer followup periods of 5–12 years are needed to detect a possible impact on overall health outcomes, such as CV morbidity and mortality.[51,91] Experts other than clinicians, such as economic analysts, social science researchers, and statisticians, can be called upon to evaluate whether individual and organizational outcomes (see Table 1) were attained.

Another part of the evaluation process is the assessment and control of factors that threaten the validity of the conclusions. The most notable factors are participation rates and attrition from the sample. Conrad, Conrad, and Walcott-McQuigg discussed sources of threat to the participation rates and internal validity of worksite intervention research.[17]

PARTICIPATION RATES

Evaluators of worksite intervention programs frequently focus only on changes among active participants, and overlook the problem of self-selection of employees into such programs. In assessing the overall benefit to the workplace, consider the number of nonparticipants, especially of those who may be at an elevated or even high risk. It is important to uncover the participation rates of low-risk and high-risk employees. Two definitions of participation rates are presented in Table 2. The second is considered a more rigorous criterion for participation. For further elaboration on the issues of participation rate see Glasgow, McCaul, and Fisher.[29]

ATTRITION FROM THE SAMPLE

Attrition from the sample constitutes a serious threat to the internal validity of most intervention studies. There is, for example, a possibility of differential attrition due to high-risk employees dropping out of the study, in which case the effectiveness of the program may be inflated. In some studies, the nonresponse to followup assessments was greater in the intervention conditions, especially in the more intensive interventions, than in the comparison condition.[39,83]

COST OUTCOMES

There are three types of assessment of cost outcomes. *Cost effectiveness* refers to the unit cost of providing a service or for achieving a specific health outcome. *Cost savings* refers to a possible reduction in actual medical care costs. *Cost-benefit analysis* compares the savings from a program, compared with the cost of providing that program.[104] Of the three cost outcomes, the one most often examined is cost effectiveness, but even this is restricted to a small proportion of the studies. Usually reported is program effectiveness in reducing cardiac risk (e.g., through hypertension control, lowering serum cholesterol levels and smoking cessation), decreased illness related to absences, cost saving to individuals and to the organization, reduced medical claims, and improved performance and productivity. Estimation of costs needed to evaluate cost effectiveness is complex, and requires consideration and recording of a multitude of parameters. Two studies have provided good examples for calculating cost-effectiveness indices.[24,115]

Cost-savings and cost-benefit analyses are less common, and their expediency has been questioned. As O'Donnel pointed out, businesses may not consider rigorous cost-benefit analyses to be a justifiable investment; such analyses may constitute a significant portion of the total program budget and may not be necessary.[78] Furthermore, besides the logical appeal, it is not totally clear that economic benefits constitute an important motivating factor for businesses to adopt health promotion programs.[112] Economists have suggested that health promotion programs are being oversold as a means of containing business costs.[112] Direct financial benefits of both reduction in medical care costs and absenteeism accrue to the employer only for those individuals with medical benefits through a self-insured plan. There are no direct changes in costs for those enrolled in community-rated health maintenance organizations (HMOs) or fully insured plans.[38] Note, too, that health care costs tend to be distributed unevenly, and a small percentage of employees incur the largest percentage of medical costs.[49] Moreover, costs may manifest most strongly in later years of life after active employees have retired.[83]

In a disease with long latency, such as heart disease, it is difficult to demonstrate reduction on morbidity and mortality resulting from prevention programs. The expected benefit may take 30–40 years to realize in the 20-year-old worker and at least 10 years in the middle-aged worker. However, CVD prevention programs may lead to worker perceptions that their company is benevolent and looking out for their interests. This might lead to substantial and immediate financial benefits to the employer by increased productivity, decreased accident costs, and lowered absenteeism. In fact, Patton argues that the impact of health promotion on productivity is the major economic benefit to the firm.[82] Other potential benefits include decreased worker turnover and enhanced ability to recruit workers.[38]

Changes in workforce size and composition as a result of turnover and changes in medical benefit plans affect costs.[83] In the dynamic, modern workplace, short-term employment is not uncommon; for example, with 15% annual turnover, 50% of the population will leave in 3 years.[38] Long-term morbidity might be an issue. Furthermore, if sick workers are not replaced or if productivity is maintained with a replacement paid by insurance, then the employer may not be concerned with the absenteeism rate or even the accident rate. In other words, improving worker's health may not translate into a cost benefit for the employer. On the other hand, firms with low employee turnover, high costs to replace or substitute an employee, and an older employee population enjoying a rich medical plan are most likely to realize economic gains from worksite health promotion.[82]

A Wider Perspective

Health promotion programs should be conceived by clinicians and others to cover first and foremost worker health, but also organizational wellness. Such programs may maximize the benefits to workers and employers alike, both in the short and long term. The physician minimizes costs from a "public health" perspective (both economic and human) by treating the sick, preventing the well from becoming sick, and creating an environment in which wellness can flourish. As Cartwright, Cooper, and Murphy state: "Organizational health can be measured in a variety of ways other than by an analysis of the profit and loss account. Profitability is a clear indicator of the success and financial health of an organization at a given point of time. However, it is not necessarily a good predictor of future performance, unless account is taken of the ability of the organization and its workforce to continue to sustain and possibly increase that level of performance over time. An automobile may be running perfectly one day, despite a neglectful owner, but it is invariably only a matter of time before a costly breakdown occurs. Similarly, the performance and financial health of an organization is dependent upon the physical and psychological health of its members."[14]

A PUBLIC HEALTH APPROACH IN CLINICAL PRACTICE *by*
June Fisher, MD and Karen Belkić, MD, PhD

Increasingly, clinicians are incorporating aspects of cardiac disease prevention into their practices—whether in primary care or cardiology. These efforts predominantly focus on personal behavior for cardiac risk reduction. It is practically unthinkable for a primary care physician or cardiologist not to take a smoking history, weigh the patient, measure the BP, and order a lipid profile. Though most of us are not trained in counseling patients regarding these risk factors, increasingly we are addressing preventive measures with our patients who are at risk. These measures may include pharmacologic agents, for patients with hypertension or lipid abnormalities, and behavioral changes such as dietary modifications, exercise, and smoking cessation. This broadening of clinical practice to include prevention of CVD is, no doubt, a consequence of the enormous public health campaign—which focuses on individual behavioral change. Ironically, while these efforts have been directed toward the workplace as a major venue to engage large numbers of people, little programmatic effort has been given to the workplace itself as a critical factor in the prevention of CVD. As pointed out by Stokols and colleagues: "These programs have emphasized risk factor reduction strategies (e.g., smoking cessation, stress management, health risk appraisal) but have not integrated disease prevention and safety programs with organizational policies to enhance the physical and social quality of the workplace."[103]

How can the clinician integrate this broader perspective into actual practice? A first and most critical step in a public health approach is to consider how the workplace could affect patients' cardiovascular (as well as overall) well-being. Taking an occupational history as it relates to the cardiovascular system is essential for all cardiovascular patients (see Chapter 8). If the history suggests that the workplace is cardionoxious, the clinical event in question should be evaluated as a potential cardiovascular sentinel event. This knowledge is indispensible for managing individual patients in a cardionoxious workplace. The next challenge is for clinicians to proactively contribute, from their unique vantage point, toward efforts to create healthy work conditions, as a key component of effective prevention.

Risk Factor Reduction and the Cardionoxious Workplace: Where Is the "Leverage Point"?

The worksite increasingly has become a key site of health promotion efforts, with implicit and often explicit focus on CV risk.[26,28,30,33,58] However, researchers have emphasized the need to incorporate a "social ecological" strategy, in which supportive environmental conditions are created to bolster individual efforts to improve their own health.[102] Similarly, Link and Phelan emphasize the importance of the social context in which individual risk factors occur.[62] These authors note that "proximate causes" of disease such as poor diet, high cholesterol, and lack of exercise, have been the major arena of epidemiologic study, while the "more distal" underlying social factors have received relatively little attention. Kok and colleagues emphasize that to be successful, the focus of risk factor modification efforts should be on the determinants of an unhealthy behavior for a given target group.[50]

Cartwright, Cooper, and Murphy apply these concepts directly to the workplace, noting that focusing on the outcome or "back-end" of the stress process offers damage limitation, but does not address the sources of stress in the organizational structure, nor the nature of the workplace.[14] Donaldson criticizes the current paradigm in worksite health promotion as failing "to consider the system of work in which employee behavior is embedded."[21] A small but emerging body of observational and controlled interventional data supports this idea, suggesting that increasing decision latitude and eliminating rapidly rotating shift work and other cardio-deleterious work stressors may be associated with favorable modification of cardiac risk factors such as smoking and hyperlipidemia.[55,80,81]

These principles also are illustrated in our own experience, as clinicians seeking to lower standard cardiac risk factors among patients with various degrees of CVD severity who work in cardionoxious jobs—most notably, professional drivers. The importance of the active role of the physician in smoking cessation efforts is well-recognized.[31,79] However, we found that despite devotion of substantial time and the use of state-of-the-art methods, our efforts among professional drivers were only minimally effective—particularly with regard to this critical cardiac risk factor—unless there was a concomitant amelioration in stressful working conditions.[7,108] Thus, we concluded: "There is a lack of attention to interventions at the workplace which could attenuate cardiac risk . . . Effective primary prevention in professional drivers requires a three-pronged approach aimed at modifiable occupational, as well as behavioral and standard risk factors."[8]

These findings were particularly important in relation to patients with advanced CVD, as well as those with highest overall cardiac risk. All of the (albeit small) groups of professional drivers who had suffered an acute cardiac event and were still smoking, and/or those who were heavy smokers (> 30 cigarettes/day), continued to smoke with the same intensity or more at 6-month followup after the physician-directed smoking cessation session. Awareness, and probably even motivation, were not the problem: nearly all of these very high-risk drivers placed smoking cessation as their first health-related priority in self-generated statements.[7] Similarly, in a cohort of San Francisco urban transit operators, even though smoking cessation was a high priority, and all operators received counseling in this regard at the time of the mandated biennial medical examinations, smoking was found to increase with length of time on the job.[89]

Wells and colleagues note that the "social-ecological approach . . . highlights the importance of high-impact leverage points" to the effectiveness of health promotion efforts.[113] Among professional drivers, our empirical data strongly implicates modifiable factors in the work environment as a "leverage point" with respect to several cardiac risk factors (CRF). Intensity and duration of exposure to this stressful occupation were associated with obesity, as well as smoking intensity. Among the cohort of San Francisco urban transit operators, body mass index (BMI) increased significantly with length of employment, after adjustment for age, race, and gender. With over 20 years on the job, the mean adjusted BMI was 27.9.[90] Multivariate analysis revealed that the total burden of occupational stressors, as assessed using the Occupational Stress Index,[8] was an independent predictor of smoking intensity, and that number of hours of professional driving per day independently predicted BMI among the professional drivers studied in Stockholm.[23] Besides finding that workplace stressors represented important determinants of baseline CRF status, some preliminary data also suggested that change in work conditions may be associated with lowering of CRF among professional drivers. It was concluded that the professional drivers who were the heaviest smokers faced the greatest load from potentially modifiable job stressors (e.g., time pressure, barriers, special hazards, long work hours), and that amelioration of at least some of these appeared to be necessary in efforts toward smoking reduction and cessation.

Further, Emdad and colleagues asserted that "long driving hours mean more sedentary time (and) may . . . trigger overeating. Drivers tend to eat a heavy meal once arriving home after a long workday. Thereafter, due to exhaustion, they often remain sedentary and then fall asleep . . . Breaking this pattern by changing the work schedule, together with dietary instruction, has resulted in notable weight reduction in individual cases."[23] Thus, in addition to intensive efforts aimed at cardiac risk factors, "modification of the work environment, with participation of the drivers themselves in formulating the modifications, would be a needed component of such a preventive intervention."[23]

Worksite health promotion effectiveness also can be improved by specific, concrete actions by the employer. For example, shared company and employee time was found to be significantly associated with long-term quit rate of worksite smoking cessation programs.[28] Physical activity could be better promoted by providing opportunities (e.g., time for exercise, proximity to the worksite). Specific recommendations have included exercise programs related to the nature of the job demands and carried out during work time, exercise activities for general fitness during breaks, and worksite exercise facilities. Empirical data indicates that social support may be a critical factor in increasing recreational physical activity among professional drivers.[23]

The Occupational Cardiology Paradigm: Acquired CV Disorders as Occupational Sentinel Health Events

There are a myriad of pathways by which work stressors can impact upon the cardiovascular system. The clinician must be on the alert for the occurrence of unexpected patterns or clusters of CVD in the workplace. Historically, in other medical disciplines, the astute clinician often has been the one who identified occupationally associated diseases, with resultant major changes in the work environment. A classic example is that of Dr. Irving Selikoff and colleagues in the relation between asbestos exposure and mesothelioma, as well as pulmonary interstitial fibrosis (asbestosis).

In contrast, cardiologists typically have not been the ones to herald the occurrence of clusters of workplace-related CVD, probably because CVD is so common. The multifactorial nature of CVD, the difficulty of evaluating psychosocial factors, and the relatively scant attention paid to the relevant occupational factors in the cardiologic literature are other major reasons why occupational cardiology remains, at best, only an incipient clinical discipline.

The concept of an *occupational sentinel health event* must be incorporated into the realm of cardiology. Markowitz cogently summarizes the fundamental role of the clinician for the implementation of the concept:

> *The occupational sentinel health event concept conveys three important and related notions. First, it is useful as a heuristic device to allow health care providers and public health authorities to sort through health events of individuals and populations to determine a priori which health events and patterns of health events are most likely to be caused by occupational factors, given current knowledge. Second, the sentinel health events concept transforms the health problems of individuals into the potential health problems of populations. To recognize the diagnosis of an occupational disease in an individual as a sentinel health event facilitates the identification of others at the workplace who are also ill or who may become ill if exposure continues. Third, the occurrence of a sentinel health event may signify the failure of a system to control known occupational hazards and thereby to prevent cases of unnecessary occupational disease.*[65]

Mullan and Murthy provided a list of 64 diseases or conditions which could be considered as occupational sentinel health events.[70] It was based on a survey of the published literature in which documentation was required concerning the etiologic agent and the occupations, industries, and/or processes which involve the noxious agent. Surprisingly, cardiovascular diagnoses are not on the list! Given the large body of data concerning the workplace and CVD, there is an urgent need to rectify the situation by systematic consideration of the multifaceted contribution of the workplace to CVD.

Invaluable clues concerning occupational sentinel health events often can be obtained from individual workers. Questions in the occupational cardiology history could include: Have you heard about a large number of your coworkers having high blood pressure, high lipid levels, or serious heart disease? Have you heard about very young coworkers developing these conditions? Queries should be made about exposure of coworkers to cardionoxious workplace factors. The scope might be broadened to include inquiries about large numbers of workers complaining of fatigue, being on sick-leave, or manifesting other nonspecific clues of exposure to cardionoxious work. It also might be illuminating to ask about relevant disorders of other organ systems; for example, musculoskeletal disorders may be repetitive motion injuries—manifestations of short-cycle, high-strain work. If these indicators suggest that a cardiovascular sentinel health event is present, a systematic followup should be triggered.

Occupational Cardiology in the Primary Care Setting: Strategies and Barriers

A suggested approach for an occupational cardiology work-up is presented in Chapter 8, with a series of strongly recommended steps as well as minimal requirements. Each of these suggestions was justified on the basis of current scientific knowledge. However, a substantial gap exists between this new diagnostic/therapeutic paradigm and established cardiologic practice. The pressing question then becomes how, in practice, to implement this paradigm, particularly within the primary care setting (Fig. 1).

Once a cardionoxious workplace is suspected, there are a number of resource persons with whom to work. An excellent resource may be a cardiologist or other clinician who sees many people from the same worksite as a result of contractual relations with the employer or the health insurer, and who has an interest in primary intervention. Besides the primary cardiology clinician, resource professionals can include: occupational health clinicians, work-stress environment specialists, industrial hygienists, and epidemiologists.

This team should work with key participants in the workplace, i.e., labor and management, in the process of hazard recognition and control. The concepts and

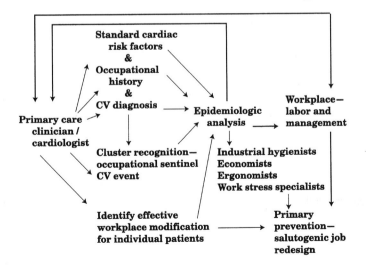

FIGURE 1.   Occupational cardiology in a primary care setting: a public health approach.

core methodology of Participatory Action Research (PAR) provide an excellent framework for this process.[22,99] Fundamentally, "the strategy involves a cyclical process of reflection and action in which the stakeholders (a) identify aspects of the system that they wish to change, (b) analyze 'causes' of system dysfunction, develop and implement action plans, and create a plan to evaluate the effects of their actions."[99] This PAR approach would be integrated with job-related monitoring of workers' health,[47] for which the clinician's role would be of paramount importance.

Some of the major barriers to implementation include: lack of training and skills in occupational health; time limitations of clinical practice; lack of access to the workplace/noncooperative management; fear on the part of management of the occupational relatedness of the CVD and the possibility of workers' compensation proceedings; employee fear of losing their jobs; and clinician reluctance to get involved in possible litigation/depositions. Many of these barriers overlap with those obstructing the implementation of preventive services, in general. Maron and colleagues emphasize the lack of perceived legitimacy of preventive medicine and the concomitant lack of incentives, including reimbursement, as key impediments to the delivery of CVD preventive services.[67]

Educational efforts, starting with structured clinical training in preventive medicine for all medical students and universal availability of combined MD/MPH programs, are critical in the long-term solution.[15] More immediately, moving from an adversarial to a cooperative interaction is essential. The authority of the clinician, whose interest is first and foremost the well-being of his or her patients, can represent a stabilizing force, promoting cooperation among the various participants in the work process (e.g., labor, management, occupational hygienists, engineers, economists).

Besides health maintenance organizations contracting primary care to a specific industry, there are a number of other settings in which an occupational cardiologic paradigm could be realized. These include: regional-geographic clinical care, referrals from coworkers because of the clinician's demonstrated interest in the workplace and CVD, contracts for mandated examinations, workers' compensation examinations, occupational health services, and screening programs (especially hypertension screening). It would be ideal to have primary care facilities for cardionoxious work staffed by clinicians whose interest and expertise is in primary CV medicine, occupational health, and work organization.

The Cardiovascular Safety of the Work Environment: Ethical Considerations

The clinician often is called upon to judge the cardiovascular work fitness of patients. This fitness-for-work assessment could be inappropriately used. The clinician should, by all means, prevent the misuse of these evaluations by the company to select "physiological super-humans" who are resistant to a cardionoxious work environment. Rather, the aim must be to foster a work environment which, *at the very least*, is not harmful to the CV system of the vast majority of persons. Achieving this goal often entails work modification to minimize factors that produce psychosocial and other forms of stress.

A crucial ethical obligation is to avoid iatrogenic disqualification. In particular, the clinician must ensure that the results of physiologic testing, e.g., ambulatory monitoring or laboratory testing of cardionoxious agents, are not misused for the purpose of identifying a "biological elite" and excluding others from the workplace, as a substitute for creating healthier working conditions. These principles are the logical extension of the health professional's basic duty "to protect confidential health information when dissemination of that information, intentional or inadvertent, can adversely affect an employee's job situation and lead to reassignment, lack of advancement, or even preferential termination.[103]

There are special circumstances (e.g., jobs whose performance may affect public safety) in which the clinician must render an estimation of risk for the occurrence of cardiac or other events which could lead to impaired consciousness (see Chapter 9). Note that many of these jobs carry with them a high cardionoxious potential, as threat-avoidant vigilant work often coupled with numerous other deleterious conditions. One of the most urgent needs is for clinicians, together with occupational ergonomists and other specialists, to have greater influence to recommend and implement cardio-protective guidelines about work conditions for these jobs. The basis for these guidelines would be integrative worksite and laboratory physiologic investigations. The clinician is continually faced with the dilemma of making a judgement about the individual's cardiovascular work fitness, knowing full well that the job *itself* is cardionoxious. A proactive approach offers the possibility of ameliorating this ethical dilemma.

The Clinician as Catalyst for Change and Advocate for Preservation of Healthy Work

The clinician's experience with the efficacy of workplace modifications for individual patients also can be invaluable in a larger context. Clearly effective changes could be extended into the public health realm, informing primary preventive workplace interventions. For example, eliminating split-shifts was associated with lowered blood pressure and behavioral changes such as smoking cessation and weight loss in a patient with borderline hypertension and other signs of the CV metabolic syndrome (see Chapter 8). If this workplace modification repeatedly yielded similar positive results in high-risk patients, a trial of eliminating split-shifts could be recommended. Here, the clinician's experience would be playing a key role in charting the exploration of potentially cardio-salutogenic workplace changes.

Another important proactive role for the clinician is to advocate for the preservation of healthy work in the face of potentially deleterious changes such as downsizing, outsourcing, and new systems of work organization, including lean production, total quality management, or modular manufacturing. Lean production has been associated with increased job demands but only minor changes in skill levels and job decision-making authority, and thus holds the potential for increasing the risk of hypertension and CHD.[54] Outsourcing has been found to be associated with cardio-deleterious catabolic changes in a small, controlled study of bus drivers.[75]

Illustrations: The Authors' Experience

The approach outlined here is grounded, in part, in our own experience as clinicians. The second author (KB) began her interest in occupational cardiology while caring for myocardial infarction (MI) patients in a coronary care unit (CCU): observing that these cardiac events were strikingly frequent among persons with stressful, cardionoxious jobs; facing the frustration of seeing those patients return to the same jobs; and often observing their repeated admission to the CCU within a short interval. These clinical impressions are corroborated by the study of Theorell, et al. demonstrating that return to high-strain work is a powerful predictor of cardiac mortality among young MI patients.[107]

The first author's (JF) research interest in stress and CVD was generated from her activities as an attending physician in internal medicine at San Francisco General

Hospital, where she and her associates performed the biennial medical examinations required by the U.S. Department of Transportation for maintenance of a commercial driver's license. Review of the first month's data suggested that there might be an elevated rate of hypertension among these transit operators. The data was then monitored for a year. Both labor and management felt that the work of a San Francisco transit operator was highly stressful, and this belief was corroborated by the clinicians' on-site observations on the buses and trolleys. Based upon these initial observations and input from labor and management, in collaboration with the University of California Berkeley's Social and Behavioral Epidemiology Program, the Northern California Center for Occupational and Environmental Health, and the Department of Medicine at the University of California, San Francisco, a major study was undertaken to investigate these observations. This study has now developed into a long-term program, not only to identify the impact of work on the operators' health status, but also to make recommendations for improving their work environment. The initial study corroborated the early observations that the transit operators had higher rates of hypertension compared to referent groups of employed persons.

Subsequently, this finding was observed to be highly consistent across various geographic and cultural settings. In-depth "triangular" investigation of the work conditions of these transit operators was undertaken, including objective observation methods to measure the barriers, obstacles, restrictive time bindings, and other stressors of urban transport operators.[35,36] A number of recommendations were made to help guarantee adequate rest time and relieve the heavily burdensome time pressure faced by the transport operators. Using the research findings and recommendations which were regularly reported back to both the company and the union, cable car operators drew up their own plan for changing the work environment. This not only increased rest times between runs, but improved productivity. More recently, these recommendations are being instituted by a joint labor-management committee on one of the most heavily travelled trolley lines. This is a pilot study for what is referred to as the Ambassador program, and will be expanded system wide.[105] A major obstacle has been a larger, political issue directly related to the underfunding of public transportation.

Technical interventions with a similar aim of improving the traffic environment in Stockholm, Sweden provide some encouraging preliminary results: trends toward lowered worksite blood pressure and heart rate levels at followup.[93]

Another result of these efforts is that U.S. Department of Transportation examinations now include an obligatory consideration of hypertension. Unfortunately, however, these do not incorporate evaluation of how hypertension specifically relates to the work environment of professional drivers. This is particularly important with regard to compliance. Hypertensive operators requiring medical treatment generally perceive that their primary care providers lack awareness of the work factors unique to their profession, and this perception hampers adherence to treatment regimens.[27] For example, many of the drivers say that the constraints of the job, e.g., not having rest breaks or easily available rest-room facilities, make them hesitant to take prescribed diuretics. They also report that many of the drugs make them feel less vigilant. This underscores the need to integratively consider the work environment from the inception of any such efforts, and the limitations of a narrowly focused, purely clinical approach.

Overall, despite the many obstacles and difficulties faced along this road, when clinicians expand their horizons to encompass a public health view of the workplace, there is a real chance of improving CV well-being of their patients, and this can be profoundly gratifying.

ACKNOWLEDGEMENT
We greatly appreciate the influence that the late Professor Bertil Gardell has had upon our perspectives and work. We would like to thank our patients and participants in research endeavors, who have provided us with insights into their work environments.

Drs. Fisher and Belkić

REFERENCES

1. Alderman MH, Marantz PR: Clinical trials as a guide to intervention. In Laragh JH, Brenner BM (eds): Hypertension: Pathophysiology, Diagnosis, and Management. 2nd ed. New York, Raven Press, Ltd., 1995, pp 2487–2500.
2. Alderman MH, Schnall PL: When to treat a patient with hypertension. In Drayer JIM, Lowenthal DT, Weber MA (eds): Drug Therapy in Hypertension. Vol. 6. New York, Marcel Dekker, Inc., 1987, pp 1–26.
3. Anderson D, Stanfacker M: The impact of worksite-based health risk appraisal on health-related outcomes: A review of the literature. Am J Health Promot 10:499–508, 1996.
4. Baldwin TT, Ford JK: Transfer of training: A review and directions for future research. Personnel Psychol 41:63–105, 1988.
5. Barrios CB, McCraty R, Cryer B: An inner quality approach to reducing stress and improving physical and emotional wellbeing at work. Stress Med 13:193–201, 1997.
6. Bauer R, Heller R, Challah S: United Kingdom heart disease prevention project: 12 year follow-up of risk factors. Am J Health Promot 121:563–569, 1985.
7. Belkic K, Emdad R, Theorell T, et al: Neurocardiac mechanisms of heart disease risk among professional drivers. Final report. Stockholm, Swedish Fund for Working Life, 1996.
8. Belkic K, Pavlovic S, Djordjevic M, et al: Determinants of cardiac risk in professional drivers. Kardiologija 13:145–149, 1992.
9. Bellarosa C, Chen PY: The effectiveness and practicality of occupational stress management interventions: A survey of subject matter expert opinions. J Occup Health Psychol 2:247–262, 1997.
10. Berridge J, Cooper CL, Highley-Marchington C: Employee Assistance Programs and Workplace Counseling. Chichester, England, John Wiley, 1997.
11. Blum TC, Roman PM, Patrick L: Synergism in worksite adoption of employee assistance programs and health promotion activities. J Occup Med 32:461–467, 1990.
12. Blumenthal JA, Thyrum TE, Siegel WC: Contribution of job strain, job status, and marital status to laboratory and ambulatory blood pressure in patients with mild hypertension. J Psychosom Res 39:133–144, 1995.
13. Carroll M: Workplace Counseling. London, Sage, 1996.
14. Cartwright S, Cooper CL, Murphy LR: Diagnosing a healthy organization: A proactive approach to stress in the workplace. In Murphy LR, Hurrell JJ, Sauter SL, Puryear Keita G (eds): Job Stress Interventions. Washington, D.C., American Psychological Association, 1995, pp 217–233.
15. Cimino JA: Why can't we educate doctors to practice preventive medicine? Prev Med 25:63–65, 1996.
16. Collins R, Peto R, MacMahon S, et al: Blood pressure, stroke, and coronary heart disease. Part 2, Short-term reduction in blood pressure: Overview of randomised drug trials in their epidemiological context. Lancet 335:827–838, 1990.
17. Conrad KM, Conrad KJ, Walcott-McQuigg J: Treats to internal validity in worksite health promotion program research. Am J Health Promot 6:112–122, 1991.
18. Copper CL, Williams S: Creating Healthy Work Organizations. Chichester, England, John Wiley, 1994.
19. DeFrank RS, Cooper CL: Worksite stress management interventions: Their effectiveness and conceptualization. J Manag Psychol 2:4–10, 1987.
20. Dejoy DM, Southern DJ: An integrative perspective on worksite health promotion. J Occup Med 35:1221–1230, 1993.
21. Donaldson SI: Worksite health promotion: A theory-driven, empirically based perspective. In Murphy LR, Hurrell JJ, Sauter SL, Puryear Keita G (eds): Job Stress Interventions. Washington, D.C., American Psychological Association, 1995, pp 73–90.
22. Elden M, Chisholm R: Emerging varieties of action research: Introduction to the special issue. Human Relations 46:121–142, 1993.
23. Emdad R, Belkic K, Theorell T, Cizinsky S: What prevents professional drivers from following physicians' cardiologic advice? Psychoth Psychosom 67:226–240, 1998.
24. Erfurt JC, Foote A, Heirich MA: The cost-effectiveness of worksite wellness programs for hypertension control, weight loss, and smoking cessation. J Occup Med 33:962–970, 1991.
25. Fauci AS, Braunwald E, Isselbacher KJ, et al: Harrison's Principles of Internal Medicine. New York, McGraw-Hill, Inc., 1998.
26. Feldman S: Today's EAP's make the grade. Personnel 68:3–40, 1991.
27. Fisher JM, Krause N, Thompson DA, et al: Study of stress and hypertension in Muni transit operators: Summary report. San Francisco, San Francisco General Hospital, Center for Municipal Occupational Safety and Health, 1991.
28. Fisher KJ, Glasgow RE, Terborg JR: Worksite smoking cessation: A meta-analysis of long-term quit rates from controlled studies. J Occup Med 32:429–439, 1990.
29. Glasgow RE, McCaul KD, Fisher KJ: Participation in worksite health promotion: A critique of the literature and recommendations for future practice. Health Educ Q 20:391–408, 1993.
30. Glasgow RE, Sorensen G, Giffen C, et al: Promoting worksite smoking control policies and actions: The community intervention trial for smoking cessation (COMMIT) experience. Prev Med 25:186–194, 1996.
31. Glynn TJ: Physicians and a smoke-free society. Arch Intern Med 148:1013–1016, 1988.

32. Goetzel RZ: Program evaluation. In O'Donnell MP, Harris JS (eds): Health Promotion in the Workplace. New York, Delmar, 1994.

33. Gomel M, Oldenburg B, Simpson JM, Owen N: Worksite cardiovascular risk reduction: A randomized trial of health risk assessment, risk factor education, behavioral counseling, and incentive strategies. Am J Public Health 83:1231–1238, 1993.

34. Green KL, Johnson JV: The effects of psychosocial work organization on patterns of cigarette smoking among male chemical plant employees. Am J Public Health 80:1368–1371, 1990.

35. Greiner BA, Krause N, Ragland DR, Fisher J: Objective stress factors, accidents, and absenteeism in transit operators: A theoretical framework and empirical evidence. J Occup Health Psychol 3:130–146, 1998.

36. Greiner BA, Ragland DR, Krause N, et al: Objective measurement of occupational stress factors—An example with San Francisco urban transit operators. J Occup Health Psychol 2:325–342, 1997.

37. Hackman JR, Oldham GR: Motivation through work design of work: Test of a theory. Organiz Behav Hum Perform 16:250–279, 1976.

38. Harris JS: The cost-effectiveness of health promotion programs. J Occup Med 33:327–330, 1991.

39. Heaney CA, Goetzel RZ: A review of health-related outcomes of multi-component worksite health promotion programs. Am J Health Promot 11:290–308, 1997.

40. Hellerstedt WL, Jeffery RW: The association of job strain and health behaviors in men and women. Int J Epidemiol 26:575–583, 1997.

41. Hurrell JJ, Murphy LR: Occupational stress intervention. Am J Ind Med 29:338–341, 1996.

42. Hurrell JJ, Nelson DL, Simmons BL: Measuring job stressors and strains: Where we have been, where we are, and where we need to go. J Occup Health Psychol 3:368–389, 1998.

43. Ivancevich JM, Matteson MT, Freeman S, Phillips J: Worksite stress management interventions: Opportunities and challenges for organizational psychologists. Am Psychol 45:252–261, 1990.

44. Johanning E, Landsbergis P, Geissler H, Karazmann R: Cardiovascular risk and back disorder intervention study of mass transit operators. Int J Occup Environ Health 2:79–87, 1996.

45. Johannson G, Johnson JV, Hall EM: Smoking and sedentary behavior as related to work organization. Soc Sci Med 32:837–846, 1991.

46. Karasek RA: Stress prevention through work reorganization: A summary of 19 international case studies. Conditions of Work Digest: Preventing Stress at Work 11:23–42, 1992.

47. Karasek RA, Theorell T: Healthy Work: Stress, Productivity, and the Reconstruction of Working Life. New York, Basic Books, 1990.

48. Kawakami N, Araki S, Kawashima M, et al: Effects of work-related stress reduction on depressive symptoms among Japanese blue-collar workers. Scand J Work Environ Health 23:54–59, 1997.

49. Kingery PM, Ellsworth CG, Corbett BS, et al: High-cost analysis: A closer look at the case for work-site health promotion. J Occup Med 36:1341–1347, 1994.

50. Kok G, Hospers HJ, den Boer D-J, deVries H: Health education at the individual level. In Orth-Gomer K, Schneiderman N (eds): Behavioral Medicine Approaches to Cardiovascular Disease Prevention. Mahwah, New Jersey, Lawrence-Erlbaum Associates, 1996, pp 185–202.

51. Kornitzer M, Dramaixs M, Thilly C, et al: Belgian heart disease prevention project: Incidence and mortality results. Lancet 1(8333):1066–1070, 1983.

52. Laflamme N, Brisson C, Moisan J, et al: Job strain and ambulatory blood pressure among female white-collar workers. Scand J Work Environ Health 24:334–343, 1998.

53. Landsbergis PA, Cahill J: Labor union programs to reduce or prevent occupational stress in the United States. Int J Health Serv 24:105–129, 1994.

54. Landsbergis PA, Cahill J, Schnall P: The impact of lean production and related new systems of work organization on worker health. J Occup Health Psychol 4:108–130, 1999.

55. Landsbergis PA, Schnall PL, Deitz DK, et al: Job strain and health behaviors: Results of a prospective study. Am J Health Promot 12:237–245, 1998.

56. Landsbergis PA, Schnall PL, Schwartz JE, et al: Job strain, hypertension, and cardiovascular disease: Empirical evidence, methodological issues, and recommendations for future research. In Sauter SL, Murphy LR (eds): Organizational Risk Factors for Job Stress. Washington, DC, American Psychological Association, 1995, pp 97–112.

57. Landsbergis PA, Vivona-Vaughan E: Evaluation of an occupational stress intervention in a public agency. J Organiz Behav 16:26–28, 1995.

58. Lechner L, De Vries H: Starting participation in an employee fitness program: Attitudes, social influence, and self-efficacy. Prev Med 24:627–633, 1995.

59. Reference deleted.

60. Reference deleted.

61. Leviton LC: The yield from worksite cardiovascular risk reduction. J Occup Med 29:931–936, 1987.

62. Link BG, Phelan J: Social conditions as fundamental causes of disease. J Health Soc Behav (Extra Issue):80–94, 1995.

63. MacMahon S, Peto R, Cutler J, et al: Blood pressure, stroke, and coronary heart disease. Part 1: Prolonged differences in blood pressure—Prospective observational studies corrected for the regression dilution. Lancet 335:765–774, 1990.

64. Maddi SR: The effectiveness of hardiness training. Consult Psychol J 50:78–86, 1998.

65. Markowitz SB: The role of surveillance in occupational health. In Rom WN (ed): Environmental and Occupational Medicine. Philadelphia, Lippincott-Raven Publishers, 1998, pp 19–29.

66. Marlatt G, Gordon JR: Relapse Prevention: Maintenance Strategies in Addiction Behavior Change. New York, Guilford Press, 1985.

67. Maron DJ, Ridker PM, Pearson TA: Risk factors and the prevention of coronary heart disease. In Alexander RW, Hurst WJ (ed): Hurst's The Heart, Arteries, and Veins. 9th ed. New York, McGraw Hill, 1998, pp 1175–1195.
68. Melamed S, Kristal-Boneh E, Harari G, et al: Variation in the ambulatory blood pressure response to daily work load—The moderating role of job control. Scand J Work Environ Health 24:190–196, 1998.
69. Melamed S, Kushnir T, Strauss E, Vigiser D: Negative association between reported life events and cardiovascular disease risk factors in employed men: The CORDIS Study. Cardiovascular Occupational Risk Factors Determination in Israel. J Psychosom Res 43:247–258, 1997.
70. Mullan RJ, Murthy LI: Occupational sentinel health events: An updated list for physician recognition and public health surveillance. Am J Ind Med 19:775–799, 1991.
71. Murphy LR: Stress management in work settings: A critical review of the health effects. Am J Health Promot 11:112–135, 1996.
72. Murphy LR: Occupational stress management: A review and appraisal. J Occup Psychol 57:1–15, 1984.
73. Murphy LR: Workplace interventions for stress reduction and prevention. In Cooper CL, Payne R (eds): Causes, Coping, and Consequences of Stress at Work. Chichester, John Wiley, 1988, pp 301–339.
74. Murphy LR, Hurrell JJ, Sauter SL, Keita GP: Job Stress Interventions. Washington, DC, American Psychological Association, 1995.
75. Netterstrom B, Hansen AM, Borritz M, Nielsen M: Outsourcing and stress: Physiological effects on bus drivers. Paper presented at the APA/NIOSH Conference on Work, Stress, and Health. Baltimore, MD, March 11, 1999.
76. Nowack KM: Initial development and validation of a stress and health risk factor instrument. Am J Health Promot 4:173–180, 1990.
77. Nowack KM: Psychosocial Predictors of Health and Absenteeism: Results of Two Prospective Studies. American Psychological Association Convention. Los Angeles, CA, 1994.
78. O'Donnell MP: Cost benefit analysis is not cost effective. Am J Health Promot 3:75–76, 1988.
79. Oldenburg B, Pope J: A critical review of determinants of smoking cessation. Behavior Change 7:101–109, 1990.
80. Orth-Gomer K: Intervention on coronary risk factors by adapting a shiftwork schedule to biologic rhythmicity. Psychosom Med 45:407–415, 1983.
81. Orth-Gomer K, Eriksson I, Moser V, et al: Lipid lowering through work stress reduction. Int J Behav Med 1:204–214, 1994.
82. Patton JP: Worksite health promotion: An economic mode. J Occup Med 33:868–873, 1991.
83. Pelletier KR: Clinical and cost outcomes of multifactorial, cardiovascular risk management interventions in worksites: A comprehensive review and analysis. J Occup Environ Med 39:1154–1169, 1997.
84. Pelletier KR, Lutz R: Healty people healthy business: A critical review of stress management programs in the workplace. Am J Health Promot 19:5–12, 1988.
85. Perloff D, Sokolow M, Cowan R: The prognostic value of ambulatory blood pressures. JAMA 249:2792–2798, 1983.
86. Perloff D, Sokolow M, Cowan RM, Juster RP: Prognostic value of ambulatory blood pressure measurements: Further analyses. J Hypertens 7 Suppl 3:S3–S10, 1989.
87. Prochaska JO, Velcier WF: The transtheoretical model of health behavior change. Am J Health Promot 12:38–48, 1997.
88. Quick JC, Quick JD, Nelson DL, Hurrell JJ: Preventative Stress Management in Organizations. Washington, D.C., American Psychological Association, 1997.
89. Ragland DR, Fisher JM, Krause N, et al: Study of stress and hypertension in Muni transit operators: Summary report. San Francisco, Center for Municipal Occupational Safety and Health, San Francisco General Hospital, 1991.
90. Ragland DR, Greiner BA, Holman BL, Fisher JM: Hypertension and years of driving in transit vehicle operators. Scand J Soc Med 25:271–279, 1997.
91. Rose G, Tunstall-Pedoe H, Heller R: United Kingdom heart disease prevention program: Incidence and mortality results. Lancet 1:1061–1065, 1983.
92. Rothman KJ, Greenland S: Modern Epidemiology. Philadelphia, Lippincott-Raven, 1998.
93. Rydstedt LW, Johansson G, Evans GW: The human side of the road: Improving the working conditions of urban bus drivers. J Occup Health Psychol 3:161–171, 1998.
94. Schnall PL, Alderman MH, Kern R: An analysis of the HDFP trial. Evidence of adverse effects of antihypertensive treatment on white women with moderate and severe hypertension. N Y State J Med 84:299–301, 1984.
95. Schnall PL, Landsbergis P, Belkic K, et al: Findings in the Cornell University ambulatory blood pressure worksite study: A review. Homeostasis 38:195–215, 1998.
96. Schnall PL, Landsbergis PA, Baker D: Job strain and cardiovascular disease. Annu Rev Public Health 15:381–411, 1994.
97. Schnall PL, Landsbergis PA, Schwartz J, et al: A longitudinal study of job strain and ambulatory blood pressure: Results from a 3-year follow-up. Psychosom Med 60:697–706, 1998.
98. Schnall PL, Schwartz JE, Landsbergis PA, et al: Relationship between job strain, alcohol, and ambulatory blood pressure. Hypertension 19:488–494, 1992.
99. Schurman SJ, Israel BA: Redesigning work systems to reduce stress: A participatory action research approach to creating change. In Murphy LR, Hurrell JJ, Sauter SL, Puryear Keita G (eds): Job Stress Interventions. Washington, D.C., American Psychological Association, 1995, pp 235–263.
100. Siegrist J, Matschinger H, Cremer P, Seidel D: Atherogenic risk in men suffering from occupational stress. Atherosclerosis 69:211–218, 1988.
101. Siegrist J, Peter R: Threat to occupational status control and cardiovascular risk. Isr J Med Sci 32:179–184, 1996.
102. Stokols D, Allen J, Bellingham RL: The social ecology of health promotion: Implications for research and practice. Am J Health Promot 10:247–251, 1996.

103. Stokols D, Pelletier KR, Fielding JE: Integration of medical care and worksite health promotion. JAMA 273:1136–1142, 1995.
104. Terborg J, Glasgow R: Worksite interventions: A brief review of health promotion programs at work. In Bauum A, McManus C, Newman S, Weinman J, West R (eds): Cambridge Handbook of Psychology, Health, and Medicine. London, Cambridge University Press, 1993, pp 45–52.
105. The MUNI Ambassador: Transport Workers Union of America, San Francisco Municipal Railway, Vol. 1, No. 1, May 1998.
106. Theorell T, Ahlberg-Hulten G, Jodko M, et al: Influence of job strain and emotion on blood pressure in female hospital personnel during work hours. Scand J Work Environ Health 19:313–318, 1993.
107. Theorell T, Perski A, Orth-Gomer K, Hamsten A, de Faire U: The effects of the strain of returning to work on the risk of cardiac death after a first myocardial infarction before age of 45. Int J Cardiol 30:61–67, 1991.
108. Ugljesic M, Belkic K, Simeunovic L, Vukajlovic M: Realizacija preventivnog plana u sprecavanju kardiovaskularnih oboljenja kod visokorizicne grupe vozaca profesionalaca (Implementation of a cardiovascular prevention plan among professional drivers: a high risk group). Srp Arh Celok Lek 120 Suppl 1:40–51, 1992.
109. van der Hek H, Plomp HN: Occupational stress management programs: A practical overview of published effect studies. Occup Med 47:133–141, 1997.
110. van Egeren LF: The relationship between job strain and blood pressure at work, at home, and during sleep. Psychosom Med 54:337–343, 1992.
111. Veterans Administration Cooperative Study Group on Antihypertensive Agents: Effects of treatment on morbidity in hypertension: Results in patients with diastolic blood pressure averaging 115 through 129 mmHg. JAMA 202:1028–1034, 1967.
112. Warner KE, Wickizer TM, Wolfe RA, et al: Economic implications of workplace health promotion programs: Review of the literature. J Occup Med 30:106–115, 1988.
113. Wells M, Stokols D, McMahan S, Clitheroe C: Evaluation of a worksite injury and illness prevention program: Do the effects of the REACH OUT training program reach the employees? J Occup Health Psychol 2:25–34, 1997.
114. Wilson MG: A comprehensive review of the effects of worksite health promotion on health-related outcomes: An update. Am J Health Prom 11(2):107–108, 1996.
115. Wilson MG, Edmunson J, DeJoy DM: Cost-effectiveness of worksite cholesterol screening and intervention programs. J Occup Med 34:642–649, 1992.

COSTS OF OCCUPATIONAL CIRCULATORY DISEASE

by J. Paul Leigh, PhD and Peter Schnall, MD

Circulatory diseases (CDs)— heart attack, stroke, and high blood pressure (BP), among others—are responsible for more deaths than any other disease or injury in the U.S. Rice, et al. estimated that these diseases generated more costs than any other disease or injury. The National Heart, Lung, and Blood Institute (NHLBI) estimated the cost to be \$189 billion in 1992[7] and \$274 billion in 1998.[20] This represents an increase in costs of more than 5% per year.

Few estimates of the numbers of deaths and costs of occupational CDs are available, however.[5,10,12,14] This is unfortunate, because we need some way to assess the magnitude of the burden. Moreover, costs have become a critical factor in the national debate on medical care. Our purpose in this study is to incorporate the best methods from prior studies to generate estimates of deaths, new disease incidence, and costs, and present a sensitivity analysis that demonstrates how our estimates vary with varying assumptions. In particular, we consider how costs vary as the allowable age ranges increase from 65 to 75, and the allowable range of diseases expands to include all circulatory diseases as opposed to just those that have been extensively studied. *Assumptions about percentage of the population exposed to job strain, vulnerable ages, and eligible ICD9 code are all new in this paper.*

METHOD

Epidemiology

There are a number of job hazards that could contribute to CD. A few chemical agents have been shown to cause or promote heart disease and hypertension. Carbon disulfide and nitroglycerin can cause or worsen ischemic heart disease (IHD). Carbon monoxide reduces oxygen supply to the heart and worsens symptoms of coronary heart disease (CHD). Lead raises BP. Second-hand (passive) smoking makes a substantial contribution. A number of nonchemical factors also have been implicated. These include noise, shiftwork, high risk of physical injury,[17] long working hours, social isolation, and physical inactivity inherent in many jobs. But the nonchemical factor that has received the most attention is job strain.

Ideally, we would like to measure how existing job hazards contribute to CD. To do so, however, requires making some assumptions that are truly heroic. We would have to: state how much of the workforce is currently exposed to job hazards that are risk factors for circulatory disease; allow for the fact that a given percent of

OCCUPATIONAL MEDICINE: State of the Art Reviews—
Vol. 15, No. 1, January–March 2000. Philadelphia, Hanley & Belfus, Inc.

the workforce changes jobs and changes exposures; state what proportion of that exposed workforce would eventually develop job-related CD; assume (guess?) when the CD would occur, i.e., 10 years or 40 years into the future; hypothesize how many of those that develop circulatory disease would die from the CD, as opposed to some other disease or injury; and make assumptions pertaining to length of exposure, length of time until a stroke, expected changes in medical treatments for the next 40 years, and so on. Given these difficulties, and in the absence of longitudinal data to address these issues, we resort to the method used by all researchers attempting to estimate the costs of CDs: we estimate diseases and deaths occurring in a recent year (1992), rather than hazard precarious forecasts of future deaths.

There are no data available that unambiguously count the number of occupational CDs. All prior studies have estimated that number by attributing a given percentage of total CDs to occupational hazards. Those percentages have ranged from below 1% to over 40%.[5,10,12,14,22] Authors of prior studies are careful to point out the inherent difficulty associated with assigning only one cause—whether it be excessive alcohol use, obesity, cholesterol, smoking, or job-related conditions—to a person with a CD. All prior authors have simply assumed that if the risk were removed, for example, if all job-related CD hazards could be eliminated, the incidence or prevalence of CD would drop by a given percent. We concur with this view. The critical issue then becomes why "given" percentages are chosen.

We are familiar with only one study of CDs that attempts to assign percents to estimate specific job-related causes (as opposed to all job-related causes). Olson and Kristensen discuss most of the factors cited above (e.g., noise, shiftwork), and they assign various percentages: for example, 1% due to noise, 7% due to shiftwork, 2% due to passive smoking, 42% due to sedentary work, and 3–13% to job strain.[22] However, percentages are not assigned to men and women equally, nor to all ages. For example, a higher percentage of women are assumed to be in high job strain positions, and only persons under 70 years of age are considered (upper age bound is 70 years). Young ages are not restricted (no lower bound), perhaps due to reasoning that CD among children and youths is relatively rare and would not alter aggregate statistics.

The only other relevant studies to assign percentages have been those by Leigh, et al (U.S.),[12] Kraut (Canada),[10] and Markowitz, et al. (New York).[14] All three assigned 1–10% in a given age range and selected group of CD. Kraut simply applied Markowitz's percents and assumptions to Canada. In Leigh, et al., coauthor Markowitz applied some earlier assumptions to generate a national rather than a New York–only estimate. Thus, although there have been three separate studies, they are strikingly similar in their assumptions.

In the most recent study, the assumed percentages were 5–10, but the age restriction (25 to 64, inclusive) was narrow.[12] Moreover, not all CDs were included. Markowitz included only hypertension, IHD, cerebrovascular disease, and atherosclerosis: ICD9 codes 401–404, 410–414, 430–438, 440. These codes cover only about 68% of all CD deaths. Since so many CDs do not manifest themselves until retirement, and since not all were considered to have job-related causes, the effective range was not 5–10%, nor was the point estimate 7.5%. The effective range became .56–1.11%, with a point estimate of .84% for job-related factors.

We believe .56%, .84%, and 1.11% represent unrealistic estimates. A lifetime spent in high job strain work may not generate clinically noticeable CD until after the person retires. Hypertension, for example, is progressive and, for most patients, irreversible. In addition, the Markowitz list excludes several "unspecified" ICD9 categories with great numbers of deaths. ICD9 code 429.2—CVD, unspecified—contained 69,379 deaths in 1992. It is likely that coroners did not have time to record these deaths in other, more precise categories, such as the ICD9 codes that Markowitz did include. Finally, although little research has been conducted on CDs and job strain associations outside of the ICD9-coded diseases included in the Leigh, et al. study, it is possible (though less likely) that job strain and other psychosocial factors play a role in other CDs as well.

Here, we alter these two assumptions about age and ICD9 codes, setting the upper age restriction at 70 in one calculation, 75 in another, and no upper limit in a third. In addition, in some calculations we restrict ICD9 codes to the narrow group in the Leigh, et al. study; in others, we consider the broad group and allow all CDs—ICD0 codes 390 to 448. Thus, for example, we include pulmonary embolism (ICD9 code 415.1), cardiomyopathy (425), cardiac dysrhythmia (427), heart failure (428), CVD-unspecified (429.2; 69,379 deaths), aortic aneurysm (441), and so on. We refer to these groups as the "short" ICD9 code list (the 68% from Markowitz[14]) and the "long" ICD9 list (100% of all ICD9 circulatory disease codes). The long list represents an outside upper limit of the psychosocial-related occupational disease burden. Some of the diagnoses in the long list currently are not believed to be related to occupation, while some (e.g., heart failure) could be a manifestation of stress-induced illness resulting from silent myocardial infarction (MI).

In 1992 the long list included 913,908 deaths, job-related and not. The short list included 623,297 deaths. The short list of diseases thus comprised 68.2% of the long list. The short list combined with the 25–65 age limit yielded 101,846 deaths, thus comprising 16.3% (101,846/623,297) of the short list. But 101,846 represents 11% of deaths on the long list. Importantly, deaths are heavily skewed towards older persons (Table 1). Roughly one-third of deaths occur at ages 0 to 74, whereas two-thirds occur after age 75.

The assumptions about which diseases to include and exclude and about age are critical. The long list combined with the least restrictive age assumption yields roughly nine times as many deaths as the short list combined with the most restrictive age assumptions (911,245 compared to 101,846).

The next assumption involves the percentage of occupationally-related deaths. Leigh, et al. assumed a 5–10% range,[12] which we believe is too conservative, especially given that odds ratios are 1.5 for CVD and hypertension when comparing workers exposed to job strain with those not exposed to job strain. Here, we consider a 5–20% range.

The same techniques could be applied to estimating the incidence of disease. However, incidence numbers are not readily available. Therefore, we rely on the estimate for the short list and least restrictive ages by Leigh, et al., who estimate that the 5% assumption results in 41,550 *job-related* new cases of CD. We use this

TABLE 1. Numbers of Deaths Regardless of Cause, Age, and ICD9 Assumptions in the U.S.

	Ages 25+[†]	Ages 25–74	Ages 25–69	Ages 25–64
All CDs (Long List)*	911,045	346,608	233,799	149,332
Only Short List**	621,344	236,390	159,453	101,846

* Includes all circulatory diseases (ICD9 codes 390 to 448); ** Only includes ICD9 codes 401–404; 410–414; 430–438; and 440
† Roughly .313% of all deaths were among those less than 25 years of age.

41,550 as an anchor and assume that all other combinations of assumptions and ICD9 codes are proportional to 41,550.

Economics

Costs are estimated using the human capital method, whereby two broad categories are constructed: direct and indirect costs. **Direct costs** include medical and administrative expenses. Medical costs include payments to hospitals, physicians, drug companies, and nursing homes. Insurance administration includes the cost of processing claims and managing financial accounts. Administrative expenses are split into administration for medical and administration for indemnity insurance.

Indirect costs include lost wages, fringe benefits, and home production. Lost wages are meant to capture not just the hardship on the person and family without the wages, but the cost to the economy in terms of lost output. Lost fringe benefits are included for the same reason as lost wages. The total economic loss is assumed to be what is required for the business to attract a qualified person to the job, including wages and fringe benefits. Home production includes time costs of nonpaid labor such as making home repairs and preparing meals.

General discussion of advantages and disadvantages of the human capital method is available.[12] Despite its weakness, it is the most popular method for estimating the costs of any illness or injury.

DIRECT COSTS

Our "top-down" approach to estimating direct costs is similar to that of Fahs, et al.,[5] Rice, et al.,[23,24] and Leigh, et al.[12] Estimates rely on ratios involving hospital days multiplied by national estimates of medical spending. These hospital day ratios act an anchors in the estimation of all direct costs. Hospitalization data are highly regarded, are collected annually, and are summarized within the same definitions, thus permitting comparisons across diseases. Similar data are not available for doctor's visits or drug use. Moreover, hospitalizations are the most expensive (broad) category of medical care, contributing 44.6% of medical costs in 1992. Doctors' services are second at 20.9%.[26] We assume that spending on all other direct costs is proportional to hospital spending.

We begin with an estimate of national expenditures on medical care—$820.3 billion or 13.6% of the gross domestic product in 1992. This is equivalent to spending $3086 per person. Medicare and Medicaid contributed 16.9% and 13.2%; other third-party government spending contributed 13.6%; direct out-of-pocket expenditures by patients and families contributed 18.9%. The remainder, 37.9%, was contributed by private health insurance and HMOs. Our estimate of $820.3 billion in healthcare expenditures includes payments for hospitalizations, doctor and dentist visits, nursing home care, drugs, and medical supplies; it also includes public healthcare expenditure, such as construction of hospitals and offices, government public health activities, and research. We include public healthcare expenditures on the grounds that without occupational circulatory disease, some portion of these public expenditures would not be necessary. We do not include cost of program administration and net cost of public health insurance in our calculations, however. We believe these figures are underestimates. The National Center for Health Statistics estimates this amount to be $39.5 billion. This would be the equivalent of roughly 5.06% of expenditures (39.5/780.8 = .506). Studies have shown that administrative costs can add up to an additional 45% to the total cost of medical care.[3,4,25,28] Cutler's estimate of 15%[3] appears to be the most reliable, and the one used in previous analyses.[12,13] We exclude the $39.5 billion, but include a 15% administrative expense to our calculations. Therefore, we use $820.3–39.5 = $780.8 to begin our calculations.

Using the National Hospital Discharge Survey[8] we then calculate the total number of days spent in the hospital by patients with a primary diagnosis for the attributable occupational CDs. Total days of hospitalization by circulatory diseases are then divided by total hospital days for all diseases and injuries in the U.S. in 1992 (190,386,000). This percent is subsequently multiplied by $780.8, which in turn is multiplied by the ratio of occupational deaths to total deaths. The procedure is displayed in Equation 1:

Med$Cir = $780.8 × (CirDays/TotalDays) × (OccCirDeaths/TotCirDeaths)
Med$Cir is our estimate of the medical dollars spent for occupational CDs; CirDays are number of days in the hospital attributed to CDs; TotalDays are the number of days in the hospital attributed to all diseases and injuries in the U.S.; OccCirDeaths are numbers of circulatory deaths attributed to occupations; and TotCirDeaths are total number of circulatory deaths due to all causes.

However, Equation 1 estimates do not account for the administrative costs. To obtain administrative costs we assume: (1) $630.2 billion was spent by insurance companies, HMOs, and governments ($150.6 billion in out-of-pocket expenditures by individuals is subtracted from $780.8 to obtain $630.2), and (2) the average of private and public insurance and HMO administrative costs is 15%.[3] Our effective multiplier is .1211 ([.15 × 630.2]/780.8) which is multiplied by the estimate above (Med$Cir) to derive the overall administrative costs. The variable OccCirDeaths itself will vary depending on our assumptions regarding age ranges and whether we use the short or long list for CDs.

INDIRECT COSTS

Indirect mortality costs were established using a standard present value equation.[13] Information for use in the present value equation was age-specific, sex-specific, and disease-specific mortality data from the National Center for Health Statistics, Vital Statistics Division, as well as life table estimates[19,27] and earnings and labor force participation data from the Bureau of Labor Statistics.

Finally, we calculated national disease-specific ratios for morbidity costs to direct costs from Rice[23,24] to obtain an estimate of the morbidity costs.

RESULTS

Results for Epidemiology

Table 2 presents results for occupationally related CD based on assumptions involving which ICD9 codes to include, which ages apply, and which percentages are appropriate. The percentages in Table 2—5%, 10%, 15%, 20%—refer to the percent of all CD deaths we assume are caused by job-related factors.

The significance of the assumptions regarding the percent attributable can now be seen. By definition, the 20% assumption provides numbers four times the size of those of the 5% assumption. If we combine the percents assumptions (5%, 10%, 15%, 20%) with the other two about including/excluding ICD9 diseases and age restrictions, we find that the numbers of deaths range from a low of 5092 to a high of 136,657—for a 36-fold difference.

Our preferred estimate is a proportion of 15%, the short list, and ages 25 through 74:35,459 deaths due to job-related factors.

TABLE 2. Occupational Circulatory Disease Deaths in the U.S.

	Ages 25+	25–74	25–69	25–64
All CDs (Long List)*				
5%	45,552	17,330	11,690	7,467
10%	91,105	34,661	23,380	14,933
15%	136,657	51,991	35,070	22,400
20%	182,208	69,320	46,760	29,868
Only Short List**				
5%	31,067	11,820	7,973	5,092
10%	62,134	23,640	15,945	10,185
15%	93,202	35,459†	23,918	15,277
20%	124,268	47,280	31,892	20,368

* ICD9 codes 390 to 448; ** ICD9 codes 401–404; 410–414; 430–438; 440
† This is our preferred estimate.

Table 3 presents similar results for the incidence of disease. Again, a 36-fold difference is apparent in comparing the least restrictive assumptions to the most restrictive (1,486,712 to 41,550). Our preferred estimate is the 15% proportion, ages 25 through 74, short list: 289,320 new diseases in 1992.

In Table 3, the factors of proportionality are ratios from Table 1. The first cell corresponding to the long list, ages 25+, is determined as follows: multiply the ratio of 911,045/101,846 by 41,550. The product is 371,678. The Leigh, et al. estimate of 41,550 new job-related cases[12] has as its counterpart in Table 1 the number 101,846. We essentially assume that the same percentage increase that "lifts" 101,846 to, for example, 911,045, also lifts 41,550 to 371,678. All other estimates are derived in a similar fashion. For example, by multiplying the ratio 346,608/101,846 by 41,550, we obtain 141,405. We assume that the same percentage increase that lifts 101,846 to 346,608 also lifts 41,550 to 141,405. In other words, we assume that the incidence of disease is proportional for all ages and all ICD9 codes.

Results for Costs

Table 4 presents our estimates of direct costs, for the two age groups (25–74 and 25–64) and the three percents (10%, 15%, and 20%). From this point on we will present a more restricted set of estimates based on these parameters. Our cost estimates are roughly proportional to those for deaths and incidence; hence, in the interest of brevity, we restrict our attention to a narrower set of assumptions.

TABLE 3. Occupational Circulatory Disease Incidence in the U.S.

	Ages 25+	25–74	25–69	25–64
All CDs (Long List)*				
5%	371,678	141,405	95,383	60,923
10%	743,356	282,810	190,766	121,846
15%	1,115,034	424,215	266,149	182,769
20%	1,486,712	565,620	381,532	243,692
Only Short List**				
5%	253,489	96,440	65,052	41,550
10%	506,978	192,880	130,104	83,100
15%	760,467	289,320†	195,156	124,650
20%	1,013,956	385,760	260,208	166,200

* ICD9 codes 390 to 448; ** ICD9 codes 401–404; 410–414; 430–438; 440
† This is our preferred estimate.

TABLE 4. Direct Costs in the U.S. (Billions)

	Ages 25–74	Ages 25–64
All CDs (Long List)*		
10%	$7.3760	$3.1778
15%	$11.0640	$4.7667
20%	$14.752	$6.3556
Only Short List**		
10%	$5.0307	$2.1674
15%	$7.5460†	$3.2511
20%	$10.0614	$4.3348

* ICD9 Codes 390 to 448; ** ICD9 Codes 401–404; 410–414; 430–438; 440
† The preferred point estimate

Again the importance of the assumption is clear. The costs in Table 4 range from $2.1674 billion to $14.752 billion. Had we included all possibilities, as in Tables 1, 2, and 3, the range between the lowest and highest would again be about 36-fold. Our preferred estimate is $7.5460 billion.

Table 5 presents our estimates of indirect costs. The range in the estimates for Table 5 is from $2.4413 billion to $15.4232 billion. Table 6 presents the total of direct plus indirect. Our preferred estimate assumes 15% of circulatory disease is due to occupation, the age range is 25–74, and the short list of circulatory diseases applies: $15.4353 billion.

Table 6 presents the total of direct plus indirect. Our preferred estimate assumes 15% of circulatory disease is due to occupations, the age range is 25–74, and the short list of circulatory diseases applies: $15,4353 billion.

DISCUSSION

Limitations

There are a number of limitations to our study. First, we did not assume any deaths or illnesses resulted from workers who worry about layoffs. As corporate restructuring continues, so do feelings of job insecurity that can lead to circulatory disease.[9,11] We do not have reliable national estimates for this association, however.

Second, disease deaths were counted as occurring in 1992. However, the exposures leading to the deaths could have occurred 20 or 30 years prior to the death. CD death rates have been slowly dropping for 20 years. On the other hand, the labor

TABLE 5. Indirect Costs in the U.S. (Billions)

	Ages 25–74	Ages 25–64
All CDs (Long List)*		
10%	$7.7116	$3.5793
15%	$11.5674	$5.3691
20%	$15.4232	$7.1586
Only Short List**		
10%	$5.2596	$2.4413
15%	$7.8893†	$3.6619
20%	$10.5192	$4.8826

* ICD9 Codes 390 to 448; ** ICD9 Codes 401–404; 410–414; 430–438; 440
† Our preferred estimate

TABLE 6.   Total Costs in the U.S. (Billions)

	Ages 25–74	Ages 25–64
All CDs (Long List)*		
10%	$15.0876	$6.7571
15%	$22.6314	$10.1358
20%	$30.1752	$13.5142
Only Short List**		
10%	$10.2903	$4.6087
15%	$15.4353†	$6.9130
20%	$20.5806	$9.2174

* ICD9 Codes 390 to 448; ** ICD9 Codes 401–404; 410–414; 430–438; 440
† Our preferred point estimate

force grows virtually every year. The point is, the true numbers are moving targets. Our estimates apply only to 1992. These numbers are likely to change in the future, but not by a great amount.

Third, several limitations suggest we underestimated costs. We did not adjust for current employment status in the present value of earnings tables; we merely adjusted for the labor force participation rate. Those currently employed are not a random sample of all persons in the labor market, and they probably have better lifetime employment prospects than all persons in the labor force. All persons in the labor force included the unemployed.

We assumed that fringe benefits were equal to 23.3% of the wage. Most studies show fringe benefits above 25%.

We ignored pain and suffering costs and quality of life issues. For example, patients can take hypertensive medications for 20 years or more with accompanying side-effects. Many patients experience shortness of breath with CHD. It is difficult to estimate these costs. Lawsuits involving nonfatal injuries almost always involve some payment for pain and suffering. A rule of thumb frequently cited in the courts is that pain and suffering equal three times the nonadministrative medical expenses. This would mean adding another roughly $22 billion to our costs. We may have *significantly* underestimated costs, since $22 billion is more than our total of $15.4 billion.

We did not include the costs of family caregiver's time nor the costs of health problems that occur among caregivers. These costs are undoubtedly large, but are difficult to estimate.[1] McFloyd and Flanagan document the deleterious psychological effects on spouses of caregiving.[16]

Critics might argue that current deaths and numbers of new disease cases do not reflect current job conditions. Rather, they reflect conditions in the workforce perhaps 40 years ago, given that sometimes CD takes 40 years to manifest. But our alternative is to develop estimates based on assumptions that many reasonable researchers would simply dismiss as fantasy, as indicated in our methods section. We generated prevalence and incidence numbers for a given year (1992) so that a general picture of the overall burden of occupational CD can be envisioned. As our ability to generate credible assumptions about the further course of CDs and their treatments improves, a study of current job hazards and exposures will become more viable. In any event, the methods and estimates we develop in our limited attempt here will likely prove useful to future researchers.

We have more confidence in our mortality and cost estimates than in the incidence estimates. Incidence numbers are notoriously hard to come by for most diseases, and this is especially true of CDs.

In estimating days of work loss for diseases, we used the Bureau of Labor Statistics' (BLS) Annual Survey data that were restricted to a 12-month calendar year. But many serious illnesses can generate work loss for much longer than 12 months. Oleinick, et al. showed that BLS data misses as much as 70% of workdays lost.[21]

Comparison to Other Studies

Studies by Markowitz, Fahs, and Leigh, et al. have received the greatest attention.[5,13,14] Their assumptions were especially conservative, however, They restricted attention to ICD9 coded diseases on our short list; they did not include any deaths or diseases in people over age 64; and they imposed a 5–10% range. The effect was to attribute less than 1% of all CDs to working conditions. We used the short list of circulatory diseases; ages 25–74, inclusive; and 15% attribution to job-related factors. Our preferred number of deaths is 35,459. We estimate nearly five times as many deaths as Markowitz[14] and Fahs.[5] If these numbers prove to be correct, job-related CD is responsible for more deaths than any other job-related disease (e.g., cancer, pulmonary disease).

Fahs preferred costs estimates were $3.5 billion to $6.0 billion. Our preferred cost estimate is $15.4 billion. Thus, we estimate costs roughly 2 to 4 times as large as Fahs. The disparity in costs is not as great as the disparity in deaths, because most deaths occur after people retire, when indirect costs are small.

NHLBI estimated 1992 costs for all CDs at $189 billion. Our estimate of $15.4 billion indicates that roughly 8.2% of these costs can be attributed to job-related factors.

Implications

We estimate 35,459 deaths and 289,320 new cases of disease. These are large numbers. In 1992, 50,067 people died from diabetes; 33,566 died of AIDS; 30,484 died by suicide; and 25,488 died from murder. Most categories of disease in government reports, in fact, record fewer than 35,000 deaths.[18] Incidence of diseases are difficult to estimate; thus, few comparisons are possible. But 289,320 per year is obviously a significant number of people newly becoming afflicted with a disease that may eventually kill them.

Assuming 8.2% also applies to the current costs of all CD, we estimate job-related CD cost to be $22.5 billion in 1998. This represents an important burden on medical care and a drain on the economy in general. Costs have become a critical factor in the national debate on the allocation of medical spending. Rarely, however, has that debate addressed job-related circulatory disease. This is a serious omission since much of this disease could be prevented.

It is likely that the lion's share of the $15.4 billion is not paid by business, but rather by workers and their families, as well as taxpayers. Most of businesses' contributions to the cost of job-related disease derive from workers' compensation (WC) premiums. Only infrequently, however, do WC systems pay for CDs. For example, firefighters and police officers in California are compensated for heart attacks whether they occur on or off the job (but not during retirement). But these are exceptions to the rule. In part, this lack of WC coverage is because the diseases do not manifest themselves until retirement, and they are assumed to have many causes other than job hazards, so that it is difficult to prove job causation. Nevertheless, some costs are absorbed by businesses in the form of high absenteeism, low morale,[2] and higher health insurance premiums. However, the specific dollar amounts have never been reliably estimated.

Most of the costs for medical care are borne by Medicare and Medicaid, i.e., by taxpayers. A significant portion of lost wages are paid for by the Social Security Administration, either through survivors' benefits or disability benefits, i.e., taxpayers. Most economic studies of the Social Security payroll tax and the Medicare tax indicate that workers pay for the tax in the form of lower wages.[12] The "workers" here refers to all workers, whether or not they develop job-related CD.

In summary, workers and taxpayers, not businesses, bear the brunt of the costs. In the language of economics, a "negative externality" exists. Businesses are not paying for the true costs of production, but are shifting the costs to others. Simple economic analysis shows that under these conditions an inefficient amount (too much) of the negative externality (job-related CD) is produced by businesses.[15] But economists have a solution: tax the negative externality. To correct this inefficiency, a tax could be imposed on those industries with jobs that are especially prone to producing CD. The proceeds from this tax could be used to defray the costs currently being absorbed by Medicare and the Social Security Administration. This **Circulatory Disease Tax Fund** could be modeled after the Black Lung Trust Fund that taxes coal companies on a per-ton-of-coal basis and uses the money to pay medical and indemnity benefits for persons with pneumoconiosis.

The Circulatory Disease Tax Fund would have two beneficial effects. First, it would resolve the equity problem. Taxpayers should not have to pay for a problem for which they are not responsible. Second, and equally as important, the tax would provide an economic incentive to businesses to decrease the causes of job-related CDs. It would encourage businesses to reassess their workplace arrangements, to decrease job strain and other job-related causes of CDs.

REFERENCES

1. Arno PS, Levin C, Memmott MM: The economic value of informal caregiving. Health Affairs 18:182–188, 1999.
2. Cooper CL, Liukkonen P, Cartwright S: Stress Prevention in the Workplaces. Assessing the Costs and Benefits to Organizations. Dublin, European Foundation for the Improvement of Living and Working Conditions, 1996.
3. Cutler DM: A guide to health care reform. J Econ Perspect 8:13–29, 1994.
4. Danzon PM: Hidden overhead costs: Is Canada's system really less expensive? Health Affairs 11:21–43, 1992.
5. Fahs MC, Markowitz SB, Leigh JP, et al: A national estimate of the costs of occupationally-related disease. Ann N Y Acad Sci 837:440–455, 1997.
6. Ferguson TW: A triple threat to California's tort bar. Wall Street Journal, April 18, 1995, p A19.
7. Fox P, Gazzaniga J, Karter A, Max W: The economic costs of cardiovascular disease mortality in California, 1991. Implications for public health policy. J Public Health Policy 17:442–459, 1996.
8. Graves EJ: Detailed diagnosis and procedures, National Discharge Survey, 1992. Vital Health Stat 13, 1994.
9. Heaney CA, Israel BA, Schurman SJ, et al: Industrial relations, worksite stress reduction, and employee well-being. J Organiz Behav 14:498–510, 1993.
10. Kraut A: Estimates of the extent of morbidity and mortality due to occupational diseases in Canada. Am J Ind Med 25:267–278, 1994.
11. Landsbergis PA, Schnall PL, Schwartz JE, et al: Job strain, hypertension, and cardiovascular disease: Empirical evidence, methodological issues, and recommendations for future research. In Sauter SL, Murphy LR (eds): Organizational Risk Factors for Job Stress. Washington, DC, American Psychological Association, 1995, pp 97–112.
12. Leigh JP, Markowitz SB, Fahs MC, Landrigan PJ: Cost of Occupational Injuries and Illness. Ann Arbor, University of Michigan Press, (in press).
13. Leigh JP, Markowitz SB, Fahs MC, et al: Occupational injury and illness: Estimates of costs, mortality, and morbidity. Arch Int Med 157:1557–1568, 1997.
14. Markowitz SB, Fischer E, Fahs MC, et al: Occupational disease in New York State: A comprehensive examination. Am J Ind Med 16:417–435, 1989.
15. Mc Connell CR, Brue SL: Microeconomics: Principles, Problems, and Policies. New York, McGraw-Hill, 1998.
16. McFloyd VC, Flanagan CA: Econcomic Stress: Effects on Family Life and Child Development. San Francisco, Jossey-Bass Inc., 1993.
17. Murphy LR: Job dimensions associated with severe disability due to cardiovascular disease. J Clin Epidemiol 44:155–166, 1991.
18. National Center for Health Statistics: Health, U.S., 1994. Hyattsville, Maryland, Public Health Service, 1995.
19. National Center for Health Statistics: Vital Statistics of the U.S., 1991. Vol. 2, Part A: Mortality. Washington DC, Public Health Service, 1996.

20. National Heart Lung and Blood Institute: Morbidity and Mortality, 1998: Chart Book on Cardiovascular, Lung, and Blood Diseases. Bethesda, MD, National Institute of Health, NHLBI, 1998.
21. Olenick A, Guire KE, Hawthorne VM, et al: Current methods of estimating severity for occupational injuries and illnesses: Data from the 1986 Michigan comprehensive compensable injury and illness database. Am J Ind Med 23:231–252, 1993.
22. Olsen O, Kristensen TS: The impact of work environment on cardiovascular diseases in Denmark. J Epidemiol Comm Health 45:4–10, 1991.
23. Rice DP, Hodgson TA, Kopstein AN: the economic cost illness: A replication and update. Health Care Financing Review 7:61–80, 1985.
24. Rice DP, MacKenzie EJ, et al: Cost of Injury in the United States: A Report to Congress. San Francisco, Institute for Health and Aging, University of California; Baltimore, Injury Prevention Center, The Johns Hopkins University, 1989.
25. Thorpe KE: Inside the black box of administrative costs. Health Affairs 11:42–55, 1992.
26. U.S. Bureau of the Census: Statistical Abstract of the United States, 1994 (114th edition). Washington, DC, 1994.
27. U.S. Department of Health and Human Services, National Center for Health Statistics: Life Tables, Vital Statistics of the U.S., 1990. Volume II, Sec. 6, Pub No. 94-1104. Washington, DC, 1994.
28. Woolhandler S, Himmelstein DU: The deteriorating administrative efficiency of the U.S. health care system. New Engl J Med 324:1535–1558, 1991.

LEGAL AND LEGISLATIVE ISSUES

LEGISLATION TO PROTECT WORKER CV
HEALTH IN EUROPE   *by Lennart Levi, MD, PhD*

The science-policy gap must be bridged, by issuing laws or decrees, agreeing on a code of practice, and educating and informing—measures based on an adequate range of scientific evidence. First, we need to consider if there is a problem to be addressed in terms of potentially noxious working conditions. If there is a problem, our second step is to review the present state of knowledge with regard to potentially noxious health effects of such conditions. If such effects are found to be likely and, in addition, qualitatively and/or quantitatively of sufficient severity, a logical third step is to discuss the need for, or existence of, legislative and other measures to modify or eliminate such conditions, in the 15 Member States of the European Union (EU) and elsewhere.

It is then up to you, the reader, to consider the applicability of these measures to the American scene.

Noxious Working Conditions?

In a major study of work conditions in the EU, which then comprised 12 Member States, the European Foundation for the Improvement of Living and Working Conditions found that 23 million workers had night work (more than 25% of their total hours worked); every third worker reported repetitive work; every fifth male and every sixth female worked under continuous time pressure; and 30% of the European workforce regarded their health at risk from work.[48]

The most recent set of representative European data come from the Second European Survey of Working Conditions, conducted by the European Foundation in early 1996. The report calls attention to the pronounced transformation of European working life from the industrial to the service sector, with a consequent change in job profile: introduction of new technology (one-third of the workforce uses computers) and more client-oriented jobs (49% indicate permanent and direct contact with clients or patients).[47] Work organization also has changed, with new management models, teamwork, just-in-time, and Total Quality management (TQM). In addition, European workers are getting older; they are working more often on fixed-term or temporary contracts; the proportion of female workers is growing rapidly; the traditional employee-employer relationship is slowly disappearing; and the unemployment rate remains very high.[47]

According to this survey, 45% of the 147 million workers in the EU Member States report having monotonous tasks; 44% no task rotation; 50% short, repetitive tasks; 35% no influence on task order; and 28% no influence on work rhythm; while 54% work at a very high speed, and 56% to tight deadlines. Thus, a considerable proportion of the workforce is exposed to a variety of work-related stressors, with likely effects on health.[54]

Health Effects?

According to a recent state-of-the-art document from the European Heart Network, there is a marked difference in CVD risk between various occupational groups: a nine-fold difference between high- and low-risk occupations in men, and a five-fold difference among women.[13] These differences are too large to be explained by conventional risk factors; factors associated with the occupation, whether physical or nonphysical, must be involved. Some of the latter are work-stress–related.

Complementing the person-environment fit model, there are two current models for predicting stress and CVD risk at work. In the **demand-control-support model**, persons in jobs with high demands and little control over decisions are in a high job-strain situation and at a higher risk of CVD.[21] Low social support at work further increases the risk.[19] According to the **effort-reward model**, people who work hard (high effort) but receive little reward (money, esteem, or status control), experience an imbalance which puts them at increased risk of CVD. Persons with a high "need for control" over their situation who are in a high effort-low reward situation are at particularly high risk.[62] Shift work and night work also increase the risk for CVD. The risk intensifies with prolonged exposure. Exposure at work to carbon disulphide, nitroglycerin, nitroglycerol, carbon monoxide, passive smoking, and possibly lead also have been shown to increase the risk for CVD.

The European Heart Network has reviewed estimates of the proportion of CVD caused by work. According to such estimates, 16% of CVD cases in men and 22% in women could be prevented by eliminating all occupational risk factors from the work environment. Job strain accounts for 6% of this risk in men, 14% in women; shift work accounts for 7% in both sexes. Inclusion of sedentary work into the calculation raises the (preventable) proportion of CVD cases caused by work to around 50%.[13]

EU Legislation and Practice

Against this background, it is reasonable to consider legislative action or other practices to protect European workers against such potentially noxious exposures. In its report on European health promotion in the workplace, the World Health Organization draws attention to such actions because they could improve the quality of life for every worker, provide return for the company, and stimulate healthier lifestyles in the population as a whole.[74] Complementary strategies fall into five categories: (1) building healthy public policies; (2) creating supportive environments for health; (3) strengthening community action; (4) developing personal skills; and (5) reorienting health services.

The most important initiative is the EU's ambitious **Framework Directive** (89/391/EEC). Under this Directive employers have a "duty to ensure the safety and health of workers in every aspect related to the work, on the basis of the following general principles of prevention:
• Avoiding risks;
• Evaluating the risks which cannot be avoided;
• Combating the risks at their source;
• Adapting the work to the individual, especially as regards the design of workplaces, the choices of work equipment and the choice of working and production

methods, with a view, in particular, to alleviating monotonous work and work at a predetermined work rate and to reducing their effect on health;

• Developing a coherent overall prevention policy which covers technology, organisation of work, working conditions, social relationships and the influence of factors related to the working environment."

According to the Advisory Committee for Safety, Hygiene, and Health Protection at Work of the European Commission, the approach taken in a number of EU countries, consistent with the Framework Directive, is first that the priority strategy for intervention is *primary prevention* and, second, that such prevention should be focused on the *organization as the generator of risk*.[14] Such an approach deals largely with foreseeable risks to health generated by the design of work and the organization's management of that work. It is not the only way forward. Not all countries nor bodies within countries have committed to such an approach. Some have placed their emphasis elsewhere, notably on employee training in coping techniques and employee assistance programs or workplace counseling.[14]

The Advisory Committee has agreed on the following recommendations with regard to action by the European Commission: *research* (development of methods; descriptive, analytic, intervention, and cost-benefit studies); *guidance* for national guidelines (to raise the awareness within Member States and to promote prevention rather than just management); *exchange of information* (through the European Agency in Bilbao, Spain, and the European Foundation in Dublin, Ireland); and *education and training* (the European Commission assisting Member States in these activities).[14] These recommendations presently are being implemented by the Commission, in accordance with the EU's recent "Constitution," the Treaty of Amsterdam. According to Article 152 of this Treaty, "a high level of human health protection shall be ensured in the definition and implementation of all Community policies and activities."

National Initiatives

It is instructive to observe how the Swedish Government has approached this task in a step-by-step manner.[32] Following a decade of intensive interactions with the scientific community, in which available information on the interrelationships between living conditions, lifestyles, and health was reviewed, the Swedish Government presented its Public Health Service Act (Act No. 560, 1985), which states:

• Our health is determined in large measure by our living conditions and lifestyle.

• The health risks in contemporary society take the form of, for instance, work, traffic and living environments that are physically and socially deficient, unemployment, abuse of alcohol and illicit drugs, consumption of tobacco, unsuitable dietary habits, as well as psychological and social strains associated with our relationship— and lack of relationship—with our fellow beings.

• These health risks . . . are now a major determinant of our possibilities of living a healthy life. This is true of practically all the health risks which give rise to today's most common disease, e.g., cardiovascular disorders, mental ill health, tumours and allergies, as well as accidents.

• Care must (therefore) start from a holistic approach . . . By a holistic approach we mean that people's symptoms and illnesses, their causes and consequences, are appraised in both a medical and psychological and social perspective.

Three years later, the Swedish Government focused in on one of the key components of the "living conditions" mentioned in its Public Health Service Act—

namely the *work environment*. It appointed a Swedish Commission on the Work Environment (SCWE) to address concern about recent trends in work-related morbidity, long-term absence due to sickness, and premature retirement.

Again based on numerous consultations with the scientific community, the SCWE presented its final report in 1990. Based on this report, the resulting amended Swedish Work Environment Act (Act No. 677, 1991) now states:

• Working conditions shall be adapted to people's differing physical and psychological circumstances.

• Employees shall be enabled to participate in the arrangement of their own job situations as well as in work changes and development that affect their jobs.

• Technology, work organization and job content shall be arranged so that the employee is not exposed to physical or mental loads that may cause ill health or accidents.

• The matters to be considered in this context shall include forms of remuneration and the scheduling of working hours.

• Rigorously controlled or tied work shall be avoided or restricted.

• It shall be the aim of work to afford opportunities for variety, social contacts and cooperation as well as continuity between individual tasks.

• It shall further be the aim for working conditions to afford opportunities for personal and occupational development as well as for self-determination and occupational responsibility.

Similar legislation has been passed in all Nordic (and some other European) countries, stating that conditions of work shall respect the physical and mental health of the workforce. Examples are the Finnish Labour Protection Act (299/1958, as amended by several Acts, including No. 1132/1997), and the Danish Work Environment Act (No. 646 of 18 December 1985, as amended by a number of subsequent Acts, including No. 867 of 13 October 1994). In April 1988, the Danish Labour Inspectorate issued its Decree on monotonous and repetitive work (No. 4.10.4), stating that work should be organized to fit the worker and his or her tasks, and proposing job rotation, job enlargement, work in semiautonomous groups, and frequent breaks as other options for workplace adaptation.

A Healthier Workplace Via Internal Control

In the United States, many decision makers seem to believe that prevention of work-related stress must be complicated, time consuming, and prohibitively expensive. This need not be so. One of the most commonsense approaches is known as internal control. Internal control simply means introducing a "self-correcting loop" into the worker-work-ecosystem. It means learning from experience, in a systematic step-by-step manner.

The first step is to identify whether there is, indeed, a problem in the working population—in terms of incidence, prevalence, and severity of work-related ill health. The next step is to try to identify working conditions causally related to this morbidity. In a third step, a package of interventions is designed and implemented in an attempt to eliminate, as far as possible, the root causes of the problem(s). Eventually, the outcomes of the interventions are evaluated, preferably in terms of (a) stressor exposures, (b) incidence and prevalence of ill health, (c) indicators of well-being, and—above and beyond internal control requirements—(d) quality and quantity of production of goods or services. Also to be considered are the costs and benefits of the intervention(s) in economic and other terms.

In two European States, Norway and Sweden, the internal control process is part of the respective Work Environment Act (WEA) and its implementation. In

Norway, the Internal Control Regulation came into force in 1992 and is now mandatory for every enterprise in the country, regardless of trade and number of employees. The Norwegian WEA states (Article 12) that work shall be organized so that it allows for the development of competence, social contacts, and opportunity to make decisions, but also avoids repetitive work and work that is paced by machine or assembly line. Internal control in this context is defined as systematic actions at the enterprise level to ensure and document that the activities for health and safety are performed in accordance with requirements specified in this WEA.

Few large-scale interventions have been evaluated. Norwegian experiences indicate that internal control as implemented in a representative sample of 915 workplaces has, indeed, contributed to increased health, improved environment and safety awareness, clearer lines of responsibility, more and/or better risk assessments, better documentation, and new strategic plans, in 42–69% of Norwegian enterprises.[53] The Swedish initiative to promote both humanization of working life and increased productivity, by applying the principles of the Swedish WEA, has been evaluated, although in a rather simplistic manner.[32] To promote practical work along these lines, the Swedish Working Life Fund was set up by a decree of the Swedish Parliament. It has distributed a total of SEK 15 billion (corresponding to roughly US $3 billion at that time) over a 6-year period aimed at a radical renewal of Swedish working life. Through financial grants to the employers, the Fund tried to promote a healthy work environment and work organization and productivity, as well as active rehabilitation programs in the workplace. The Fund was used for some 25,000 work life programs covering approximately 3 million of Sweden's 4 million employees. Evaluation was carried out by a survey administered to 20% of a random sample of 7500 of the major programs. The survey was addressed to key persons in each program, both management and labor. In *service sector programs*, waiting time for customers decreased by > 10% in 34% of cases; performance time decreased by > 10% in 33% of cases; costs went down by at least 10% in 23% of cases because of better understanding of customer needs; and performed work per employee went up by 10% or more in 42% of cases. In *industrial programs* included in the sample, production errors went down by > 10% in 45% of cases; time for delivery decreased by > 10% in 52%; readjustment time decreased by > 10% in 34%; and productivity increased by > 10% in 45%. Across sectors, physical job strain decreased by > 10% in 59%, employee codetermination (decision latitude) increased in 64% of all cases, and employee work satisfaction and motivation increased in 71% of the cases. Virtually no negative effects were reported. Ratings by management and labor union representatives were almost equal.

CHEMICAL AND PHYSICAL EXPOSURE REGULATIONS IN THE U.S. *by Lawrence Fine, MD, PhD*

Both NIOSH and OSHA have established exposure limits for several of the definite or suspected chemical exposures associated with adverse CV effects.[40] For **carbon disulfide** the OSHA exposure limit is 10 ppm, while NIOSH recommends an exposure limit of 1 ppm (3 mg/m³). The exposure limits, unless specified for a short time period, are expressed as the time-weighted average (TWA) exposure for an 8-hour working shift within a 40-hour work week. The NIOSH short-term exposure level of 15 minutes (STEL) for carbon disulfide is 10 ppm, while the ceiling value limit for OSHA is 100 ppm for a 30-minute maximum peak exposure.

In addition to exposure limits based on the level of a chemical in the air, there also are biological exposure limits based on the concentration of a chemical or metabolic byproduct in the breath, blood, or urine. The American Conference of Governmental Industrial Hygienists (ACGIH) has developed the concept of the biological exposure index (BEI).[34] Exposure to carbon disulphide can be assessed by determining the concentration of 2-thiothiazolidine-4-carboxylic acid in the urine. The biological exposure index recommended by the ACGIH is 5 mg/g creatinine.[44]

For **carbon monoxide** (CO) the OSHA TWA exposure limit is 50 ppm (55 mg/m^3). NIOSH recommends a TWA exposure limit of 35 ppm (40 mg/m^3) with a ceiling (peak) level of 200 ppm (229 mg/m^3). Workers exposed during an 8-hour period at the OSHA exposure limit may achieve a carboxyhemoglobin level of 5% or more, levels comparable to those often found in moderate to heavy cigarette smokers. Levels of nonexposed nonsmokers generally are below 1%. The BEI for CO is a carboxyhemoglobin level of 3.5%.

Methylene chloride OSHA exposure limit is 500 ppm with a ceiling level of 1000 ppm and 2000 ppm (5-minute peak in any 2-hour period). One could use the CO BEI for methylene chloride, since it is metabolized into CO. **Nitroglycerin and ethylene glycol dinitrate** OSHA ceiling levels are both 0.2 ppm (0.1 mg/m^3), while NIOSH short-term is 0.1 mg/m^3. Skin absorption is the most important route of exposure.

The NIOSH recommended TWA level of **lead** in the air is 0.1 mg/mg^3; the OSHA TWA is 0.05 mg/mg^3. One of the goals of the OSHA lead standard is to reduce blood lead levels below 40 mg/dl. Blood lead levels do not always correlate with the amount of lead stored in the bones of the body. Therefore, the blood lead may not be an accurate measure of total body lead burden and may not reflect recent exposure. The EDTA lead mobilization test was used extensively to assess body lead burden, but it has been replaced by the less invasive in vivo x-ray fluorescence for determination of bone lead content.[33]

NIOSH has now evaluated the latest scientific information for **noise**. Its 1998 recommendations go beyond attempting to conserve hearing by focusing on preventing occupational noise-induced hearing loss (NIHL). The NIOSH recommended exposure limit (REL) for occupational noise exposure (85 A-weighted decibels [dBA] as an 8-hour TWA) was re-evaluated using contemporary risk assessment techniques and incorporating the 4000-hertz (Hz) audiometric frequency in the definition of hearing impairment. The new risk assessment reaffirms support for the 85-dBA REL. With a 40-year lifetime exposure at the 85-dBA REL, the excess risk of developing occupational NIHL is 8%—considerably lower than the 25% excess risk at the 90-dBA permissible exposure limit currently enforced by OSHA and the Mine Safety and Health Administration (MSHA). Exposures at or above 85-dBA REL are hazardous.

NIOSH previously recommended an exchange rate of 5 dB for the calculation of TWA exposures to noise. However, NIOSH now recommends a 3-dB exchange rate, which is more firmly supported by scientific evidence. The 5-dB exchange rate is still used by OSHA and MSHA, but the 3-dB exchange rate has been increasingly supported by national and international consensus.

NIOSH recommends an improved criterion for significant threshold shift: an increase of 15 dB in the hearing threshold level at 500, 1000, 2000, 3000, 4000, or 6000 Hz in either ear, as determined by two consecutive audiometric tests. The new criterion has the advantages of a high identification rate and a low false-positive rate. In comparison, the criterion NIOSH recommended in 1972 has a high false-positive rate, and the OSHA criterion (called the standard threshold shift) has a relatively low identification rate.

The noise reduction rate (NRR) is a single-number, laboratory-derived rating that the U.S. Environmental Protection Agency requires to be shown on the label of each hearing protector sold in the U.S. In calculating the noise exposure to the wearer of a hearing protector at work, OSHA derates the NRR by one-half for all types of hearing protectors. In 1972, NIOSH recommended the use of the full NRR value; however, in this document, NIOSH recommends derating by subtracting from the NRR 25%, 50%, and 70% for earmuffs, formable earplugs, and all other earplugs, respectively. This variable derating scheme, as opposed to OSHA's straight derating scheme, considers the performances of different types of hearing protectors.

This document also provides recommendations for the management of hearing loss prevention programs for workers whose noise exposures equal or exceed 85 dBA, including program evaluation. For further information, see NIOSH's Criteria for a Recommended Standard, Occupational Exposure to Noise (June 1998), http://www.cdc.gov/niosh/98-126.html.

SHIFT WORK REGULATIONS *by Kyle Steenland, PhD*

Kogi recently reviewed international regulations on the organization of work, principally the recommendations of the International Labor Organization (ILO) dating from 1990, and the directive of the European Council of 1993 which (at least in theory) must be enforced within the European Economic Community.[22] These regulations apply more generally to all work organization, but a number of points are directly relevant to shift work. The ILO recommendations call for: (1) advice to the worker at regular intervals on how to cope with shift work, (2) transfer to a similar day job when the worker is found unfit for shift work, (3) special compensation for shift work, (4) consultation between worker and employer in the details of the shift work, and (5) at least 11 hours of rest in each 24-hour period (no consecutive full-time shifts). The European directive is similar. It calls for: (1) a minimum daily rest period of 11 hours in a 24-hour period, (2) a rest period of at least 35 consecutive hours per 7-day period, (3) maximum of 48 work hours per week, and (4) transfer to day work when problems with night work are recognized.

In the United States there are no general regulations covering shift work, although there are some regulations for particular sets of transportation workers (i.e., pilots, truck drivers, and railroad workers). NIOSH has published guidelines for shift work.[51]

U.S. REGULATIONS FOR WORK ORGANIZATION
by Nick Warren, ScD

Despite the growing body of evidence for a relationship between work organization, job characteristics, and CVD, little occupational health legislation or regulation addresses workplace risk factors. One approach is legislation to ensure adequate staffing levels in hospitals and nursing homes, both to ensure patient safety and moderate job demands, thus reducing employee stress. Proposals to this effect have been introduced by healthcare worker unions in California and New Jersey in 1999.

A potentially broader approach to regulation of work organization is directed toward regulation of ergonomic hazards and reduction of risk for work-related musculoskeletal disorders (MSDs). The body of research linking work organization and musculoskeletal disorders is much smaller than the research on work organization and CVD, having begun later.[3,7,23,31,37] However, ergonomics is one of the few areas in which regulatory efforts have addressed issues of work organization and psychosocial job characteristics. These efforts have been general, sometimes inadvertent, and have met with considerable resistance. But they represent a first step to which future regulatory initiatives may refer.

Review of the Standards and Programs

CALIFORNIA

The California Standard on Repetitive Motion Injuries (RMIs) is the only standard currently enacted.[11] Despite several challenges, it currently stands in its original 1997 wording (awaiting the results of a case on appeal). However, the standard is quite short (1 page) and limited, referring only to injuries "predominantly caused by a repetitive job, process, or operation." If more than one employee in a workplace has experienced an RMI, the standard requires establishment and implementation of a program including worksite evaluation, control, and training. The only wording relevant to work organization issues in this Standard is requirement that "the employer shall consider engineering controls . . ., and administrative controls, such as job rotation, work pacing, or work breaks." These simple aspects of work organization are seen only as factors that can affect intensity and duration of a biomechanical exposure. However, attention to these controls also could result in beneficial reductions of psychosocial stressors, such as job strain, by increasing job variety and control.

NORTH CAROLINA

The Draft Ergonomic Standard for the State of North Carolina is similar in its approach.[41] Although the standard would require attention to a broader range of biomechanical stressors (called "ergo stressors") than the California standard, there is no reference to any psychosocial or work organization issues. Employers are required to solicit early reports of symptoms from employees. After a 30-day period that either allows temporary symptoms to subside or allows determinations of work-relatedness, the employer must implement controls to limit exposure "to the maximum extent practicable." Controls listed include engineering changes to the workstation and equipment, work practice controls, and administrative controls, primarily of the work hardening and exercise variety. The work practice controls include work breaks, job rotation, changing the order of work, and "changing the way work is done." This ambiguous last phrase, combined with the requirement that "the employer, *in consultation with the affected employee* (italics added), shall implement one or more of the . . . controls" seems to provide a limited arena in which employee control of the work process could be increased.

WASHINGTON

Although not a regulation, the Washington State Department of Labor has produced a valuable reference for employers, Fitting the Job to the Worker: An Ergonomics Program Guideline (1995). Given the possibility that nonmandatory program guides might someday serve as a basis for part of an ergonomic standard, the information is relevant. The main body of the document, outside of a strong recommendation to involve employees in all stages of the program, does not specifically address work organization or psychosocial stressors. However, "work rates" are identified as potential stressors, including increased over-time and piecework. As in the state regulations, job rotation and rest breaks (low-level work organization changes) appear as possible controls. Appendix C does recommend self-pacing as a way to reduce high rates of repetition. Self-pacing also could increase work variety and possibly reduce job strain.

Appendix F, Psychosocial Risk Factors, begins by stating, "Psychosocial risk factors arise from the interaction of the individual (psychological) and the business' culture and attitudes toward employees (sociological)." It notes that these risk factors are difficult to incorporate into a program but "can be serious and costly in terms of employee discomfort, increased absenteeism, and loss of productivity." This guide is the only document that acknowledges that effects of psychosocial stressors can be both psychological and physical (specifically noting fatigue, heart rate changes, and changes in sleep or appetite). Employers are encouraged to consider controls specifically targeted towards psychosocial stressors: implementing procedural changes (not specified); listening to employees and providing regular positive feedback; soliciting employee input on changes that affect their work; ensuring adequate staffing and resources or reducing expectations; training to help reduce risk factors, including job design, stress reduction, and communication/interaction skills.

AMERICAN NATIONAL STANDARDS INSTITUTE (ANSI) Z-365

The draft ANSI Ergonomic Standard (1997, 1998) is a much more extensive document than the state standards. The first four sections tend to focus only on biomechanical workplace exposures. Section 2, Definitions, lays out an interesting distinction between psychosocial and work organization factors. Psychosocial factors are defined as work environment characteristics that affect interpersonal relationships (including the employee to the organization). By contrast, work organization factors receive a lengthy and very broad and useful definition, one that invites the reader to consider the multifactorial and multilevel assessment of risk for which recent research argues.[23,72,73] In part: "These factors broadly consider various aspects of job content (e.g., workload), organizational characteristics (e.g., tall vs. flat organizational structures), interpersonal relationships at work (e.g., supervisor-employee relationships), temporal aspects of the work and task (e.g., shift work, changing risk factor conditions such as equipment maintenance, raw materials and quality control), financial and economic aspects (e.g., pay, benefits), community aspects (e.g., prestige and status) and physical aspects of work (e.g., thermal or chemical exposure)."

However, this promising early entry in the standard does not appear again in the rest of the document. Elsewhere, the ANSI standard conceives of work organization factors as workplace characteristics that "can alter the characteristic properties or effects of physical stress exposure," such as magnitude, repetition, duration, and recovery time. Oddly, the proposed standard then proceeds: "It is not understood how to intervene with psychosocial and work organization factors." And later (in section 6.8.2.3): "It is not feasible in this standard to provide recommendations on specific work organization factors such as wage incentive systems or workplace conflict resolution." We are referred to the TQM literature. However, the standard does present a list of "specific work organization factors," which addresses aspects of job demands and job control (thus, by implication, heart disease risk) and, to an extent, supervisor support, but not coworker support, skill discretion, and larger issues like job security. The administrative controls presented in section 6.8.2. specifically recommend reducing these hazards: close performance monitoring, wage incentives, machine-paced work, absence of employee latitude in how the job is performed, time pressure and overload, unaccustomed work, overtime/extended work hours, and work allocation.

Finally, the ANSI Z-365 draft standard contains an extensive rationale for employee involvement in the ergonomic program, a blueprint for involvement in all phases, and mandatory language to ensure involvement. The range of involvement proposed does not by itself guarantee that employees will have substantial influence in the program, but it lays the ground rules within which that influence could evolve. Thus, even if work organization stressors are narrowly conceived as "altering the characteristic properties" of physical exposures, the control tactics and strategies recommended could be used to substantially alter some of the most stressful job characteristics, and thereby reduce the risk of heart disease.

OSHA 1995

More extensive and well thought-out references to work organization appeared in the 1995 OSHA Draft Ergonomic Protection Standard, which did not achieve standard status. In the mandatory portion of the standard, machine-paced work (a classic example of high job strain) is the only work organization variable that achieves entry into the checklist, and work organization is addressed only once in the body text, under "definitions." The definition notes six aspects of work organization, similar to those seen in the ANSI standard: inadequate work-rest cycles, excessive work pace and/or duration, unaccustomed work, lack of task variability, machine-paced work, and piece rate.

In the nonmandatory appendices, the standard presents extensive and thoughtful analysis of work organization factors, suggesting that physical "workplace risks can be intensified by work organization characteristics," a formulation similar to the first ANSI proposed mechanism. Appendices A and B contain a detailed review of several work organization risk factors and their ramifications. Unlike the ANSI standard, this document clearly proposes possible control tactics—tactics which could reduce exposure to job strain and thus CHD risk:

• Work recovery cycles—alternate task types, task cycles, introduce variation, change scheduling

• Excessive work pace—let employee set pace, especially in very demanding jobs, job rotation, no overtime for hard tasks unless redesigned, breaks

• Unaccustomed work—break-in periods, effective maintenance and repair

• Lack of task variability—increased recovery periods, alternate tasks, job enlargement, job rotation

• Changing postures

• Machine-paced work—self-paced is preferable, provide buffers, increase cycle time, provide adjustability of line speed ("Increases in line speed should be discussed with the workers on the line and the equipment suppliers to determine safety concerns.")

• Piece rate and incentive systems should be avoided if possible.

Addendum B-5 proposes the following:

• Provide clear job descriptions

• Avoid monotony, fast cycle times, low variety, and boring tasks

• Create clear and unambiguous lines of reporting—avoid conflicting supervision

• Train supervisors to manage and develop better interpersonal skills, to reduce tension

• Schedule work to avoid recurrent deadline stress—anticipate and communicate peak workloads; prepare work ahead in slack times.

• Avoid excessive overtime by replacing workers who are absent for extended periods of time.

• Communicate with workers about work monitoring practices to reduce tension.

• "Resolving organizational issues usually requires the involvement of people who frequently interact with the area. Problem-solving teams have been used successfully to develop creative solutions and to facilitate implementation."

Although this draft standard was never enacted, the review of work organization stressors (which are, of course, pertinent to CHD risk) and possible control tactics and strategies remains the most comprehensive attempt to date to regulate work organization risk factors.

OSHA 1999

By contrast, the 1999 OSHA Draft Ergonomics Program Standard, a much more restricted document, only mentions work organization at the very end, in its tables listing specific workplace conditions. The tables list three aspects of work organization: work recovery cycles, work rate, and task variability. The standard does not state the theoretical reasons for including these three factors, but they appear similar to the ANSI factors thought to increase the characteristics of exposure (duration, magnitude, etc.). Correspondingly, possible administrative controls for MSD risk in the draft include "employee rotation, rest breaks, alternative tasks, job task enlargement, redesign of work methods, and adjustment of work pace."

Probably of more import to the control of psychosocial stressors at work are the two basic elements in the ergonomics program requirement: (1) hazard identification and hazard awareness, and (2) management leadership and employee participation. The standard spells out employer responsibility for soliciting and aiding employee participation in hazard identification, developing control measures, training, and program evaluation. In the presence of committed management and labor organizations, these could be the conditions for a substantially altered psychosocial work organization in the company. However, nothing in the standard guarantees this level of employee influence.

OSHA SAFETY AND HEALTH RULE

Though not an ergonomic standard, the OSHA Draft Proposed Safety and Health Program Rule proposes to reduce work-related fatalities, illnesses, and injuries by requiring employers to establish a workplace safety and health program. This program would ensure compliance with OSHA standards and the General Duty Clause of the OSHA act. The elements of the program are almost an exact duplicate of the provisions in the Draft Ergonomics Program Standard, described above. Hence, the requirements for management leadership and employee involvement present the same set of reasons for hope and pessimism, concerning the possibility of reducing psychosocial stressors in the workplace.

Conclusions

It is not surprising that ergonomics is the one area in which regulatory efforts address issues of work organization. Ergonomics programs may be unique in recognizing the effect of work environment because the effect of poor work organization on musculoskeletal disorders is so apparent. The different standards and programs reviewed present different theoretical reasons for attending to work organization factors. In general, most documents use a limited definition, seeing negative work organization factors as altering the characteristics of physical (biomechanical) exposure (magnitude, duration, repetition, and recovery time, in the ANSI formulation). However, if an employee's control over the job is increased in the interests of improving the rest schedule, this still represents increased decision latitude and has implications for reduced job strain beyond the reduction of MSDs.

Institution of an ergonomics program may itself be a positive psychosocial intervention. The "word on the corporate street" is that ergonomics programs work (i.e., reduce injuries and save money) and that the most effective way to institute an ergonomics program is through a joint labor/management ergonomics team (as is recommended in all standards). However, none of the requirements for employee participation come close to insuring substantial employee influence on the program.

There is tremendous resistance to the focus on work organization and psychosocial stressors in ergonomic regulations, because their control, much more than the control of physical exposures, may alter **political and power relationships** within companies. For ergonomics programs to be truly successful in reducing rates of disease, it appears that management must distribute or share some power and information. Other forces also require this redistribution within companies: market demands for innovation and creativity, flexible and customized production, and more responsive and effective customer service—all of which are driving organizational change (within certain sectors). It is possible that the confluence of these market forces with new types of and approaches to regulation could result in the gradual reduction of workplace psychosocial stressors and the concomitant improvement in worker health, satisfaction, and well-being.

WORKING LIFE IN JAPAN *by Teruichi Shimomitsu, MD, PhD, and Yuko Odagiri, MD, PhD*

Japan is known among industrial and cardiovascular health circles for having identified and brought to the attention of the world *karoshi*—death from overwork. *Karoshi* is sudden death from ischemic heart disease or cerebrovascular disease due mainly to physiologically demanding work conditions such as long working hours or shift work.[60] *Karoshi* may be thought of as an occupational "sentinel health event" (see Chapter 8) focusing attention on a particular problem of the workplace.

Japan has had difficulty in setting standards for an appropriate number of working hours. Employees, especially middle managers, are often required to work long overtime hours without compensation.[59] Complicating this already difficult situation is the Japanese economic recession of the 1990s, which has forced drastic, systematic reorganization. The unique Japanese employment system, including the lifetime employment system and seniority-constrained wage and promotion systems, is now falling apart. Companies are trying to reorganize by removing layers of management. These reorganizations have brought the workers more work and responsibility, without corresponding increases in pay, as well as a feeling of job insecurity.

According to statistics from the Policy Planning and Research Department of the Ministry of Labor, the percentage of workers who complained of anxiety, worry, and stress in their working lives gradually increased from 50.6% in 1982 to 62.8% in 1997. Another recent report, based on 1998 data, from the Ministry of Health and Welfare says the number of those who died from suicide has dramatically increased to 25.3/100,000 persons from 18.8/100,000 persons in 1997. It is especially high among men in their 50s and has grown by more than 50% among this group in just 1 year. It is speculated that the severe economic situation and physical and mental overload are the main reasons for the high suicide rate.

To protect workers from extreme burdens, the government has taken legislative action and has presented several strategies for dealing with issues of work-related stress and health. In 1972, the **Industrial Safety and Health Law** (ISH Law) was enacted to assure the safety and health of workers in the workplace. The law stipulates that employers must offer an annual physical examination to all workers, which they are required to attend. The goal of the exam is secondary prevention through the early detection and treatment of noncommunicable diseases.

The Ministry of Labor enacted the **Total Health Promotion Plan** in 1988, to deal with the rapid aging of the population and to prevent noncommunicable diseases. It was designed to improve the total health of employees. The goal of this plan is not only early detection and treatment of noncommunicable diseases but also health promotion and disease prevention. Each company has an occupational physician who conducts a medical examination, lifestyle evaluation, and exercise test. An exercise prescription and lifestyle consultation are based on the results. In some cases, mental health care and nutritional guidance also are provided.

A 1992 amendment to the ISH Law included a commitment to facilitate the promotion of a "comfortable" working environment. Here, "comfortable working environment" refers not only to the actual physical workplace but also to the whole working environment.

In 1993, the government established prefectural Industrial Health Promotion Centers and Local Industrial Health Centers in all parts of Japan to support health care, including mental health care, for the employees of smaller firms, which are not able to offer the same healthcare services as larger firms.

With the revision of the ISH Law in 1996, occupational physicians now possess the right to act as direct advisors to employers on working conditions and worker health to prevent occupational illnesses like *karoshi*, and promote health. Conversely, the employers have an obligation to consider the recommendations of the occupational physicians.

In 1998, the Japan Ministry of Labor established the **9th Industrial Accident Prevention Plan**, which includes strategies for managing increasing mental stress: (1) promotion of interdisciplinary research and investigation to prevent stress-related ill health among all workers, especially white-collar workers, (2) maintenance of a high standard of training for managers and supervisors, (3) provision of information to workers to control or manage their own work-related stress, (4) implementation of stress-related consultation systems, and (5) promotion of stress management at the workplace.

Unfortunately, these strategies may not be sufficient to protect workers from ill health. The Tokyo Declaration emphasizes that it is vital to identify ways to overcome current difficulties and prevent foreseeable future difficulties, while at the same time maximizing the tremendous potential inherent in this period of dramatic transformation.[68] It also mentions that there is a great need for the exchange of experiences and increased cooperation between all relevant actors from the world's three leading postindustrial settings, the European Union, Japan, and the U.S., with regard to (1) implementation of information on prevention, (2) surveillance and monitoring, (3) education and training of occupational and other key professional groups, (4) methodological development, and (5) creation of a clearing house for all relevant information using state-of-the-art technology.

We hope policy-makers and decision-makers throughout the three settings utilize the Tokyo Declaration as a framework for healthier work in healthier workplaces.

WORKERS' COMPENSATION: WORKPLACE STRESS AND THE CVD CONNECTION *by Mark Kimmel, PhD*

Workers' compensation (WC) laws and regulations were established at the beginning of the 20th century to address work-related injuries. Prior to the establishment of the WC system, employees sued employers with only occasional success. However, after exposés by writers (e.g., *The Jungle* by Upton Sinclair), mine disasters, and the 1911 Triangle Shirtwaist Factory fire in New York, there were demands for greater workplace safety and compensation for injured workers. In addition, lawsuits against employers started being won due to jury sympathy.[16] WC laws were trade-offs, limiting employers' liability but providing treatment and benefits for their injured employees; employees were prohibited from suing for additional damages. These laws were designed as part of a "no fault" system. Employees did not have to prove negligence, and employers paid lower benefits. Also beneficial to employers was the fact that cases were not heard in regular law court, where there are potentially more generous liability rules.

One of the theories underpinning WC is that industry pays for the cost of goods production, including injuries sustained by workers and medical treatment costs. These costs are not shifted to society in general nor to the injured workers and their families (what economists call "externalities of costs").[52]

Throughout the 20th century, ongoing political struggles have shaped the definitions of illness, impairment, and disability under WC laws. Moreover, it appears that the political strength of various groups has been an important factor in determining their ability to obtain presumptions of disability under the law.

During the last decade there has been a national effort by employers and insurance companies to reduce benefits and tighten eligibility standards for WC claims.[67] The justification for limiting stress claims has been based, in part, on the contention that many stress claims are fraudulent and result in unacceptably high costs for employers. In addition, there has been a historical tendency to view stress injuries as "soft" and intangible, especially when compared to the "hard" findings of orthopedic injuries. In California (CA), the legislature revised and restricted WC laws in 1993 for psychiatric injuries after employers threatened to move their businesses to more "employer-friendly" states. The new laws prevented employees from filing claims for "good faith personnel actions," and created a higher threshold for compensability. Today only some states compensate injured workers for psychiatric stress or "mental stress" claims.

The California Case

In WC, distinctions are made between "mental-mental," "mental-physical," and "physical-mental" cases. The mental-mental cases typically are psychiatric cases in which a worker alleges harassment, conflicts, discrimination, or work overload. Physical-mental cases include the psychological consequence of a physical injury, such as when a worker sustains an orthopedic injury and has accompanying pain and depression. Mental-physical cases are those where mental stressors (i.e., psychological) give rise to physical disorders such as a heart attack. Physical injuries sustained as a result of mental stress do not have to meet the higher threshold requirements of the CA Labor Code (LC) 3208.3. for mental-mental cases.

It is important to make the distinction between the overlapping concepts of stress and psychiatric disorders. Stress is defined as an individual's perception of and management of challenges and demands that he or she faces in the environment.

These demands can be physical, psychological, or both. Stress-related disorders range in intensity from the mild and sub-clinical to the acute and disturbing post-traumatic stress disorders. The implications of stress-related disorders for the WC system are enormous, both in the costs they represent to employers and the toll they take on workers when they go untreated.

Psychiatric injuries (mental-mental claims) due to hostile work environments, sexual harassment, personnel actions, and demands placed on employees (which are perceived as unfair or discriminatory) often result in depression, anxiety, and/or pain disorders. Typically, workers do not file claims for work overload or re-engineering, but rather focus on some negative aspect of their work environment. In CA, for example, psychiatric claims that are substantially (at least 35%) caused by "lawful, nondiscriminatory, good-faith personnel actions" are prohibited. This has shielded many businesses from the effects of downsizing, re-engineering, or what is euphemistically called "creative destruction."

Employees in these "leaner and meaner" organizations face higher demands and longer hours, which may be associated with mild and subclinical signs and symptoms such as anxiety or depression. The law, at least in CA, requires a worker to prove that the actual events of employment were the "predominant cause" (presumed to be more than 50%) among all the other causes of the psychiatric injury. While this has been difficult to prove until recently, more objective analysis of jobs and work environments may hold promise in documenting "actual events."

This more objective approach to assessment is consistent with the Albertson Inc. vs. WCAB 1982 case where a worker's psychiatric stress was based on a misperception of workplace matters. The court ruled that for a psychological injury to be compensable "the employment itself must be a positive factor influencing the course of the disease." In this case the mere perception of psychiatric stress was not sufficient to be considered compensable.

CVD AND WC: LEGAL ASPECTS

The CA Constitution established the WC system to adequately provide "for the comfort, health and safety, and general welfare of any and all workers and those dependent upon them for support to the extent of relieving from the consequences of any injury or death incurred" (Article XIV, Section 4, 1917). This language is broad and flexible in its intent and suggests that as the nature of work changes and our understanding of the consequences of work develops, new medical conditions will be considered compensable.

The labor codes were created to determine whether an injury is work related. The first question is, did the injury "arise out of employment" (AOE), and the second question is did the injury "occur in the course of employment" (COE). There is a requirement to provide a "reasonable link" between exposures and resultant impairments. As part of this linkage "actual events" or tangible exposures and incidents must be present. In certain industrial accidents there is no question that the injury is work related; however, in some cumulative injuries the relationship between workplace risk factors and activities and the resulting disease is equivocal and controversial. There are some well-documented relationships between specific exposures such as vinyl chloride and angiosarcoma of the liver, and there has been a growing consensus about the link between repetitive motion, poor ergonomics, and musculoskeletal disorders. However, medical research has yet to define precisely the causal factors associated with many other occupational illnesses. As noted in the *Physician's Guide to Medical Practice in the California Workers' Compensation*

System, "there are many exposures, pathologies, and diseases that have not been fully investigated, or for which the causal mechanism is not known."

AOE and COE are somewhat overlapping concepts. AOE relates the workplace incident(s), exposures, and risk factors to the damage that a worker has incurred. COE means that the activities are work-related. Therefore, AOE explains what the *nature* of the condition is, and COE pinpoints *where and how* the condition occurred. For example, when an employee goes to the post office to buy stamps for the employer, the task is COE. However, if the employee stops for a personal errand, COE is disrupted.

Note that if a worker has pre-existing CVD that is nondisabling, and the workplace aggravates the condition and causes impairment and disability, the employer is responsible for treatment and/or benefits. The employee (the applicant) must show by the "preponderance of evidence" that the illness or disorder is related to the employment, but it does not have to be the sole source of the injury. The landmark case Liberty Mutual vs. Calabresi (1946) found that the employer was responsible for the resultant disability when a laborer performed heavy lifting with pre-existing CVD. If a workplace accelerates or precipitates symptoms to the point of impairment, the injury is compensable.

When an injury aggravates a pre-existing condition, resulting in permanent disability, **apportionment** (i.e., assignment of causation and responsibility for benefits) becomes an issue. Apportionment does not require an employer to pay for the effects of a pre-existing injury or condition. This is especially relevant in CVD, which may take a number of years to manifest and may have a number of causes. Often, apportionment is difficult because the physician cannot estimate the level of disability that would have existed absent the most recent injury.

In CA and several other states, WC law distinctions are made between illness, impairment, and disability. One may have an illness such as hypertension and not be impaired. Impairment refers to a loss of function. Disability refers to an inability or reduced ability to compete in the open labor market as a result of impairment. Therefore, a disabled worker may have an impairment that interferes with his or her ability to compete in the open labor market, but does not interfere with the current job.

CURRENT TRENDS IN WC FOR JOB STRESS

The recent national effort by employers and insurance companies to reduce benefits and tighten eligibility standards for WC claims[67] has led to decreases in benefits paid, minimal changes in insurance premiums, and increases in the overall profitability of WC carriers.[10] It is within this context that many states also have passed laws that establish more stringent criteria for psychiatric stress claims. Due to supposed abuses in psychiatric cases, the CA legislature has established a higher threshold for psychiatric claims for injuries on or after July 16th, 1993. For these claims an injured worker must prove that the actual events of employment were the predominant cause of the psychiatric injury (more than 50%). From January 1990 till July 16th, 1993 there was a 10% threshold for compensability. For psychiatric injuries that result from a violent act, the actual events of employment must have been a substantial cause (35% of the causation from all other sources combined) (LC 3208.3) of the injury.

The revised CA labor codes also prohibit claims for psychiatric injuries that are caused by "lawful, nondiscriminatory, good faith personnel actions." (Similar changes to the law occurred in New York State.) Apparently there were complaints that many employees filed WC claims after receiving poor performance evaluations;

they claimed that they had been harassed. The difference between a good-faith personnel action and an abusive management practice may depend on whose point of view you take, the employee or the manager.

The revised CA psychiatric labor codes have saved employers large sums of money; however, there are significant costs to workers and society in general when mental or physical illness due to job stress is not recognized and treated (see Chapter 11). If one adds the cost of medical care, lost time from work, and morbidity and mortality from new systems of work organization that pressure employees to increase productivity, then productivity gains may not be as impressive as we are led to believe (if they remain at all).[30] By reducing WC benefits and thereby externalizing the costs onto individuals, their families, and health insurance plans, only an illusion of cost reduction and efficiency is created.

Occupational Stress, CVD, and Workers' Compensation

These medical/legal distinctions and definitions are particularly problematic when applied to occupational stress. First, job stress-related disorders may not become manifest for many years. As Selye noted, an individual may be able to resist a stressor for a long period of time before he/she becomes exhausted.[56] Since workers change jobs and employers more frequently than in the past, it is more difficult to attribute a chronic stress condition to a current employer. Apportionment again applies in these cases. However, there is another principle that the employer "takes the employee as he finds him," which means that compensation will not be denied "even though the worker was 'predisposed' to injury or a previous condition made it more difficult for the worker to heal from the injury." Second, many stressors may cause some physical strain without an individual necessarily being aware of it. This is sometimes the case in hypertension (which is generally an asymptomatic condition). Third, stress often has been conceived as a mediated process whereby the individual's coping repertoire either predisposes him to or shields him from health risks. This has led many practitioners to focus on individual factors of resilience or vulnerability (mediators) rather than work-related stressors (primary causes). An extreme form of this approach is illustrated in Millon's analogy of personality as a kind of immune system that buffers individuals from psychological disorders.[36] This personal characteristics hypothesis holds that persistent, adverse psychological reactions after exposure to stressors represent exacerbations of pre-existing character pathology or indicate predisposition to such reactions.

CVD is a multifactorial medical condition. However, for the most part, physician evaluators have tended to focus on nonindustrial causes such as obesity, family history, smoking, and lack of exercise. While these factors undoubtedly contribute to CVD, the basic principle in WC law that the employer "takes the employee as he finds him" applies here also. This principle implies that the employer is responsible for a work-related impairment even if the employee has unhealthy habits, unless and except to the extent the nonindustrial factors caused actual pre-existing disability or would in the absence of industrial injury. Thus, if a work-related psychosocial factor is accepted as a risk factor for hypertension or CVD, even if other risk factors (e.g., obesity) are present, the employer is held responsible for any impairment resulting from exposure to that risk factor.

HIGH-RISK OCCUPATIONS

Work stress has been recognized as a cause of CVD in WC labor codes for many years. Police officers, fire fighters, and other law enforcement groups who have developed heart diseases have been presumed to have compensable occupational illnesses under CA WC laws. Although there is an intuitive logic that those faced with violence and unpredictable social conflicts experience a kind of stress not found in other occupations, these assumptions are not well documented, nor necessarily even well founded in empirical research. Why are fire fighting and law enforcement presumed compensable for CVD while other types of work are not? When these groups were first made eligible for WC for CV events there was little epidemiologic evidence that they were at high risk. Possible reasons are public sympathy for individuals in these occupations and the political strength of police and fire unions. Today, there is a growing body or research that suggests that there may be other occupational groups who are at equal risk for developing CVD. Acknowledgment of this information would enable workers in other occupations to be recognized as having legitimate WC claims.

JOB STRAIN, HYPERTENSION, AND CVD

Within the past two decades a number of workplace psychosocial stressors have been identified. One such exposure is job strain, the consequence of physical and psychological demands placed on workers who do not have adequate control over their tasks. Additional work-related stressors include effort-reward imbalance, shift work, and work overload. Job strain has been found to be associated with a variety of health risks, including CVD,[21,55] and job stress in general has been associated with musculoskeletal disorders.[4,7]

The growing body of epidemiological research that shows an association between job strain, high blood pressure, and CVD is rarely discussed in WC cases. Physicians evaluating employees for WC cases generally are unaware of the job strain data and rarely conduct an analysis of the workplace or job to ascertain levels of exposure to job strain. Most often they rely on the worker's self-report regarding tasks and activities, or on a job description, which is vague and imprecise. Rarely, physicians compare blood pressure readings over time to see if they correlate with the individual's self-reported experience of stress. They also may draw conclusions about work-related stress by measuring blood pressure after a person has been off work or on vacation to check for decreased pressure. Unfortunately, one of the insidious aspects of hypertension is that individuals with this condition are unaware of it and do not experience stress. In some research on job strain, individuals who report having jobs high in demand and low in control fail to report any subjective distress associated with work.

For the most part, physicians tend to overlook the industrial contribution to a patient's illnesses unless the patient complains of stress at work. Frequently, both the illness (hypertension) and the cause (job strain) do not produce obvious symptoms. The physician, unaware that a particular patient has an "at risk" occupation, tends to attribute medical problems to lifestyle or idiosyncratic causes.

The consequence of having a high-strain job is that the worker is subjected to what can best be described as **microtrauma** on a daily basis. This microtrauma may be imperceptible to the worker, who may feel pressure to perform or meet deadlines, but is not subjectively experiencing high levels of distress. In addition, there is evidence that a lack of perceived supervisory support in those facing job strain can exacerbate illness risk.

If one considers these high-job-strain environments to be subjecting workers to microtrauma, then many workers have potentially compensable WC claims. In WC law the term "actual events" refers to whether something tangible and identifiable occurred in the work environment. Typically, "actual events" refers to exposures to chemicals or, in psychiatric claims, to discrete incidents. Were society to recognize that workplace stressors, such as job strain, caused repeated microtraumas that over time lead to impairment and disability, then many CVD cases would be compensable. (The methodology for assessing actual events [microtrauma] is described in Chapter 2.)

COLLECTIVE BARGAINING TO REDUCE CVD RISK FACTORS IN THE WORK ENVIRONMENT   *by Paul Landsbergis, PhD*

Most collective bargaining agreements include limits on exposure to CVD risk factors such as chemical and physical hazards, shiftwork and long work hours, and psychosocial stressors. Contracts can help to moderate job demands, increase employee job control and job skills, and provide a more supportive atmosphere, through provisions on job security, work standards, work assignments, performance evaluations, technological change, harassment, discrimination, staffing, comparable worth, skills training, and career development.[2,57,61] By providing employees with a voice in improving working conditions and protection from arbitrary decisions through seniority provisions, a grievance procedure, or labor-management committees, collective bargaining agreements can help reduce job stress.[29] In addition, by raising income and offering promotion opportunities, such contracts can increase the socioeconomic status (SES) of employees and thereby reduce the risk of CVD associated with low SES. Examples of contract language for two sectors are provided below, followed by language designed to limit exposure to specific job hazards.

Sectors

Clerical and Computer Work.   An agreement between Yale University and Local 34, the clerical employees union, provides for greater employee decision-making authority, resources, and support: a labor-management health and safety committee; rules for schedule changes and flex-time; forums for employee participation; day care; leaves of absence; and an employee assistance program.[76] Elsewhere, computer operators have bargained for workstation improvements, ergonomic training, and rest breaks.[42] For example, the American Federation of Teachers (AFT) Local 1521 and the Los Angeles Community College District agreed that "every employee actively working at a video display terminal shall be required to take a 15-minute work break every hour away from the terminal to accomplish other work."[27] There is evidence that greater job decision latitude (control over schedule, regular breaks, and work variety) may help prevent repetitive strain injuries.[37]

Health Care.   Nurses' desire for professionalism at work can be thwarted through understaffing (leading to increased workload demands), lack of autonomy, or an authoritarian climate.[49] Collective bargaining can be an important means of achieving professionalism. Unions have bargained for clinical career ladders for nurses in various specialties, joint physician-nurse committees, and greater in-service education.[28] The California Nurses Association recently negotiated a contract with Kaiser Permanente to create 18 new "quality liaison" positions—union-appointed nurses who will monitor conditions, such as understaffing, that affect the quality of patient care as well as increase employee stress.[18] The Service Employees International Union has negotiated contract language on minimum

staffing guidelines, patient care classification, staffing and patient care committees, limits on non-nursing duties, and distribution of workload. Nurses' unions
and associations also have negotiated the process and timing of hospital restructuring, have sometimes refused to delegate nursing work to inadequately trained
aides, and have protested nurse layoffs through public demonstrations and legislative testimony.[1,8,17,50,75]

Hazards

CHEMICAL, PHYSICAL, AND SAFETY HAZARDS

Many contracts contain provisions to control chemical, physical, and safety hazards. For example, the contract of the Pacific Coast Marine Firemen and the PAC
Maritime Association states that "employers agree not to use carbon tetrachloride or
other toxic compounds or chemicals that are considered harmful and hazardous to personal health. Refusal to use harmful compounds will not be deemed refusal of duty."[27]

The United Auto Workers (UAW) Local 2244 and the New United Motor
Manufacturing, Inc. agreed that "the company will continue to administer a Noise
Control and Hearing Conservation Program. . . . A noise abatement plan will be developed on an annual basis and reviewed with the local Union . . . The company will
make its best efforts to achieve an 80 dB standard. . . ."[27]

AFT Local 1521 and the Los Angeles Community College District agreed that
"during hours of darkness, or when an employee's workstation is in a remote area,
Clerical/Technical unit employees may request that campus police provide a security escort for them."[27]

Oil, Chemical, and Atomic Workers Union (OCAW) Local 8-149 and Berlex
Laboratories agreed that it is company policy "to provide safe and sanitary working
conditions including . . . necessary safeguards on all machinery and equipment in
conformity with all Federal, State and Local Regulations . . ." The International
Longshoremen's and Warehouse Union and the Pacific Maritime Association agreed
that "longshoremen shall not be required to work when in good faith they believe
that to do so is to immediately endanger health and safety."[27]

SHIFTWORK

European unions have negotiated various provisions for reducing the stress of
shiftwork, including fewer work hours and early retirement.[15] The civil air traffic
agency in Italy and union representatives drew up several agreements between 1982
and 1991 to improve working conditions.[12] Modifications include:

• Modernizing radio systems and automating aeronautical information, flight
data processing, and air traffic management. These advances make information more
reliable, allow more time for making decisions, eliminate many risky traffic peaks,
and provide a more balanced workload.

• Reducing work hours. The operative work week is now 28–30 hours.

• Changing shift schedules: rapid shift rotation (one day on each shift); one
night shift followed by 2 days rest; length of shift adjusted to workload (5–6 hours
for morning, 7 hours for afternoon, 11–12 hours for night); provision for short naps
on the night shift; keeping a regular shift rotation for personal, family, and social
life; having a long break (45–60 min.) for a meal during work shifts.

• Reducing environmental stressors, such as decreasing noise and increasing
light.

• Improving physical fitness by providing gyms in the largest facilities.

PSYCHOSOCIAL STRESSORS

Effects on Work and Family. The OCAW Local 8-149 Work and Family Program established committees whose members negotiated with management to improve employer policies that have a stressful effect on union members' personal lives and family responsibilities, e.g., mandatory overtime, no advance notice of overtime, access to a telephone during worktime, and lack of parental leave.[35] The Communications Workers of America (CWA) negotiated a policy in their contract with Bell Atlantic that allows workers to return to work on a reduced schedule for up to 12 months after the birth or the adoption of a child. When on reduced schedule, the employee returns to the same status and benefits as before the leave.[24] Paid maternity leave is guaranteed in many European countries.

New Technology and Performance Monitoring. Some contracts have language that require bargaining over the introduction of new technology.[57,61] Job redesign can also be a joint labor-management process. For example, CWA members at an Arizona facility, together with AT&T management, "eliminated individual measurement and remote secret observation." Average work time was measured only for the whole group. "Service observation was performed by small groups of peers by the old-fashioned 'jack-in' method, where the observer sits beside the person being monitored, listens to a few calls and then discusses the results with the employee." As a result, there were fewer customer complaints, and both the grievance rate and absenteeism were lower.[43] A 1989 contract provision between the CWA and U.S. West, which is still in effect, bans individual electronic performance monitoring.

Stress and Speed-Up. The standard office building agreement of the Southern CA Service Employees International Union stipulates "There shall be no speed-up or increase in the work load so as to impose an undue burden upon any employee . . . . or where the effect of such speed up or increase in the work load is to diminish the work force or lessen the total number of hours worked at any location."[57]

Acutely Stressful Traumatic Events. An agreement between AFSCME Local 3999 and the City of Santa Fe calls for "appropriate and adequate Critical Incident Stress Debriefing."[27]

New Systems of Work Organization, including Lean Production. Unions also have negotiated terms for new systems of work organization, which have been introduced by employers throughout the industrialized world to improve productivity, product quality, and profitability. Such new systems have taken a variety of forms and names, including lean production, total quality management, team concept, cellular or modular manufacturing, re-engineering, and patient-focused care. Responses to stressful lean production systems have included strikes, OSHA inspections, surveys to document conditions, and collective bargaining. Such efforts have modified lean production, to some extent, by moderating work demands (via more staff; control over line speed and job standards), increasing job control (e.g., by allowing election of team leaders, transfer between jobs, formation of joint committees), creating ergonomics programs, and expanding access to training.[30]

For example, a 1994 strike by General Motors (GM) workers in Flint, Michigan occurred, according to the UAW, due to increased workload caused by lean production methods, increased overtime, and decreased break time and vacation time—particularly difficult for a work force averaging 47 years of age. They argued that the result was increased stress, sick leave, and repetitive motion injuries. The settlement included: 779 new hires; many workload grievances settled; union approval over workshops on new manufacturing techniques; a rehabilitation center for injured workers; and an ergonomics agreement.[26,69]

Worker Participation Programs

In some cases, joint labor-management negotiation and implementation of team programs[20] appear to have resulted in improved working conditions. Such programs, sometimes called **High-Performance Work Organizations**, have been established to both increase business competitiveness and "sustain good jobs" within the protection of a union contract.[70] For example, the International Association of Machinists and Maine Iron Works approved a contract giving workers a voice in running the company. This contract bases pay raises on workers learning new skills and contains a no-layoff clause, but also eliminates many work rules.[6]

The GM-UAW creation of the Saturn Auto Company was based on a concept of extensive worker participation and increased worker decision latitude. Workers can decide how to divide up work and rotate tasks within their team, hire new team members, and schedule vacations and other time off.[5] Recently, however, there has been conflict over the scope of teams' latitude and over shiftwork,[25] and in 1999 a new local union leadership was elected pledging to end rotating shifts.[64]

Some agreements (e.g., the United Food and Commercial Workers and Iowa Beef Processors) provide for trained **ergonomic monitors**, employees who conduct workplace surveys and inspections and recommend solutions.[27] Expanding the role of such monitors to include psychosocial work stressors may be a useful component of a workplace surveillance program to detect and reduce CVD risk factors.

The collective bargaining approach is one of the primary strategies used by working people to improve their work environment. It has the advantage of mandating work reforms through a legal document, not easily subject to change due to one manager's whim or management turnover. According to a report from the U.S. Departments of Labor and Commerce, employee participation efforts "in unionized settings in which the union is involved as a joint partner with management are particularly likely to survive."[71] "Over 80% of American workers want a say in decisions affecting their jobs and how their work is performed . . . Outside of union settings, employees have little independent means for initiating these efforts."[71] The ability of employees to apply this strategy is dependent on the proportion of the workforce that belongs to unions (currently only about 15% in the U.S.), the strength of the labor movement in a particular country, and the willingness of unions and management to negotiate over work organization. Collectively bargained efforts also need to be much more extensively evaluated for impact on CVD risk.

REFERENCES

1. American Nurses Association: The Report of Survey Results: The 1994 ANA Layoffs Survey. Washington DC, ANA, 1995.
2. Arndt R: Coping with job stress: The role of the union safety and health committee. Labor Studies J 6:53–61, 1981.
3. Bernard B: Musculoskeletal Disorders and Workplace Factors. Pub. No. 97-141. Washington DC, U.S. Department of Health and Human Services, National Institute for Occpational Safety and Health, 1997.
4. Bernard B, Sauter S, Fine L, et al: Job task and psychosocial risk factors for work-related musculoskeletal disorders among newspaper employees. Scand J Work Environ Health 20:417–426, 1994.
5. Bluestone B, Bluestone I: Workers (and managers) of the world unite. Technology Review 30–40, 1992.
6. BNA Current Developments. August 23, 1994, p A3.
7. Bongers PM, de Winter CR, Kompier MAJ, Hildebrandt VH: Psychosocial factors at work and musculoskeletal disease. Scand J Environ Health 19:297–312, 1993.
8. Brannon RL: Restructuring hospital nursing: Reversing the trend toward a professional workplace. Int J Health Serv 26:643–654, 1996.
9. Brulin G, Nilsson T: Arbetsutveckling och forbattrad produktivitet (Work development and improved productivity). Stockholm, School of Business Research, 1995.

10. Burton J: Workers' Compensation Monitor 10 (July-August), 1997.
11. California Code of Regulations: Title 8, Section 5110. Repetitive Motion Injuries. 1997.
12. Costa G: A seven-point programme to reduce stress in air traffic controllers in Italy. Conditions of Work Digest: Preventing Stress at Work, Vol. 11. Geneva, International Labor Office, 1992, pp 172–183.
13. EHN: Social Factors, Work, Stress, and Cardiovascular Disease Prevention in the European Union. Brussels, European Heart Network, 1998.
14. EU: Report on Work-Related Stress. The Advisory Committee for Safety, Hygiene, and Health Protection at Work. Luxembourg, European Commission, 1997.
15. European Foundation for the Improvement of Living and Working Conditions. Compensation for shiftwork. Bulletin of European Shiftwork Topics. No. 4. 1991.
16. Gersuny C: Work hazards and industrial conflict. Hanover, New Hampshire, University of New England, 1981.
17. Grenier A: Cost and quality matters: Workplace innovations in the health care industry. Washington DC, Economic Policy Institute, 1995.
18. Gruelle M: California nurses win battle at Kaiser over health care. Labor Notes, May 1998.
19. Johnson JV, Hall EM: Job strain, workplace social support, and cardiovascular disease: A cross-sectional study of a random sample of the Swedish working population. Am J Public Health 78:1336–1342, 1988.
20. Kaminski M: Wayne integrated stamping and assembly plant, Ford Motor Co./UAW local 900. In Kaminski M, Bertell D, Moye M, Yudken J (eds): Making Change Happen: Six Cases of Unions and Companies Transforming Their Workplaces. Washington DC, Work and Technology Institute, 1996, pp 25–44.
21. Karasek R, Theorell T: Healthy Work: Stress, Productivity, and the Reconstruction of Working Life. New York, Basic Books, 1990.
22. Kogi K: International regulations on the organization of shift work. Scand J Work Environ Health 24 Suppl 3:7–12, 1998.
23. Kourinka I, Forcier L: Work-Related Musculoskeletal Disorders: A Reference Book for Prevention. London, Taylor & Francis, 1995.
24. Labor News for Working Families. Vol. 6, issue 4, Fall 1998.
25. Labor Notes. January 3, 1995.
26. Labor Notes. November 1994.
27. Labor Occupational Health Program: Collective Bargaining for Health and Safety: A Guidebook for Unions. Berkeley, LOHP, University of California, 1999.
28. Landsbergis PA: Occupational stress among nurses: New developments in theory and prevention. In Humphrey (ed): Human Stress: Current Selected Research, Vol. 3. New York, AMC Press, 1989, pp 173–195.
29. Landsbergis PA, Cahill J: Labor union programs to reduce or prevent occupational stress in the United States. Int J Health Serv 24:105–129, 1994.
30. Landsbergis PA, Cahill J, Schnall P: The impact of lean production and related new systems of work organization on worker health. J Occup Health Psychol 4:108–130, 1999.
31. Leino PI, Hanninen V: Psychosocial factors at work in relation to back and limb disorders. Scand J Work Environ Health 21:134–142, 1995.
32. Levi L: Stress management and prevention on a European Community level: Options and Obstacles. In Kenny D (ed): Stress and Health—Research and Clinical Applications. North Ryde, Australia, Fine Arts Press, 1999, pp 279–294.
33. Loghman-Adham M: Renal effects of environmental and occupational lead exposure. Environ Health Perspect 105:928–939, 1997.
34. Lowry LK: The biological index: Its use in assessing chemical exposures in the workplace. Toxicology 47:55–69, 1987.
35. May L: Work and family committees. Conditions of Work Digest: Preventing Stress at Work, Vol. 11. Geneva, International Labor Office, 1992, pp 164–171.
36. Millon T: Disorders of Personality. New York City, Wiley Press, 1981.
37. Moon SD, Sauter SL: Beyond Biomechanics: Psychosocial Aspects of Musculoskeletal Disorders in Office Work. London, Taylor & Francis, 1996.
38. National Safety Council: ASC Z-365 Draft Ergonomic Standard, Section 6, 1998.
39. National Safety Council: ASC Z-365 Draft Ergonomic Standard, Sections 1–4, 1997.
40. NIOSH: NIOSH Pocket Guide to Clinical Hazards. Pub. No. 94–116. Cincinnati, OH, U.S. Department of Health and Human Services, National Institute for Occupational Safety and Health, 1994.
41. North Carolina Department of Labor: Draft Section. 0600. Ergonomic Standard, http:www.dol.state.nc.us/news/ergostd.htm, 1999.
42. NYC unions win safety pact. VDT News 7:5, 1990.
43. Office of Technology Assessment: The Electronic Supervisor: New Technology, New Tensions. OTA-CIT-333. Washington DC, U.S. Government Printing Office, 1987.
44. Omae K, Takebayashi T, Nomiyama T, et al: Cross-sectional observation of the effects of carbon disulphide on arteriosclerosis in rayon manufacturing workers. Occup Environ Med 55, 1998.
45. OSHA: Draft Ergonomics Program Standard. Occupational Safety and Health Reporter, Vol. 28. Washington DC, Bureau of National Affairs, 1999.
46. OSHA: Draft Proposed Ergonomic Protection Standard. Special Supplement of the Occupational Safety and Health Reporter, Vol. 24. Washington DC, Bureau of National Affairs, 1995.
47. Paoli P: Second European Survey on Working Conditions 1996. Dublin, European Foundation for the Improvement of Living and Working Conditions, 1997.
48. Paoli P: First European Survey on the Working Environment 1991–1992. Dublin, European Foundation for the Improvement of Living and Working Conditions, 1992.
49. Ponack AM: Unionized professionals and the scope of bargaining: A study of nurses. Ind Labor Rel Rev 34:396–407, 1981.

50. Richardson T: Reengineering the hospital: Patient-focused care. In Parker M, Slaughter J (eds): Working Smart. Detroit, Labor Education and Research Project, 1994, pp 113–120.
51. Rosa R, Colligan M: Plain Language about Shift Work. Cincinnati, DHSS/NIOSH Pub. No. 97-145, 1997.
52. Russo R, Attorney at law, Former president of the California Applicant Attorney's Association. Personal Communication, 1999.
53. Saksvik PO, Nytro K: Implementation of internal control of health, environment, and safety in Norwegian enterprises. Safety Science 23:53–61, 1996.
54. Sauter SL, Hurrell JJ Jr, Murphy LR, Levi L: Psychosocial and Organizational Factors. Introduction, Chapter 34.2. Encyclopaedia of Occupational Health and Safety. Geneva, International Labour Office, 1998.
55. Schnall PL, Landsbergis PA, Baker D: Job strain and cardiovascular disease. Annu Rev Public Health 15:381–411, 1994.
56. Selye H: The general adaptation syndrome and the diseases of adaptation. J Clin Endocrinol 6:117, 1946.
57. Service Employees International Union: Stress: Contract Provisions. Washington DC, SEIU, 1983.
58. Service Employees International Union: Nurse Staffing Kit. Washington DC, SEIU, 1998.
59. Shimomitsu T: Occupational health and stress in Japan. Asian-Pacific Newsletter on Occupational Health and Safety 6:16–19, 1999.
60. Shimomitsu T, Levi L: Recent working life changes in Japan. Eur J Public Health 2:76–86, 1992.
61. Shostak AB: Union efforts to relieve blue-collar stress. In Cooper CL, Smith MJ (eds): Job Stress and Blue-Collar Work. New York, Wiley, 1985, pp 195–205.
62. Siegrist J: Adverse health effects of high-effort/low-reward conditions. J Occup Health Psychol 1:27–41, 1996.
63. Sinclair U: The Jungle. Bantam Classics, 1981.
64. Slaughter J: 'Partnership' takes a hit at Saturn. Labor Notes, April 1999.
65. State of California Department of Industrial Relations: Physician's Guide to Medical Practice in the California Workers' Compensation System, 2nd ed. Sacramento, California DIR, 1997.
66. State of Washington Department of Labor: Fitting the Job to the Worker: An ergonomics program guideline. http://www.ergoweb.com/Pub/Info/Std/fjw.html, 1995.
67. Tarpinian G, Tuminaro D, Shufro J: The politics of workers' compensation in New York State. New Solutions, Summer:35–45, 1997.
68. The Tokyo Declaration. J Tokyo Med Univ 56:760–767, 1998.
69. Time: October 24, 1994.
70. Turner BJ: Getting to high performance workplaces. In Kaminski M, Bertell D, Moye M, Yudken J (eds): Making Change Happen: Six Cases of Unions and Companies Transforming Their Workplaces. Washington DC, Work and Technology Institute, 1996, pp 1–2.
71. U.S. Departments of Labor and Commerce: Fact Finding Report. Commission on the Future of Worker-Management Relations. Washington DC, U.S. Departments of Labor and Commerce, 1994.
72. Warren N: The Organizational and Psychosocial Bases of Cumulative Trauma and Stress Disorders. UMI Number 9726279. Lowell, University of Massachusetts, 1997.
73. Warren ND, Dillon CD, Morse T, et al: Biomechanical, psychosocial, and organizational risk factors for WRMSD: Population-based estimates from the Connecticut Upper-Extremity Surveillance Project. (Revised and resubmitted to J Occup Health Psych, 2/99), 1999.
74. WHO: Health Promotion in the Workplace. Strategy Options. European Occupational Health Series No. 10. Copenhagen, World Health Organization Regional Office for Europe, 1995.
75. Wunderlich GS, Sloan FA, Davis CK: Nursing staff in hospitals and nursing homes: Is it adequate? Washington DC, National Academy Press, 1996.
76. Yale University & Local 34–Federation of University Employees: Agreement. New Haven, CT, 1988.

WORKPLACE INTERVENTION STUDIES
by Tage S. Kristensen, DrMedSci

WHY INTERVENTION RESEARCH?

Intervention research and programs are particularly relevant and important in the field of CVD prevention for two reasons: First, we know more risk factors for CVD than for any other major disease.[18,24,25,27,29] Second, CVD is the major cause of death in many countries and will continue to be so in the foreseeable future.[30]

In most textbooks on empirical methods, research designs are ordered in a hierarchy with case reports at the bottom and randomized trials at the top (Table 1). It generally is assumed that the most conclusive evidence regarding causality is gathered from randomized trials, while case studies can be used only for generating hypotheses. This hierarchy can be useful, but the randomized trial is not the only road to causal evidence. Rather, we should regard the randomized trial as a basic paradigm or model to keep in mind when we discuss and evaluate empirical research. Conclusions on causal evidence should be based on the total body of empirical evidence with relevance for a causal hypothesis, be it experimental or observational.[4,40]

The intervention study is a strong design. The three main reasons for doing intervention research are: (1) strong causal evidence, (2) demonstration of feasibility, and (3) the power of the practical example. In those cases where an intervention study is possible, the evidence usually is considered as strong support—or falsification—of a causal hypothesis. However, bear in mind that causal evidence is of little practical importance if the intervention is not feasible. While etiologic studies try to answer the question: "Does the pill have (the desired) effect?", feasibility studies try to answer the equally important question: "Does the patient take (the intended) pill?"[42] It does not help that the patient takes the pill, if it has no effect, and it is equally superfluous that the pill has a beneficial effect, if the patient does not take it. Therefore, both etiologic research and feasibility studies are of paramount importance. Feasibility studies are particularly important in the occupational setting, because of the large number of barriers against implementation of research findings in this environment.

The power of the practical example is its demonstration that a given intervention is possible and has the intended effect. Usually the power of the practical example is strongest when the example comes not only from the same country but also from the same type of industry. English union representatives and management from the car industry are easier to convince if a given intervention has proved to be effective in another English car factory than if the example is taken from a kindergarten in San Francisco!

TABLE 1.   The Hierarchy of Research Designs

Intervention studies:	Randomized trials
	Quasi experiments
	Natural experiments
Observational studies:	Longitudinal studies
	Case-control studies
	Prospective studies
	Cross-sectional studies
	Case-only studies
	Case reports

TYPES OF INTERVENTION STUDIES

There are five main types of intervention studies: laboratory experiments, clinical trials, field trials, community trials, and natural experiments. Sometimes, the term "quasi experiment" is used to describe intervention studies without a comparison group. Work environment intervention studies usually are classified as field trials (the participants are healthy individuals), community trials (the unit of intervention is not the individual but the worksite), or natural experiments (in those cases when the interventions are not planned by the researcher or are part of a systematic evaluation program).

Dramatic changes often occur in the working environment without any evaluation of short- or long-term effects on the health of the employees. Such changes may involve new chemical or physical substances, new shiftwork systems, new ways of organizing work, or new methods in biological engineering. As a rule, changes at the workplaces are introduced to reduce production costs and/or to increase productivity, not to improve the health of the employees. In many countries, however, increasing attention is being paid to the possible long-term consequences for employee health and psychological well-being, and the dual goal of increased productivity and improved workers' health is being pursued.

The role of the employees in workplace interventions varies dramatically. At one end of this spectrum, changes or interventions are introduced by management without any participation of the employees or their representatives. In some cases the workers are not even aware of the changes or of the possible health consequences. At the other end are the participatory intervention projects (also called Participatory Action Research), in which the workers and/or their representatives take active part in all phases.[14] To some degree, the nature of the collaboration between researchers, workers, and management reflects national norms and traditions. In Scandinavia, for example, where more than 90% of all employees are unionized, the workers almost always are involved in worksite intervention projects. A strong participatory element is especially important when the organizational intervention study focuses on work organization, communication, or interpersonal relations.[22]

INTERVENTION RESEARCH IN CARDIOVASCULAR WORKPLACE EPIDEMIOLOGY

Some of the following examples are natural experiments, which may not normally be considered as interventions, but they are included to illustrate the great potential of this type of research.

Interventions Concerning Physical and Chemical Factors

THE FINNISH STUDY OF VISCOSE RAYON WORKERS
EXPOSED TO CARBON DISULFIDE

This study is perhaps the most famous and also the best executed CV occupational intervention study: 343 exposed workers were compared with 343 control persons working at a paper mill in the same town. After 5 years of followup a relative risk of 5.6 for IHD was observed among the exposed. This alarming result was discussed with management and the workers, and a number of measures were taken to reduce the risk. Workers with long exposure and/or symptoms of IHD were transferred to other departments without exposure; the concentration of carbon disulfide in the air was monitored closely; and personal protective equipment was used during peak exposures. During the 3 years after this vigorous intervention, the same number of IHD deaths were observed in the exposed and comparison groups. After 15 years of followup the Finnish research team concluded that the high excess risk among the carbon disulfide–exposed workers had been eliminated (Fig. 1).[11–13,33,34]

As a result of this research, the whole world was convinced about the role of carbon disulfide in IHD. The study had a clear design and produced strong results. It shows what it takes to perform a convincing study: a relatively small exposed group, a well-chosen comparison group of the same size, a vigorous reduction of the exposure, and a lot of patience. Psychosocial intervention studies could in principle reach the same level of clarity and conclusiveness. This implies that the methods and designs used in psychosocial studies have high quality and validity.

Interventions Related to Work Schedules

A large number of epidemiological studies have demonstrated that the incidence of IHD is increased among shift workers and other employees working at odd hours.[2,24] The mechanisms that explain the increased risk are not fully understood,

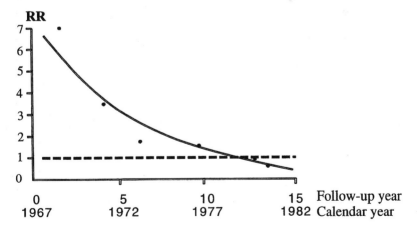

FIGURE 1. Relative risk of ischemic heart disease among Finnish workers exposed to carbon disulfide, compared with controls. (From Nurminen M, Hernberg S: Effects of intervention on the cardiovascular mortality of workers exposed to carbon disulfide: A 15-year followup. Brit J Ind Med 42:32–35, 1985; with permission.)

but disturbances in the physiological circadian rhythm of the organism seem to play an important role.

ORTH-GOMÉR'S STUDY OF POLICEMEN

Orth-Gomér studied the possible detrimental effects of shift work by performing a cross-over intervention study. A group of 46 Stockholm policemen were divided into two groups of 23. One group started to work according to a "clockwise" rotation schedule, while the other group worked according to the usual "counterclockwise" rotation schedule. Under the clockwise system, the policemen started a bit later every day, which is more in accordance with biologic rhythmicity since the spontaneous circadian period has been shown to be approximately 25 hours. After 4 weeks of work and some days of rest, the two groups switched schedules for another 4-week period. Questionnaire data and measures of a number of physiologic factors were collected before, during, and after each schedule.

Triglycerides, systolic blood pressure, serum glucose, and serum uric acid levels were lower during clockwise rotation. No differences were found in cholesterol and diastolic blood pressure (BP). Self-rated health, length of sleep, and quality of sleep also were better during clockwise rotation. Orth-Gomér concluded that the clockwise system reduced CV risk and also improved the quality of life of the policemen.[35,36]

This study has a number of strong features. It employed questionnaire data as well as physiologic measures, and it used a design in which the participants were their own controls. In this way a number of relatively clear results were achieved in spite of the small group of participants. Interestingly, the policemen chose the old system (the counter-clockwise) instead of the new system, when the study was finished. This was due to the simple fact that a counter-clockwise system gives longer coherent periods of time off than the clockwise system where the free time "disappears" during the regular working days. Thus, the policemen chose to have more time with their families and sacrificed their health and personal well-being. Some months later, however, the policemen changed their minds. After a new ballot they decided to adopt the more healthy system: the clockwise schedule.

THE JAPANESE STUDY ON OVERTIME WORK BY HAYASHI, ET AL.

It is well known that Japanese workers sometimes are exposed to excessive levels of overtime work. Compared with other countries, the Japanese experience could be perceived as a natural experiment in itself. The Japanese expression *karoshi*, or death from overwork, has received considerable attention in the scientific as well as the popular literature. Hayashi, et al. studied the effects of overwork on a number of health-related endpoints, including BP and heart rate.[10] In one part of this study, workers with more than 60 hours of overwork per month were compared with "unexposed" workers with less than 30 hours of overwork. Among workers without hypertension, systolic and diastolic BP and heart rate were higher in the group with a high level of overwork. In another part of the study, the workers were used as their own controls. They were followed during a busy period with almost 100 hours of overwork per month and in a control period with approximately 40 hours of overwork per month. Workers had higher diastolic BP and heart rate during the period with excessive overwork. The workers also experienced fewer hours of sleep and more fatigue symptoms during this period.

THE STUDY OF TAX ACCOUNTANTS BY FRIEDMAN, ET AL.

In this classic study on serum cholesterol and blood clotting time, accountants were followed over time and served as their own controls.[7] During the high-stress periods, before the delivery of the tax returns, the accountants worked as much as 70 hours per week, as opposed to as little as 30 hours during the quiet periods. The high-stress periods were characterized not only by long working hours, but also by a sense of urgency and conflicting demands from the clients. The average serum cholesterol level of the accountants was significantly higher during these periods, and the blood coagulation time was significantly shorter—both factors that indicate a higher risk of CVD.

These three examples demonstrate that the field of work schedules and working hours is particularly well suited for studies with a clear experimental design. In some cases the researcher may be able to influence the design of the intervention, while in other cases a natural experiment may be the only possibility. Competition due to the "global economy" makes it very likely that nonstandard working hours and very long work periods will be widespread phenomena in the future, which means that this type of research should be given high priority.

Interventions on Psychosocial Job Characteristics

A DANISH PSYCHOSOCIAL INTERVENTION STUDY

In 1996, a large psychosocial intervention study was initiated in Copenhagen by the National Institute of Occupational Health (Intervention Project on Absence and Wellbeing; IPAW).[28] Worksites and departments from three different sectors participate: Nursing homes, technical services of the Copenhagen City, and a large pharmaceutical company. Of the worksites, 22 are high-absence intervention (N = 1181), 14 are high-absence control (N = 535), and 15 are low-absence control (N = 351). The goal of the study is to increase influence, predictability, meaning of work, and social support at work (the intermediate end-points) by changing the organization of work at each of the intervention sites. With regard to job demands, the goal is to establish a situation with optimal demands (not too high, not too low). After the baseline questionnaire study, the intervention work sites started a process of change together with professional consultants (not the research team). The most important end-points are absence from work, labor turnover, mental health, and general health of the workers. The worksites will be followed for 5 years, and the employees will fill out questionnaires three times. Furthermore, the participants will be followed in national hospital and death registries with regard to CVD.

This study was intended to have many of the features of the controlled trial. It is difficult, however, to follow strict research plans when working with "real worksites" over a long period of time. The work sites are not run by researchers, and management does not give high priority to agreements with researchers if these agreements are in conflict with current management plans. At the present stage, we have learned two major lessons. First, it is difficult to choose intervention and comparison workplaces in anything close to a "random" fashion in an organizational intervention study. Such a study requires enthusiasm and willingness to change deeply rooted ways of running the workplace, and it is impossible to allocate workplaces to enthusiasm versus no enthusiasm in a randomized way. Second, we have found it difficult to assess the actual interventions at the intervention workplaces. This is the "black box" problem of psychosocial intervention. We know what we intended the intervention to be like, but we have great difficulties in reproducing the actual course of events in the participating worksites.

A SWEDISH INTERVENTION STUDY

It is well known that urban bus drivers comprise a high-risk group, with high rates of CVD, low back pain, lung cancer, gastrointestinal disorders, and other health problems.[21,45] In Stockholm, Johansson, Evans, and Rydstedt carried out a well-designed intervention study to investigate possible effects of improving working conditions for bus drivers.[6,17,41] The intervention centered on physical design changes in the bus routes and a number of technological improvements to decrease traffic congestion, lessen passenger demands, and ease bus operation in general. Bus drivers working on the intervention route were compared with matched drivers on similar control routes. The study showed decreased CV activation at work, fewer on-the-job hassles while driving, and less perceived stress at work among the interventional drivers. In the intervention group, the systolic BP decreased 10.7 mmHg, diastolic BP decreased 3.5 mmHg, heart rate was reduced 3.7 beats per minute (bpm), and the index for perceived stress went down 0.4 points. In the control group the corresponding reductions were 4.3 mmHg, 1.2 mmHg, 0.5 beats, and 0.1 points. The differences were statistically significant, except for diastolic BP. Further analyses showed that the reduction in job hassles could explain the positive effect in the intervention group. Among these were illegally parked cars blocking the buses, risky driving behaviors of drivers of other vehicles, risky behavior of pedestrians/cyclists, delays because of passenger obstruction on bus, and delays because of passenger information inquiries. The study used questionnaires, observational methods, and physiological measures, and is a convincing demonstration of the positive health effects of a systematic improvement in working conditions. The study confirms the hypothesis that minor hassles are an important source of stress in the daily lives of people. The basic assumption is that minor hassles have adverse effects on health and psychological well being because they are uncontrollable, frequent, and rather impervious to individual coping efforts.

Netterstrøm's Observational Study of Copenhagen Bus Drivers

In a prospective study of IHD among bus drivers, Netterstrøm and Juel analyzed the mortality and incidence of IHD among drivers who worked at routes with different traffic intensity.[31] The routes were classified by an experienced driver, who did not know the purpose of the study. After control for relevant factors, the relative risk (RR) for IHD was 2.7 among the drivers on high-intensity routes compared with the drivers on low-intensity routes. When only the time as bus driver was analyzed, the RR was 6.2. Similar results were found for bus drivers in two large provincial towns. Other researchers have found the same pattern in London and Stockholm bus drivers.[1,39]

This study can be regarded as a natural experiment. The drivers were, in fact, randomized to high or low traffic intensity routes, since they could not apply for work on specific routes. New drivers were allocated to the routes when this was necessary to run the bus lines, and moves from one line to another were not common. Thus, the Copenhagen bus lines at that time were almost operating as a large double-blind randomized trial. Today the situation has changed considerably because of the great interest in stress and disease among bus drivers. Both management and drivers are aware of stress issues, which means that a similar study performed today would have to deal with substantial problems due to information and selection bias.

A Norwegian Study of Rumors about Factory Closure

Erikssen and colleagues monitored the BP and pulse of 225 male workers at a ferro-alloy plant.[5] The hypothesis was that there would be an association between heat exposure and BP. This hypothesis was not confirmed, but the researchers noticed a remarkable pattern when they analyzed the trend of BP and pulse over time.

During 1982–84 these measures were at a constant level, but then a rather dramatic rise took place: the average systolic BP increased 15 mmHg, the diastolic about half as much, and the pulse increased 7 bpm. This pattern could not be explained by differences in measurement methods, changes in exposure, or changes in the composition of the work force. On the contrary, the analyses showed that the pattern was the same for all age groups and for heat-exposed as well as nonexposed workers.

The authors could find only one plausible explanation. From 1985 to 1987 the factory experienced serious financial difficulties, and there were many rumors about factory closure. Some of the workers were asked to retire at an early age, and a number of meetings were held to inform the workers about the serious problems of the company. Alternative employment opportunities in the small town were scarce. In short, the workers were experiencing a period of low control and low predictability. The authors concluded that the rise in BP and pulse was caused by this prolonged period of stress.[5]

This was a natural experiment and it resembles the study by Iversen, et al. (see below) in a number of ways. Four major differences are that the workers did not experience actual unemployment; the endpoint was not IHD, but pulse and BP; the researchers discovered the stressor long after it had ceased to exist; and there was no control group. In this case the lack of control group is not a major problem, because we know the normal level and trend of BP and pulse in a population. It is unlikely that the average systolic BP increases by 15 mmHg in a group of 200 workers without any reason.

A STUDY OF BELGIAN BANK EMPLOYEES

About 500 employees from a private bank and 800 from a semi-public savings bank were followed for 10 years with regard to morbidity and mortality.[23] After 5 years and 10 years, an almost doubled risk of IHD was observed among the private bank employees, compared with the employees in the savings bank. This finding could not be explained by differences in well-known risk factors such as serum cholesterol, tobacco, or high BP. The researchers had noticed a striking difference between the two groups when they attended the medical examination: "Cohort I (private bank) subjects were in a hurry and were worried, as their daily program was tight, whereas subjects of cohort II (public savings bank) seemed more relaxed."[20] The authors tested the job stress hypothesis through a retrospective questionnaire about job conditions in the two cohorts. The results confirmed that the employees of the private bank experienced a higher level of job stressors than did the savings bank employees. The difference was significant among clerks as well as executives.[20,23]

Again, this might be called a natural experiment. As with the Norwegian study of BP, the researchers were not aware of the "exposure" until they had found a remarkable pattern in the results. Thus, the explanation was ex post facto, which is always unsatisfactory from a scientific point of view. On the other hand, such studies are excellent for generating hypotheses, and they show that alert researchers are just as important as alert clinicians for generating new and interesting hypotheses. In this case the "control group" was a perfect choice. The two groups had the same type of job, the same age, the same social class, and worked only 500 meters apart.

IVERSEN'S STUDY OF A SHIPYARD CLOSURE

Iversen and colleagues studied the effects of becoming unemployed by following two groups of Danish shipyard workers: one group (N = 887) worked at a shipyard that closed in 1983, and the comparison group (N = 441) worked at a similar shipyard without (threats of) closure. The incidence of hospital admissions due to CVD among the workers from the closed shipyard was compared with the control group during three distinct periods. Before the closure (1979–80) the RR was 0.80, during closure (1981–83) it was 1.04, and after closure the RR was 1.60. This means that the RR doubled during the study period. For IHD alone the RR was 2.6 during the period after closure. Hospital admissions due to other diseases did not increase among the unemployed. In fact, the opposite trend was observed for accidents and diseases of the digestive system.[16]

This is a natural experiment. The researchers could re-establish the hospital admissions of the two historical cohorts through the National Register of Patients by using the personal registration numbers of the shipyard workers. This method can only be used in Nordic and a few other countries. Of course, randomization is impossible in cases like this, but Iversen quickly established a comparison group, and both groups were followed after closure using questionnaires and hospitalization data.

These six psychosocial interventions illustrate the significance of the central dimensions of stressors at work. The significance of high demands is illustrated in the studies on bus drivers, in the bank study, and in the Danish IPAW intervention study. Control is an important dimension in all the studies, with the bank study as a possible exception. Predictability plays a significant role in the Norwegian study of rumors, in the Iversen study on unemployment, and in the IPAW study. Furthermore, social support and meaning of work are central dimensions in the IPAW study. Finally, effort-reward imbalance seems to be a stressor in the bus driver studies and in the two studies on (threats of) unemployment. Future intervention studies in the psychosocial field should be theory based to increase scientific validity and generality.

All of the aforementioned intervention studies are extremely different with regard to exposure, endpoints, duration, design, study base, and setting. Nevertheless, these examples demonstrate the broad range of possibilities for research and practice in the field of CV health at the worksite. Any difficulties due to the fact that the worksite is the "arena of research" should be seen as challenges for the researcher. For example, the researcher should be ready when opportunities for studying natural interventions present themselves. In the case of Iversen's study of unemployment, the rumors about a possible factory closure were mentioned in the news, and Iversen contacted the shipyard a few days later, ready to start his project. Situations like that cannot be planned, but research institutions can be ready to act by preparing themselves for the unexpected and by maintaining good relationships with relevant workplaces as well as management and union representatives.

These studies do have one important factor in common: none is based on a representative sample of individuals from a geographical area or country. In CV epidemiology, the sampling of individuals has been a strong tradition since the Framingham studies started in the 1940s. This tradition has resulted in a strong orientation towards individual risk factors in CV epidemiology and prevention. In studying the role of work environmental factors, the use of representative samples has a number of negative consequences: (1) the jobs of the respondents are poorly described, (2) many of the respondents have medium exposure or low exposure, which gives low statistical power, (3) most occupational titles are much too broad, which results in heterogeneous groups, and (4) superficial knowledge about the jobs makes it difficult to suggest improvements of the work environment.[26] In the study of occupational risk factors (observational as well as interventional), it is of paramount importance to use a focused study design and to identify exposed/nonexposed groups rather than "representative" individuals. A closer look at the examples presented here illustrates the point: None of the risk factors, such as carbon disulphide, rumors about factory closure, working in a private bank, or driving a bus in the city, could have been identified in a large representative study.

It could be argued that many of the examples mentioned (such as the studies of Belgian bank employees and Copenhagen bus drivers) are not intervention studies, but ordinary observational studies. This is, of course, correct from a formal point of view, but the intervention paradigm is not only the recipe of a study design; it is a way of looking at and analyzing a study. Society sometimes performs experiments which the researcher would not be allowed to perform. It was by looking at the different sources of water supply in London in the middle of the 19th century that John Snow discovered the association between contaminated water and cholera.[43] The situation was close to an experiment, because some households received clean water from one company while others did not. Snow analyzed this pattern correctly, and his results could be used immediately for prevention.

LEVELS OF INTERVENTION

Within the field of occupational intervention, it is customary to distinguish between three levels of intervention: the individual level, the individual/group interface level, and the organizational level (Table 2). The issue of intervention level has caused discussion and controversy in occupational medicine and disease prevention for many years. When physical and chemical exposures are the focus, the issue is "personal protection" versus "improvements of the work environment." Employers argue that it is unnecessary to spend millions of dollars to reduce the noise level at a workplace when the same effect can be achieved by using cheap and uncomplicated earplugs. Employees argue that earplugs (and other types of personal protective equipment) are not safe and may cause accidents, and that it is the responsibility of the employer to provide a safe workplace.

When psychosocial factors and stress are the focus, the issue is equally controversial. NIOSH uses the following careful wording: "Nearly everyone agrees that job stress results from the interaction of the worker and the conditions of work. Views differ, however, on the importance of worker characteristics versus working conditions as the primary cause of job stress. These differing viewpoints are important

TABLE 2. Examples of Interventions at Three Different Levels in the Workplace

The individual level:
　　Using personal protective equipment (such as mask or earplugs)
　　Practicing meditation or relaxation techniques
　　Eating a healthy meal during lunch
　　Attending a company fitness program after working hours

The individual/group interface level:
　　Respecting the nonsmokers when smoking at the workplace
　　Creating peer groups to help victims of harassment or bullying
　　Using support groups of workers in health promotion programs to keep colleagues from resuming
　　　smoking
　　Teaching the workers to solve conflicts at work through assertion training

The organizational level:
　　Enforcing company policy on passive smoking
　　Changing the organizational structure of the workplace to increase workers' control and skill
　　　discretion
　　Reducing workplace noise levels
　　Changing the shiftwork system from a counter-clockwise to a clockwise schedule

because they suggest different ways to prevent stress at work . . . Although the importance of individual differences cannot be ignored, scientific evidence suggests that certain working conditions are stressful to most people. Such evidence argues for a greater emphasis on working conditions as the key source of job stress, and for job redesign as a primary prevention strategy."[32]

Recent reviews have found that most studies on workplace stress interventions have analyzed the effects of interventions at the *individual* level (Table 3). This situation is deplored by many researchers because they feel that intervention research should focus more on the fundamental causes of stress at work.[8,19,44] Almost all reviews on the topics of stress management, organizational interventions, and stress intervention conclude that there should be much more intervention research at the organizational level. However, few authors analyze the explanations for the present situation. There seems to be an implicit understanding that the researchers should "know better," and the situation could be changed through a common decision to do other types of research. Rather than "blaming the researcher," consider some of the main obstacles related to organizational interventions:

• Organizational interventions are time-consuming and expensive because they involve many employees.

• Organizational interventions are difficult to describe, control, and evaluate.

• Management dislikes the idea of an intervention study because they view the organization of the workplace as their responsibility. They give up some power by participating in a research project.

• Management may think that possible mistakes or unpopular actions taken by company leaders during the intervention will be made public to the employees or to the media.

• The workers (and/or unions) may be opposed to some organizational interventions because they believe they interfere with the collective bargaining system at the workplace.

• Management also may be afraid of losing a monopoly on information.

• Organizational interventions may raise the expectations of the workers and may increase job dissatisfaction if those expectations are not met.

• If the intervention is a failure, it may cause internal as well as external troubles.

Many of these points should be quite obvious to researchers of social phenomena. Doing intervention research requires mutual confidence and respect of all the parties involved. Workplace participants may get the impression that researchers lose interest in the problems as soon as they have collected the data they need for their project. Before starting an organizational intervention project is is a good idea to have a formal agreement in which the obligations and rights of all participants are

TABLE 3. Distribution of Stress Management Studies According to Level
of Intervention and Level of Outcome

Level of Interventions	Level of Outcome Measures		
	Individual	*Individual/Organization Interface*	*Organization*
Individual	20	11	3
Individual/organization interface	2	1	
Organization	2	1	2

Note: one study could include several types of interventions.
From van der Hek H, Plomp HN: Occupational stress management programmes: A practical overview of published effect studies. Occup Med 47:133–141, 1997; with permission.

clarified. (For a further discussion of the questions related to the "individualistic bias" of psychosocial interventions, see references 15, 22, 38, and 44.)

In connection with the prevention of CVD, it would be extremely interesting to see more organizational intervention studies related to shift work, job strain, social support at work, effort-reward imbalance, job stress in general, noise, chemicals, and passive smoking. Furthermore, organizational level changes should be included in workplace health promotion and rehabilitation studies.

Primary, Secondary, and Tertiary Prevention

The question of primary versus secondary or tertiary prevention often is confused with the level of intervention, so that organizational interventions are considered "primary" while the interventions at the individual level are considered "secondary" or "tertiary." This is not necessarily a correct distinction. Most textbooks define primary prevention as interventions with the purpose of preventing the occurrence of disease among healthy individuals; secondary prevention as early diagnosis and treatment; and tertiary prevention as treatment to limit consequences of disease. Individual and organizational level interventions can benefit healthy as well as "ill" persons. Much of the confusion probably originates from a basic confusion related to the concept of disease. Most studies do not distinguish sharply between symptoms, signs, risk factors, illness, and disease. If symptoms such as stress or fatigue and risk factors such as high cholesterol or hypertension are considered "diseases," then it follows that almost all employees have a disease, and, hence, that most prevention is secondary.

Since this book is about CV diseases, I find it most fruitful to limit the definition to these diseases and not consider stress, hypertension, or other risk factors as diseases. Reduction of stress, treatment of hypertension, and smoking cessation are primary prevention activities.

In CV epidemiology it is common to distinguish between mass intervention strategy and high-risk intervention strategy. The high-risk strategy aims at reaching individuals with high risk (e.g., those with high cholesterol level or tobacco smokers), while the mass intervention strategy aims at reducing the risk of everyone a little bit, thereby reducing the whole burden of disease in the population. There is a third strategy in occupational and environmental medicine: the environmental strategy.

The workplace can play an important role in the prevention of CVD and other diseases by combining different prevention strategies. The workplace should be a healthy environment, promote a healthy lifestyle according to the cultural and social norms of the society, and play an active role in the rehabilitation of employees with (previous) CVD. These three strategies are not mutually exclusive; they can supplement and strengthen each other to achieve these goals (Fig. 2). For example, the workplace should have a clear policy on passive smoking so that nobody is exposed (the environmental approach); help smokers in their efforts to quit smoking through an active health promotion plan (the health promotion approach); and contribute to the rehabilitation of workers with CVD (or lung diseases) by providing a job without air pollution (the rehabilitation approach). Stress management and health promotion programs focusing on the individual or on individual risk factors often have been accused of blaming the victim, and with good reason. Under an integrated prevention program, the workers feel that the workplace contributes to their health and well being, and the employer will notice that the employees contribute to their own health, as well.[3]

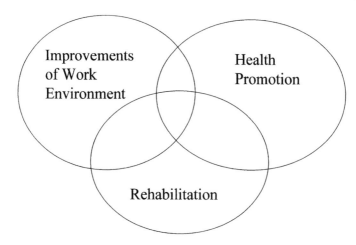

FIGURE 2. A model of integrated prevention of CVDs at the workplace.

CONCLUSIONS

The key word for intervention studies and programs at the workplace is integration: integration between interventions at different levels; between primary, secondary, and tertiary prevention; between mass, high-risk, and environmental approaches; and between different disciplines. Although occupational intervention research can be criticized for methodological and theoretical weaknesses,[9] it is still a fact that the quality has improved appreciably during recent years.[15,22] Intervention research and practical intervention programs give us insight regarding etiology as well as feasibility that cannot be gained in any other way: Which types of interventions result in desired changes with regard to health and well-being, and which types of interventions are possible to implement at the workplaces? Intervention research requires collaboration between researchers and individuals at the worksite, and researchers should realize that the learning process in this teamwork goes both ways. Intervention research tends to be more complicated than observational research, but the benefit with regard to scientific and practical insight is considerable. Therefore, the alert researcher should always look for windows of opportunity to perform intervention research together with workers (and their representatives) and employers.

REFERENCES

1. Ahlbom A, Theorell T: Hjartinfarkt hos trafikpersonal vid Storstockholms lokaltrafik (Myocardial infarction among personnel in the Greater Stockholm traffic system). Lakartidn 77:3472–3473, 1980.
2. Boggild H, Knutsson A: Shift work, risk factors, and cardiovascular disease. Scand J Work Environ Health 25:85–89, 1999.
3. Dejoy DM, Southern DJ: An integrative perspective on worksite health promotion. J Occup Med 35:1221–1230, 1993.
4. Elwood JM: Causal Relationships in Medicine. A Practical System for Critical Appraisal. Oxford, Oxford University Press, 1988.
5. Erikssen J, Knudsen K, Mowinckel P, et al: Blodtrykksstigning hos stresseksponerte industriarbeidere (Increase in blood pressure among stress-exposed industrial workers). Tidsskr Nor Laegeforen 110:2873–2877, 1990.
6. Evans GW, Johansson G, Rydstedt L: Hassles on the job: A study of a job intervention with urban bus drivers. J Org Behav 20:199–208, 1999.
7. Friedman M, Rosenman RH, Carroll V: Changes in the serum cholesterol and blood clotting time in men subjected to cyclic variations of occupational stress. Circulation 17:852–861, 1958.
8. Ganster DC, Schaubroeck J: Work stress and employee health. J Management 17:235–271, 1991.
9. Goldenhar LM, Schulte PA: Methodological issues for intervention research in occupational health and safety. Am J Ind Med 29:289–294, 1996.

10. Hayashi T, Kobayashi Y, Yamaoka K, Yano E: Effect of overtime work on 24-hour ambulatory blood pressure. J Occup Environ Med 38:1007–1011, 1996.
11. Hernberg S, Partanen R, Nordman C-H, Sumari P: Coronary heart disease among workers exposed to carbon disulphide. Br J Ind Med 27:313–325, 1970.
12. Hernberg S, Nurminen M, Tolonen M: Excess mortality from coronary heart disease in viscose rayon workers exposed to carbon disulphide. Work Environ Health 10:93–99, 1973.
13. Hernberg S, Tolonen M, Nurminen M: Eight-year follow-up of viscose rayon workers exposed to carbon disulphide. Scand J Work Environ Health 2:27–30, 1976.
14. Israel BA, Schurman SJ, Hugentobler MK: Conducting action research: Relationships between organization members and researchers. J Appl Behav Science 28:74–101, 1992.
15. Ivancevich JM, Matteson MT, Freeman S, Phillips J: Worksite stress management interventions: Opportunities and challenges for organizational psychologists. Am Psychologist 45:252–261, 1990.
16. Iversen L, Sabroe S, Damsgaard MT: Hospital admissions before and after shipyard closure. Br Med J 299:1073–1076, 1989.
17. Johansson G, Evans GW, Rydstedt LW, Carrere S: Job hassles and cardiovascular reaction patterns among urban bus drivers. Int J Behav Med 5:267–280, 1998.
18. Karasek R, Theorell T: Healthy Work: Stress, Productivity, and the Reconstruction of Working Life. New York, Basic Books, 1990.
19. Kasl SV, Serxner S: Health promotion at the worksite. Int Rev Health Psychol 1:111–142, 1992.
20. Kittel F, Kornitzer M, Dramaix M: Coronary heart disease and job stress in two cohorts of bank clerks. Psychother Psychosom 34:110–123, 1980.
21. Kompier MAJ, di Martino V: Review of bus drivers' occupational stress and stress prevention. Stress Med 11:253–262, 1995.
22. Kompier MAJ, Geurts SAE, Grundemann RWM, et al: Cases in stress prevention: The success of a participative and stepwise approach. Stress Med 14:155–168, 1998.
23. Kornitzer MD, Dramaix M, Gheyssens J: Incidence of ischemic heart disease in two Belgian cohorts followed during 10 yr. Eur J Cardiol 9:455–472, 1979.
24. Kristensen TS: Cardiovascular diseases and the work environment. A critical review of the epidemiologic literature on nonchemical factors. Scand J Work Environ Health 15:165–179, 1989.
25. Kristensen TS: Cardiovascular diseases and the work environment. A critical review of the epidemiologic literature on chemical factors. Scand J Work Environ Health 15:245–265, 1989.
26. Kristensen TS: The demand-control-support model: Methodological challenges for future research. Stress Med 11:17–26, 1995.
27. Kristensen TS, Kronitzer M, Alfedsson L: Social Factors, Work, Stress, and Cardiovascular Disease Prevention. Brussels, The European Heart Network, 1998.
28. Kristensen TS, Nielsen ML, Smith-Hansen L: The Intervention Project on Absence and Well-being (IPAW): Theoretical and methodological background. Scand J Work Environ Health (in preparation), 1999.
29. Marmot M, Elliot P: Coronary Heart Disease Epidemiology: From Aetiology to Public Health. Oxford, Oxford University Press, 1992.
30. Murray JL, Lopez AD: The Global Burden of Disease. Geneva, WHO, 1996.
31. Netterstrom B, Juel K: Impact of work-related and psychosocial factors on the development of ischemic heart disease among urban bus drivers in Denmark. Scand J Work Environ Health 14:231–238, 1988.
32. NIOSH: Stress at work. DHHS (NIOSH) Publication No. 99-101. Cincinnati, OH, NIOSH, 1999.
33. Nurminen M: Studying the occurence of occupational health problems: Illustrative dissections. Helsinki, Department of Public Health Science, 1984.
34. Nurminen M, Hernberg S: Effects of intervention on the cardiovascular mortality of workers exposed to carbon disulfide: A 15-year followup. Brit J Ind Med 42:32–35, 1985.
35. Orth-Gomer K: Intervention on coronary risk factors by adapting a shift work schedule to biologic rhythmicity. Psychosom Med 45:407–415, 1983.
36. Orth-Gomer K, Olivegard-Landen R: Ar det mojligt att lindra de ogynnsamma effekterna av skiftarbete? (Is it possible to reduce the detrimental effects of shift work?) Lakartidn 80:2426–2430, 1983.
37. Orth-Gomer K, Eriksson I, Moser V, et al: Lipid lowering through work stress reduction. Int J Behav Med 1:204–214, 1994.
38. Parkes KR, Sparkes TJ: Organizational Interventions to Reduce Work Stress. Are They Effective? A review of the literature. London, HSE Books, 1998.
39. Rosenman RH, Friedman M: The possible relationship of occupational stress to clinical coronary heart disease. Calif Med 89:169–174, 1958.
40. Rothman KJ: Causal Inference. Chestnut Hill, MA, Epidemiology Resources, 1988.
41. Rydstedt LW, Johansson G, Evans GW: The human side of the road: Improving the working conditions of urban bus drivers. J Occup Health Psychol 3:161–171, 1998.
42. Skov T, Kristensen TS: Etiologic and prevention effectiveness intervention studies in occupational health. Am J Ind Med 29:378–381, 1996.
43. Snow J: On the Mode of Communication of Cholera. London, Churchill, 1855.
44. van der Hek H, Plomp HN: Occupational stress management programmes: A practical overview of published effect studies. Occup Med 47:133–141, 1997.
45. Winkleby MA, Ragland DR, Fisher JM, Syme SL: Excess risk of sickness and disease in bus drivers: A review and synthesis of epidemiological studies. Int J Epidemiol 17:255–262, 1988.

THE WORKPLACE AND CARDIOVASCULAR HEALTH: CONCLUSIONS AND THOUGHTS FOR A FUTURE AGENDA

by Karen Belkić, MD, PhD, Peter Schnall, MD, Paul Landsbergis, PhD, and Dean Baker, MD

We argued in the introduction that to adequately address the CVD epidemic, there is a need for a social epidemiologic approach that focuses on the workplace. Here, we briefly review the empirical, theoretical, and biological evidence presented earlier to demonstrate "convergent" validation that the relationship between workplace stressors and CVD risk is causal. The empirical findings are consistent with and predicted by the theoretical models, and the linkage between them is demonstrated to be plausible via biological mechanisms and experimental research. We then elaborate on new strategies, presented in the latter part of this book, for enhanced prevention and clinical management, workplace interventions, and social policy to reduce the impact of CVD.

EMPIRICAL EVIDENCE OF WORKPLACE EFFECTS ON CVD

In Chapter 2, we presented a substantial body of findings concerning the impact of workplace psychosocial, chemical, and physical conditions on CVD. The most consistent evidence is provided by research on sources of psychosocial stress at work, which are also the most prevalent risk factors. The most highly studied of these is work with high psychological demands coupled with low decision latitude, i.e., job strain. On the basis of empirical reviews focused on men and on women, as well as the recent review by the European Heart Network,[34] and notwithstanding some studies with null results, the conclusion of Schnall, Landsbergis, and Baker that "a body of literature has accumulated that strongly suggests a causal association between job strain and cardiovascular disease" has been corroborated and strengthened. The data relating job strain to AmBP and decision latitude to CVD outcomes are particularly compelling.

Besides consistency of association among studies, other evidence supporting causality has emerged. There are now data, albeit limited, suggesting a dose-response relationship between exposure to job strain or its major dimension(s) and both CVD and BP. New job strain cohort studies further confirm that exposure precedes outcome in time. Overall, of ten such studies in men, six show an increased CVD risk due to job strain or its components, and an additional two provide mixed results. Of five cohort studies among women, four demonstrate an elevated CVD risk related to job strain or its components.

Epidemiologic evidence of the plausibility of the relationship between job strain and CVD has expanded. Cross-sectional, as well as some longitudinal data, linking exposure to job strain with elevated AmBP in men and women suggests one major mediating mechanism for this process. There are now cohort data demonstrating that a change in job strain exposure is associated with a change in BP.[58] Furthermore, some data suggests an association between job strain and/or its major dimensions and other CVD risk factors, primarily smoking intensity in men, and possibly increased coagulation tendencies.

The magnitude of association between job strain and CVD typically range from risk ratios (RR) of about 1.2–2.0 for studies using imputed job characteristics (with resulting nondifferential misclassification bias towards the null), to 1.3–4.0 for studies using self-reported job characteristics. Associations are more consistent and stronger among blue-collar workers, with RR as high as 10. Systolic BP at work (as measured with an ambulatory monitor) among employees facing job strain is typically 4–8 mmHg higher than among those without job strain.

Another model of work stress, the Effort-Reward Imbalance (ERI) Model, also has been studied cross-sectionally and longitudinally, primarily in men. There are significant positive associations between high effort/low reward and elevated lipid levels, hypertension, and CVD, with magnitudes of effect similar to or even greater than in self-report job strain studies. A British study indicates that the effects of job control and ERI are statistically independent of each other in the prediction of CHD,[6] and a currently unpublished Swedish study finds that the combined effects of exposure to job strain and to ERI on CVD are much stronger than the separate effects of each model.[51]

There are also data indicating a relationship between threat-avoidant vigilant work and CVD. For example, in studies comparing occupations, professional driving, particularly urban transportation, emerges as the occupation with the most consistent evidence of elevated risk of CHD and hypertension (see Chapter 2). Such psychosocial factors may help to explain the nine-fold difference between high and low CVD risk occupations in men and a five-fold difference in women.

In addition to psychosocial job stressors, there is some evidence that work schedules and physical and chemical workplace hazards may increase the risk of CVD. Notwithstanding the difficulties involved in researching this area, a substantial body of longitudinal data implicates shift work as an independent CVD risk factor; however, there are also some well-designed cohort studies with null findings. Investigations of long work hours are more sparse, but quite consistently show a relationship to elevations in ambulatory and casual BP, and to CVD. In three fairly recent papers, the effect of long work hours independently of other workplace stressors was demonstrated with respect to increased BP and risk of MI. Finally, some support exists for a significant association between physical factors—most notably cold, heat, noise, and passive smoking—and hypertension and/or CVD. While sedentary jobs have been linked to CVD risk, certain patterns of workplace physical activity (e.g., irregular episodes of heavy physical exertion alternating with sedentary work), also are implicated in risk of MI. As to other physical factors, such as vibration and heavy lifting, physiologic data suggests that these may have an untoward effect on the CV system; however, epidemiologic data is extremely limited. Cardionoxious chemical agents include: carbon disulfide (a well-established risk factor for CAD), nitrate esters (sudden cardiac death), carbon monoxide (myocardial ischemia, MI, sudden death, CHD mortality), lead and arsenic (possible risk factors for hypertension), and solvents (dysrhythmias, with methylene chloride giving a clinical picture similar to carbon monoxide).

Population Attributable Risk, Occupational Factors, and CVD

Psychosocial, chemical, and physical exposures at the workplace, along with sedentary work, represent a major public health burden on working populations. We can calculate the population attributable risk (PAR%)—i.e., the reduction of incidence if the population were entirely unexposed to occupational risk factors for heart disease—to estimate the degree to which work-related factors account for the epidemic of hypertension and CVD. The PAR% calculations depend on two assumptions: (1) the prevalence of exposure, and (2) the strength of association between exposure and the outcome of interest. Thus, the PAR% results will vary greatly among population groups and study results, engendering some difficulty in generalization.

Since there is excellent data available for job strain, we can calculate some representative results. Using data from the Cornell Worksite and Ambulatory BP Study[59] with an exposure rate to job strain of 20% and an odds ratio (OR) of 3 between job strain and hypertension, 28.6% of hypertension among working men in New York City could be attributed to job strain.* PAR% also have been calculated for European data on job strain and CVD. The European Heart Network[34] cites Olsen and Kristensen, who used exposure to monotonous, high-paced occupations as a proxy measure for job strain, taking a very conservative estimate, and calculated PAR% for CVD as 6% for men and 14% for women in Denmark.[48] However, when they estimated a total CVD burden for Danish workers due to occupational factors—job strain (but not ERI), sedentary work, physical and chemical exposures, and shift work—the PAR% was greater than 50%. A PAR% of 15.3% for CVD mortality due to isostrain in the Swedish male working population can be calculated based on a reported OR of 1.9 and 20% exposure rate to isostrain.[26] In Europe as a whole the exposure to job strain may be as high as 30%,[9] which would yield a similar or higher PAR% to that calculated for Sweden. A full discussion of the number of cases and the costs of CVD in the U.S. for various estimates of PAR% due to job strain is found in Chapter 11.

While the empirical evidence and PAR% calculations presented above demonstrate the effect of CVD of psychosocial risk factors, and there is additional data for work hours, shift work, and chemical and physical exposures, studies examining the combined or interactive burden of these factors are lacking. There is some evidence of an interaction between psychosocial stressors, such as between job strain and low social support,[11,25] job strain and ERI,[51] and high work demands and low economic rewards.[39] However, we know little about the possible synergistic effects of combinations of various types of risk factors, except for a few studies such as that of Alfredsson, et al. showing an increased SMR for heavy lifting plus hectic work.[2] Nonetheless, even without this knowledge, the evidence to date indicates that workplace risk factors account for an important burden.

THEORETICAL PLAUSIBILITY OF A PSYCHOSOCIAL CONNECTION

Psychosocial Models

The occupational health movements of the latter part of this century raised the concern that the modern work environment caused serious illness and injury. In the

---

* PAR% = Pe (RR-1)/1 + Pe(RR-1) where Pe is the exposure rate in the population as a whole, and RR is the risk ratio. OR may be substituted for RR.

1970s, psychosocial researchers began to address this issue with respect to CVD. As posed by Karasek and Theorell: "Did the social organization of work also cause serious physical illness? Without scientific evidence of such associations (evidence of job dissatisfaction would not suffice) the same political will to redress worker hazards could not easily be mustered. This evidence would be much more difficult to accumulate, however. In the case of physical occupational health hazards, such as in coal mining, the cause of injury was often obviously environmental, but for psychosocial risks work-related and nonwork-related factors were interlocked."[29] A critical obstacle was the theoretical conceptualization and modeling of workplace stressors.

A pioneering breakthrough came in 1979 with the publication of the Job Strain Model, based upon the premise that strain occurs when there is excessive psychological workload demands together with low job decision latitude[30] (see Chapter 3). This appears to provoke arousal, as well as distress, activating both the sympathoadrenomedullary and adrenocortical axes, a highly deleterious combination.[13,14]

A third dimension, social support, was added later to the model.[25] It was found that lack of social support at work interacted with job strain to substantially increase the risk of CVD. A variety of investigations, including cross-sectional and longitudinal observational population studies, intervention research, and animal experiments, have shown that social isolation and lack of social support are harmful to CV health.[4,21,49]

More recently, the ERI Model was introduced by Siegrist and colleagues.[60,61] In comparison to the Job Strain Model with its emphasis on moment-to-moment control over the work process (i.e., decision latitude), the ERI model provides an expanded concept, emphasizing macro-level long-term control through rewards such as career opportunities, job security, esteem, and income. The ERI Model posits that work stress results from an imbalance between these rewards and effort. Effort is seen to stem both extrinsically from the demands of the job and intrinsically from the individual's tendency to be overly committed to these work demands.

Key dimensions are shared by the Job Strain and ERI Models: both control as well as challenge (demands) are an integral part of each. However, control varies— from micro (task) level in the former, to macro level in the latter. The nature of the challenge varies from model to model, but there is a challenge of some kind in each.

In addition to these two models, which have been well developed theoretically and empirically confirmed in relation to CVD, other promising formulations are emerging. One is the concept of threat-avoidant-vigilant work, which seems particularly relevant in understanding the stress of certain occupations at high CVD risk. Such work is onerous since it requires continuous maintenance of a high level of attention, in order to avoid the disastrous consequences that could occur with a momentary lapse or a wrong decision.

Social Class, Workplace Factors, and CVD

There is a considerable and consistent body of evidence of an inverse association between socioeconomic status (SES) and incidence and prevalence of CVD, primarily CHD (see Chapter 2). The higher CVD risk among men and women in lower SES groups, e.g., blue-collar workers, began to appear in the 1950s[17,40,79] and has risen progressively over the period 1960–1993.[17]

These changes in CVD mortality rates among the blue-collar workers are paralleled by increasing income inequality, which differs greatly among countries, and is measured by the size of the income gap between the rich and the poor. Income inequality profoundly affects overall mortality,[27] although only a modest direct effect has been heretofore demonstrated for CVD.[33,42] In the industrialized world, "It is not the richest countries which have the best health, but the most egalitarian."[75] In the U.S., the "earnings distribution among workers has widened greatly and is the most unequal among developed countries."[71] The role of work in relation to income inequality as a potential contributor to adverse health outcomes is an important area for future research. ERI would be a particularly suitable model to investigate these relationships.

As pointed out by Johnson and Hall, not only do "those in the upper levels of the professional and managerial hierarchy enjoy ample financial remuneration, they also have the right to exercise authority over others, to expect obedience and even subservience, and to enjoy prominent social position, the privileges of voluntary action and association, and the many ineffables of an affluent lifestyle."[24] These authors elaborate that work control "varies systematically as a function of social class." SES usually is operationalized by education, income, and occupational status. The latter two factors are features of work. In fact, status at work, variety and scope for use of initiative and skill, and ability to exercise authority and control are some of the main ways by which SES is defined. In the Whitehall study, the distribution of job control was the major factor contributing to the socioeconomic gradient in CHD risk across civil service employment grade.[32,41] In contrast to low job control, job strain has a weaker and, in some studies, null association with SES. However, job strain appears to interact with low SES. Job strain has a stronger association with CVD and with BP in workers of lower SES.

Not only are psychosocial workplace stressors, most notably low decision-making latitude or control, more prevalent among workers of lower SES, but these workers also are more frequently exposed to physical and chemical hazards that can impact upon the CV system. Shift work generally is more common among blue-collar compared to white-collar workers. Standard cardiac risk factors such as smoking, obesity, and lack of recreational physical activity also are more prevalent among those in the lower SES groups.[28] These risk factors can be affected by an unhealthy workplace.

Thus, low SES is associated with a number of workplace factors that can impact upon CVD risk. These include low job control, exposure to shiftwork, and physical and chemical hazards. Persons in low socioeconomic strata disproportionately receive inadequate wages and salaries, lack promotion prospects, and may face downward mobility. These factors likely contribute to an increased ERI among those in lower SES groups. Exposure to job strain is associated with a greater CVD risk among blue-collar, as compared to white-collar workers. Standard cardiac risk factors, often related to an unhealthy workplace, also are more prevalent in the former. These interrelations, explored in detail in Chapters 2 and 3, render the conclusion of Johnson and Hall that the realities of social class and work are "inextricably linked,"[24] of profound relevance to CV well-being.

Insights from Cognitive Ergonomics and Brain Research

Constructs such as job strain and ERI are based heavily on sociological theory. Cognitive ergonomics and brain research provide insights that complement these models, and provide a deeper understanding of dimensions such as psychological demand, control, and conflict. Thus, for example, when speaking of mentally demanding work, we can go far beyond queries about "working hard" and "working fast." With a more quantitative, objective appraisal of the burden of work processes, and a better grasp of the possibilities and limitations of the human central nervous system, a more rational approach to work design emerges. By analyzing tasks in terms of allocation of mental resources, we can better determine what is too much (leading to overload), what is too little (leading to underload), what is incoherent or contradictory (leading to conflict), etc. A critical ratio is that between "knowledge-based" labor processes, which require conscious attentional resources, and those that are "skill-based," which can be performed in parallel and feature rapid, smooth, learned, and highly integrated patterns.[15,47] We also can pinpoint how to promote the worker's autonomous control, not only to meet the moment-to-moment exigencies of the situation, but, ideally, to be in harmony with his/her own needs, as well. Simply stated, this knowledge can help humanize the work process. Examples of the practical implementation of this approach are provided in Chapters 3 and 6.

Cognitive ergonomics and brain research also illustrate that emotional dimensions of human labor impact profoundly on mental burden. For survival reasons, our nervous systems are constructed to selectively allocate mental resources to potentially harmful stimuli, even if the threat is purely symbolic. It is essential to take into account the often hidden burden represented by threat-avoidant vigilant activity. Neurophysiologic studies demonstrate that imminent threat of an accident in the symbolically represented traffic milieu is associated with an unusually high level of selective attention. To avoid such situations, compensatory allowance, especially increased time allocation, must be included in the work planning "equation."

There is a need for psychometric tools that account for the total burden of work stressors, using a cognitive-ergonomic approach, and with relevance to CVD risk. The Occupational Stress Index[3] represents one such possible tool. Potential multiplicative interactions and higher-level terms should be explored within that model and more generally. The burden of unpaid labor, which is disproportionately performed by women, also must be considered.

BIOLOGICAL PLAUSIBILITY OF A WORKPLACE–CVD RELATIONSHIP

A large body of evidence indicating that occupational stressors can profoundly impact numerous pathophysiologic processes, resulting in CV dysfunction and disease, has been presented. As described in Chapter 4, experimental animal studies implicate central stress mechanisms in cardiac electrical instability, as well as in hypertension, disorders of heart beat dynamics, and atherogenesis. The reader also is referred to the very recent paper by Rozanski, Blumenthal, and Kaplan, which reviews how psychosocial factors can affect the pathogenesis of CVD.[56]

Stressors most often provoke a defense response, and, in extreme cases, the defeat reaction. These responses, which in the worst situation may both be operative in turn, can activate the sympatho-adrenomedullary and hypophyseal-adrenocortical pathways, respectively. Empirical studies have demonstrated an association between numerous work stressors and elevations in catecholamines and cortisol.

Direct empirical confirmation, based on epidemiologic and field studies at the workplace, is not available for all of the pathways. Of the processes discussed in Chapter 5, the most attention has been paid to exposure to job strain in relation to elevation in BP and development of hypertension. Here, cross-sectional and longitudinal ambulatory BP data clearly show that hypertension can arise as a result of chronic exposure to job strain. Plausible stress mechanisms that can lead from elevations in BP to chronic hypertension include changes in vascular resistance, as well as renal mechanisms. The relationship among chronic exposure to job strain, elevations in workplace AmBP, and increased left ventricular mass also has been empirically confirmed.

Metabolic changes, including hyperlipidemia and heightened coagulation tendency, together with an increased progression of carotid atherosclerosis, have been linked to aspects of stressful work, especially ERI. A risk for the combined occurrence of hypertension and hyperlipidemia, characteristic of CV metabolic syndrome, has been associated with ERI. CV metabolic syndrome appears to be driven by augmented sympathetic outflow. Further attention is needed to the relation between work stressors and the occurrence of hemodynamic and biochemical abnormalities characteristic of this syndrome.

As to myocardial ischemia, the biological mechanisms generally are well-defined, and many are related to workplace factors (e.g., increased double product [heart rate × SBP], left ventricular hypertrophy, atherosclerosis). Mental stress in the laboratory has been consistently shown to provoke myocardial ischemia in patients with stable ischemic syndromes. However, field studies of myocardial ischemia in relation to workplace stressors are exceedingly sparse.

We also know quite a bit about the stress mechanisms that can lower cardiac electrical stability. Until recently, however, the possibilities for noninvasive ambulatory monitoring to detect the electrically vulnerable myocardium before sudden cardiac death occurred were limited. Neither the quantity nor the pattern of ventricular extrasystolic activity proved sufficiently predictive. With more advanced technologies, it is now feasible to simultaneously follow several ECG parameters that impact on cardiac electrical stability (ST segment, heart rate variability, QT interval), together with ventricular arrhythmias, during work. Furthermore, studies of patients with automatic implantable cardioverter defibrillators (AICD) could examine job-related exposures, providing direct information about the potential for workplace factors to trigger life-threatening tachyarrhythmias. We do know that AICD fire significantly more on Mondays,[52] suggesting a relation to work activity.

There is some empirical evidence of a septadian overrepresentation of Mondays vis-à-vis cardiac events.[53,77] The early morning hours, during which several preconditions for plaque rupture and thrombus formation are present, are known to be the period of highest risk for these events.[16,46] In the morning hours after waking, systolic BP increases by about 20–30 mmHg, heart rate and vascular tone rise, platelets are hyperreactive, while fibrinolytic activity is at its low.[67] Sympathetic activation occurs upon assuming the upright position, and in the early morning cortisol is at its peak. This can result in a glucocorticoid-related increase in coronary-artery sensitivity to catecholamine-mediated vasoconstriction.[67,76] The epidemiologic and biological data, taken together, indicate that the stress of work after a weekend of respite may precipitate acute cardiac events among working patients.[38,76] Psychosocial, physical, and chemical factors, along with long and irregular work hours, can chronically promote the underlying pathological processes, as well as act as trigger mechanisms for acute cardiac events.

CONVERGENT VALIDATION OF THE CAUSAL LINK

The theoretical constructs of how workplace factors affect the development of CVD are corroborated by the large body of empirical data confirming this relationship. We have suggested the term "econeurocardiology" (see Chapter 4) to represent the biological paradigm by which social factors, such as work stress, are perceived and processed by the central nervous system, resulting in pathophysiological changes that increase CVD risk. All told, the biological and theoretical plausibility of this view, coupled with the empirical evidence, provides convergent validation for the conclusion that environmental stressors from the workplace play an important role in the development of CVD.

There is a need for intervention studies as the strongest evidence for causality. These studies also provide practical experience and techniques for implementing changes at the worksite and evaluating their effectiveness. More longitudinal data with assessment of cumulative exposure and changes in exposure is needed, as well. To know where to intervene, the prevalence of both cardionoxious exposures and CVD must be mapped—i.e., **surveillance**. Such a map will facilitate the identification and management of individual exposed workers with varying CVD severity, who may benefit from clinical intervention.

There remain a number of methodologic issues for resolution (see Chapters 6 and 7). These include the need for refined measurement tools of the Job Strain and ERI Models. Improved reliability and validity of exposure assessment would be obtained through "triangulation"—the use of self-report methods complemented by imputation—and by data from observers, whenever possible. Improved outcome assessments with earlier detection at the preclinical level can now be realized by new noninvasive monitoring techniques applicable in field studies at the workplace. More examination also is warranted as to how circumstances of occupational life affect behavior patterns, such as hostility and overcommitment, which can in turn, affect CVD risk.

CURRENT STATUS AND FUTURE DIRECTIONS

Implications for Clinical Practice: Advancing the Discipline of Occupational Cardiology

Unlike several other medical subspecialties (e.g., pulmonology), for cardiology the workplace has yet to become an integral consideration. Consequently, there are few guidelines (with the exception of those related to physical activity levels) to help clinicians make informed recommendations concerning occupational factors, as these pertain to patients with various degrees of CVD severity. In Chapters 8 and 9, we offer physicians and allied health professionals a practical set of tools for the evaluation and management of working people at risk. First, taking an occupational history as it relates to the CV system is imperative, and an approach is outlined to help clinicians accomplish this. Next, a graded, risk-stratified algorithm is proposed for an occupational cardiologic assessment of patients whose jobs could be harmful to the CV system. High-risk, but still preclinical patients are identified, and a set of diagnostic steps is proposed. This work-up can serve to guide clinicians in making specific recommendations concerning working conditions. Ambulatory monitoring is particularly helpful for objectively determining which workplace modifications are most conducive to the patient's CV well-being.

Return to work (RTW) after cardiac events (see Chapter 9) is an especially delicate question. The cardiologic caregiver must evaluate the full clinical picture, including symptoms and morphological and functional status, as well as address complex personal, psychological, social, economic, legal, and ethical issues. The importance of job characteristics is illustrated by the existing, albeit limited, longitudinal data, showing that return to high-strain work is a significant predictor of mortality in young men post-MI, independent of clinical indices.[65] Notwithstanding the need for large-scale clinical investigations of this type, these findings should prompt the clinician to raise the question posed by Theorell and Karasek: "Should heart attack patients return to stressful jobs?"[66] A similar query could be relevant, as well, to patients with hypertension (see Chapter 10), especially in light of the Cornell Worksite Ambulatory Blood Pressure Study, which indicates that changing from a high- to low-strain job was associated with a sizable fall in AmBP among such patients.[58]

Workers whose cardiac status represents a public safety issue (see Chapter 9) raise another difficult issue, frequently related to RTW. The clinician must render an estimation of risk for the occurrence of cardiac or other events that could lead to impaired consciousness. Airline pilots have received the most stringent evaluation in this regard, but these issues also pertain to operators of ground transport and other heavy machinery and to workers whose jobs entail threat-avoidant vigilant activity. An expanded occupational **public health role of the clinician** could be crucial in this particular realm. Clinicians, together with occupational ergonomists and other specialists, must have greater influence to recommend and implement cardio-protective guidelines about work conditions for these jobs. As it stands now, the clinician is repeatedly faced with the dilemma of making a judgement about the individual's CV work fitness, often knowing full well that the job itself is cardionoxious. A more proactive approach offers the possibility of ameliorating this ethical dilemma.

A public health perspective is vital for the clinician to effectively protect his/her patients exposed to cardionoxious work. The clinician must be on the alert for the occurrence of unexpected patterns or clusters of CVD. Historically, in other medical disciplines, the physician often has been among the first to identify occupationally associated diseases, with resultant major changes in the work environment. However, for a number of reasons (see Chapter 10) clinicians typically have not been the ones to herald the occurrence of clusters of job-related CVD. There is an urgent need to incorporate the concept of an **occupational sentinel health event** into the mainstream of cardiology.

The clinician also can play an important role in evaluating CV health impact of changes in the work environment and worksite health promotion programs, including individual stress management. The physician may be in a unique position to help transform an adversarial situation to a cooperative relationship, and thereby to represent a stabilizing force. Cooperation among the various participants in the work process (e.g., labor, management, occupational hygienists, engineers, economists) can be promoted by the authority of the clinician, whose interest is first and foremost the well-being of his or her patients.

Current Trends in Working Life

As we embark upon the 21st century in the United States, despite a booming economy, much prosperity, and relatively low unemployment rates, there is a large and growing income disparity, and working conditions are deteriorating for many. Working men and women are putting in longer work weeks and are increasingly exposed to job conditions that can undermine CV health.[36a] In Europe, in 1996, 23% of those employed were working more than 45 hours/week.[73] In the U.S., average weekly work hours increased by 3.5 to 47.1 hours from 1977 to 1997.[5] Workers in the U.S. have now surpassed Japanese workers in total number of hours worked per year, and work longer hours than in any other industrialized country.[22]

Substantial changes in job characteristics have occurred over the past generation in industrialized countries. In Europe, surveys indicate an increase in "time constraints" (i.e., workload demands) between 1977 and 1996.[9] Similarly, in the U.S., increases between 1977 and 1997 were reported for "working very fast" (from 55%

to 68%) and "never enough time to get everything done on my job" (from 40% to 60%).[5] Somewhat augmented job decision latitude also has been noted. In Europe, the proportion of workers reporting a measure of autonomy over their pace of work rose from 64% in 1991 to 72% in 1996.[73] In the U.S. "freedom to decide what I do on my job" increased from 56% in 1977 to 74% in 1997, and "my job lets me use my skills and abilities" rose from 77% in 1977 to 92% in 1997.[5] However, at least in Europe, increases in autonomy were not sufficient to compensate for heightened work intensity. The combination of augmented demands and little or no rise in control over the work process results in an increased exposure to job strain. The proportion of high-strain jobs in Europe increased from about 25% in 1991 to about 30% in 1996.[9] Unfortunately, there is no published data on the percentage of the U.S. working force experiencing job strain currently. However, as described above, employed men and women are working harder and longer today than they did 25 years ago.[36a]

Paralleling these trends in working conditions, and in large part responsible for them, new systems of work organization have been introduced by employers throughout the industrialized world to improve productivity, product quality, and profitability. Such efforts have taken a variety of forms and names, including lean production (e.g., Japanese Production Management), total quality management, cellular or modular manufacturing, and high-performance work organizations. These new systems have been extolled as reforms of Taylorism and the traditional assembly-line approach to job design.[36a]

According to a report from the U.S. Departments of Labor and Commerce, over "80% of American workers want a say in decisions affecting their jobs and how their work is performed."[71] The traditional method by which employees have influenced working conditions, including job stressors, is through the establishment of labor unions.[36] This is an example of the exercise of "collective control"[33] a strategy often utilized when prospects for exerting control individually at work are limited. However, in the U.S. the proportion of employees who are members of labor unions has declined sharply in the past 40 years.

Perhaps one explanation for the rapid increase in lean production techniques is the weakened position of labor unions.[36] As a consequence, the labor movement in the U.S. has not been able to greatly influence the enactment of legislation to improve psychosocial working conditions/reduce job strain, such as was accomplished in Scandinavia, nor has it been able to prevent the decline in real income for lower SES employees.[74,80]

Weakened unions also have been unable to prevent employers from implementing aspects of lean production such as downsizing, outsourcing to low-wage suppliers, 24-hour operations, compressed work weeks, increased overtime, contingent work, and workforce flexibility.[36a] Such trends may help explain increases in time constraints and workload demands reported in European and U.S. surveys over the past 20 years. Downsizing[12,54,72] and excessive overtime[8,10,19,68,70] can have dramatic negative effects on employee health. These trends, which result in increased job strain and ERI, contribute to CVD risk differences between upper and lower SES groups[17] and to the minimal or no recent decline in CVD incidence,[18,55,64,78] especially among lower SES workers.[18,69]

One of the consequences of lean production is the progressive disappearance of "passive" and "relaxed" jobs, with the four quadrants of the Job Strain Model collapsed into two: active versus high-strain jobs. Previously passive jobs are now accelerated (e.g., housekeepers in hotels carry phone equipment and upon completion of a task must immediately report to a supervisor for the next assignment; security workers are routinely assigned to other tasks while simultaneously being on guard). Those who had relaxed jobs, such as some college professors/scientists, now face increasing teaching loads and incessant deadlines for grant proposals. This process of work intensification, if unchecked, may well contribute to a further sharpening of class boundaries: people will tend to be in one of two types of occupations—characterized by high or low levels of decision authority but *all* with high demands. According to the U.S. Departments of Labor and Commerce, "The stagnation of real earnings and increased inequality of earning is bifurcating the U.S. labor market, with an upper tier of high-wage skilled workers and an increasing 'underclass' of low paid labor."[71] At the same time, traditionally autonomous self-employed workers (e.g., physicians and attorneys in private practice, single shop owners) are disappearing. Physicians are working harder and are experiencing progressive loss of their decision-making authority in the setting of corporate managed care.

Leisure time is eroding, and work and home life are blending.[36a] The average U.S. married-couple family worked 247 more hours in 1996 than in 1989.[44] The quality of family life is severely compromised under these circumstances. According to a national U.S. survey in 1997, "Employees with more difficult, more demanding jobs and less supportive workplaces experience substantially higher levels of negative spillover from work into their lives off the job—jeopardizing their personal and family well-being."[5]

Implications for Public Health Policy

The evidence that psychosocial exposures are important in the etiology of hypertension and CVD and that these exposures may well be on the increase has serious implications for public health. These exposures also can affect a range of other health outcomes, including repetitive motion injuries[45]; alterations in the immune system[20]; adverse pregnancy outcomes,[7] including pregnancy-induced hypertension[37]; and negative psychological effects, such as anxiety,[62] burnout,[35] passivity,[29,31] and depression.[30] Increased rates of disorders such as repetitive motion injuries could be the "canary in the coal mine"—a possible warning of future hypertension and CVD.

SURVEILLANCE

According to the authors of the recent Tokyo Declaration, we need to institute a program of "surveillance at individual workplaces and monitoring at national and regional levels in order to identify the extent of work-related stress health problems and to provide baselines against which to evaluate effects at amelioration. They recommend that workplaces assess both workplace stressors and health outcomes known to result from such exposures . . . on an annual basis."[1]

Worksite screening should obtain prevalence data on cardionoxious exposures (e.g., job strain) and on work-related CVD. Worksite point estimates of BP (see Chapter 7) would be particularly useful, being inexpensive and relatively simple to obtain, with ambulatory BP monitoring performed whenever possible. Holter monitoring is needed to survey the prevalence of silent myocardial ischemia, and to assess other sensitive, noninvasive parameters such as heart rate variability. Carotid ultrasound is also an invaluable screening tool. The incidence of CVD events and standard cardiac risk factors should be systematically registered. Since many large companies require annual physical exams and collect much of the relevant data, it should be a relatively simple task to enter this information into a database and make it available to those concerned with worker health. Appropriate precautions to protect employee confidentiality must always be observed.[63]

INTERVENTIONS

Worksites identified as high risk for CVD should be targeted for interventions (see Chapter 13). Primary interventions would focus on creating a healthy workplace. For example, high-strain jobs could be redesigned to provide optimal levels of employee decision-making latitude and skill discretion, and workloads could be realistic, compatible with human capacity. Since the workplace appears to be a "leverage point" with regard to standard CVD risk factors (see Chapter 10), such interventions could have the additional benefit of lowering these risk factors.

A number of worksite intervention studies have specifically focused on reducing stressful features of work organization, and several have measured changes in CVD risk factors. Two Swedish studies exemplify interventions with some successes:

1. Employees of a large government agency participated in an intervention which included worker committees that developed and carried out action plans to reduce sources of workplace stress. A significant decrease in apolipoprotein B/apolipoprotein AI ratio occurred in the intervention group but not in the control group, an effect which could not be explained by smoking, eating, exercise, weight or other lifestyle factors. Stimulation from and autonomy over work significantly increased in the intervention group but remained the same in the control group.[50]

2. Researchers examined a new auto assembly work organization which contained small autonomous work groups having much greater opportunities to influence the pace and content of their work than either traditional assembly work or the Japanese management method of "lean production." Workers in the flexible sociotechnical systems organization did not show increases in systolic BP, heart rate, and adrenaline during their work shift as did workers on a traditional assembly line. In addition, catecholamines showed more rapid "unwinding" (toward non-workday baseline levels) after work in the flexible organization, particularly for female workers.[43]

The workplace is also a good setting for interventions aimed directly at traditional risk factors, e.g., dietary interventions by improved nutrition in cafeterias, exercise programs, and medical treatment (e.g., for hypertension).

LEGISLATION

We will need societal measures to support the above initiatives. Japan and much of Western Europe have taken the lead in passing legislation making certain forms of work stress illegal and mandating healthy work. An example is the *Swedish Work Environment Act (Act No. 677, amended in 1991)* which states:

• Working conditions shall be adapted to people's differing physical and psychological circumstances.

• Employees shall be enabled to participate in the arrangement of their own job situations as well as in work changes and development that affect their jobs.

• Technology, work organization, and job content shall be arranged so that the employee is not exposed to physical or mental loads that may cause ill health or accidents.

• The matters to be considered in this context shall include forms of remuneration and the scheduling of working hours.

• Rigorously controlled or tied work shall be avoided or restricted.

• It shall be the aim of work to afford opportunities for variety, social contacts, and cooperation, as well as continuity between individual tasks.

• It shall further be the aim for working conditions to afford opportunities for personal and occupational development as well as for self-determination and occupational responsibility.

A prerequisite to implementing a "healthy work" policy is the establishment of a system of workplace surveillance to identify high-risk work environments. This, however, remains to be achieved on a broad scale.

Secondly, we may need legislation intended to provide companies with incentives to accomplish these goals. This could include a national tax on companies with excess levels of job-related risk factors and/or CVD outcomes (see Chapter 11). In this way, businesses would be encouraged to reassess their workplaces to lower job strain and other cardionoxious exposures.

Finally, in the U.S. we will need national legislation mandating a healthy workplace, similar to the laws passed in Europe and Japan (see Chapter 12).

We concur with the conclusions of the European Heart Network on Social Factors, Work, Stress, and Cardiovascular Disease in the European Union that "the substantial scientific basis of the association of psychosocial factors and cardiovascular disease risk . . . (should) ensure that social, occupational, and individual factors will not be left off the health agenda."[34] These protective steps are important to reduce the likelihood that working men and women are exposed to cardionoxious risk factors at the workplace. They recognize that today's stressful jobs are the result of human design and thus amenable to change. But taken as a totality the steps outlined above are basically a defensive strategy which fails to address the human need for fulfilling work, work that satisfies human needs for dignity, creativity, and a sense of worth.

We have now reached the point where it is possible to design work that promotes health and well-being. It is not demanding work per se that is harmful, but work without control over how one meets the job demands or uses one's skills. Tomorrow's jobs will be deliberately crafted to allow the full development of the human spirit through work which encourages—not discourages—human potential. This means creating a work environment that is conducive to human mental and physical health. A key characteristic of a "health-liberating" work environment will be the full participation of all working people in the decision-making processes surrounding the organization of work.

Note: Some material adapted by permission from Landsbergis, et al; reference 36a. Copyright 1999 by the Educational Publishing Foundation.

REFERENCES

1. The Tokyo Declaration. J Tokyo Med Univ 56:760–767, 1998.
2. Alfredsson L, Spetz C, Theorell T: Type of occupation and near-future hospitalization for myocardial infarction and some other diagnoses. Int J Epidemiol 14:378–388, 1985.
3. Belkic K, Savic C, Theorell T, et al: Mechanisms of cardiac risk among professional drivers. Scand J Work Environ Health 20:73–86, 1994.
4. Berkman L: The role of social relations in health promotion. J Psychosom Res 57:245–254, 1995.
5. Bond JT, Galinsky E, Swanberg JE: The 1997 National Study of the Changing Workforce. New York, Families and Work Institute, 1998.
6. Bosma H, Peter R, Siegrist J, Marmot M: Two alternative job stress models and the risk of coronary heart disease. Am J Pub Health 88:68–74, 1998.
7. Brandt LPA, Nielson CV: Job stress and adverse outcome of pregnancy: A causal link or recall bias? Am J Epidemiol 135:302–311, 1992.
8. Cooper C: Working hours and health. Work Stress 10:1–4, 1996.
9. European Foundation: Time constraints and autonomy at work in the European Union. Dublin, European Foundation for the Improvement of Living and Working Conditions, 1997.
10. Falger PRJ, Schouten EGW: Exhaustion, psychologic stress in the work environment, and acute myocardial infarction in adult men. J Psychosom Res 36:777–786, 1992.
11. Falk A, Hanson BS, Isacsson SO, Ostergren PO: Job strain and mortality in elderly men: Social networks, support, and influence as buffers. Am J Public Health 82:1136–1139, 1992.
12. Ferrie JE, Shipley MJ, Marmot M, et al: The health effects of major organizational change and job insecurity. Soc Sci Med 46:243–254, 1998.

13. Forsman L: Individual and group differences in psychophysiological responses to stress with emphasis on sympathetic-adrenal medullary and pituitary-adrenal cortical responses. Stockholm, Department of Psychology, University of Stockholm, 1983.
14. Fredriksson M, Sundin O, Frankenhaeuser M: Cortisol excretion during the defense reaction in humans. Psychosom Med 47:313–319, 1985.
15. Gaillard AWK: Comparing the concepts of mental load and stress. Ergonomics 36:991–1005, 1993.
16. Genes N, Vaur L, Renault M, et al: Rythme circadien des infarctus du myocarde en France: resultats de l'etude USIK (Circadian patterns of myocardial infarction in France: Results of the USIK study). La Presse Medicale 26:603–608, 1997.
17. Gonzalez MA, Artalejo FR, Calero JR: Relationship between socioeconomic status and ischaemic heart disease in cohort and case-control studies:1960–1993. Int J Epidemiol 27:350–358, 1998.
18. Hallqvist J, Diderischsen F, Theorell T, et al: Is the effect of job strain on myocardial infarction due to interaction between high psychological demands and low decision latitude? Results from Stockholm Heart Epidemiology Program. Soc Sci Med 46:1405–1415, 1998.
19. Hayashi T, Kobayashi Y, Yamaoka K, Yano E: Effect of overtime work on 24-hour ambulatory blood pressure. J Occup Environ Med 38:1007–1011, 1996.
20. Henningsen GM, Hurrell JJ, Baker F, et al: Measurement of salivary immunoglobulin A as an immunologic biomarker of job stress. Scand J Work Environ Health 18 Suppl 2:133–136, 1992.
21. House JS, Landis KR, Umberson D: Social relations and health. Science 241:540–545, 1988.
22. International Labour Office: Key Indicators of the Labour Market 1999. Geneva, International Labour Office, 1999.
23. Johnson JV: Collective control: Strategies for survival in the workplace. Int J Health Services 19:469–480, 1989.
24. Johnson JV, Hall EM: Class, work, and health. In Amick B, Levine S, Tarlov AR, Walsh DC (eds): Society and Health. New York, Oxford University Press, 1995, pp 247–271.
25. Johnson JV, Hall EM: Job strain, workplace social support, and cardiovascular disease: A cross-sectional study of a random sample of the Swedish working population. Am J Public Health 78:1336–1342, 1988.
26. Johnson JV, Hall EM, Theorell T: Combined effects of job strain and social isolation on cardiovascular disease morbidity and mortality in a random sample of the Swedish male working population. Scand J Work Environ Health 15:271–279, 1989.
27. Kaplan G, Pamuk E, Lynch JW, et al: Inequality in income and mortality in the United States: Analysis of mortality and potential pathways. Br Med J 312:999–1003, 1996.
28. Kaplan GA, Keil JE: Socioeconomic factors and cardiovascular disease: A review of the literature. Circulation 88:1973–1998, 1993.
29. Karasek R, Theorell T: Healthy Work: Stress, Productivity, and the Reconstruction of Working Life. New York, Basic Books, 1990.
30. Karasek RA: Job demands, job decision latitude, and mental strain: Implications for job redesign. Adm Sci Q 24:285–308, 1979.
31. Karasek RA: Job socialization and job strain: The implications of two related psychosocial mechanisms for job design. In Gardell B, Johansson G (eds): Working Life. London, Wiley, 1981.
32. Kawachi I, Marmot M: What can we learn from studies of occupational class and cardiovascular disease? Am J Epidemiol 148:160–163, 1998.
33. Kennedy BP, Kawachi I, Prothrow-Stith D: Income distribution and mortality: Cross-sectional ecological study of the Robin Hood index in the United States. Br Med J 312:1004–1007, 1996.
34. Kristensen TS, Kronitzer M, Alfedsson L: Social factors, work, stress, and cardiovascular disease prevention. Brussels, The European Heart Network, 1998.
35. Landsbergis PA: Occupational stress faced by health care workers: A test of the job demand-control model. J Organiz Behav 9:217–239, 1988.
36. Landsbergis PA, Cahill J: Labor union programs to reduce or prevent occupational stress in the United States. Int J Health Services 24:105–129, 1994.
36a. Landsbergis PA, Cahill J, Schnall P: The impact of lean production and related new systems of work organization on worker health. J Occup Health Psychol 4:108–130, 1999.
37. Landsbergis PA, Hatch MC: Psychosocial work stress and pregnancy-induced hypertension [see comments]. Epidemiology 7:346–351, 1996.
38. Lown B: Sudden cardiac death: Biobehavioral perspective. Circulation 76 Suppl I:I186–I195, 1987.
39. Lynch J, Krause N, Kaplan GA, et al: Workplace demands, economic reward, and progression of carotid atherosclerosis. Circulation 96:302–307, 1997.
40. Marmot M, Rose G, Shipley M, et al: Employment grade and coronary heart disease in British civil servants. J Epid Commun Health 32:244–249, 1978.
41. Marmot MG, Bosma H, Hemingway H, et al: Contribution of job control and other risk factors to social variations in coronary heart disease incidence. Lancet 350:235–239, 1997.
42. McIsaac SJ, Wilkinson RG: Income distribution and cause-specific mortality. Eur J Public Health 7:45–53, 1997.
43. Melin B, Lundberg U, Soderlund J, Granqvist M: Psychophysiological stress reactions of male and female assembly workers: A comparison between two different forms of work organization. J Organiz Behav 20:47–61, 1999.
44. Mishel L, Bernstein J: The state of working America. Washington, DC, Economic Policy Institute, 1998.
45. Moon SD, Sauter SL: Beyond Biomechanics: Psychosocial Aspects of Musculoskeletal Disorders in Office Work. London, Taylor & Francis, 1996.
46. Muller JE, Ludmer PL, Willich SN, et al: Circadian variation in the frequency of sudden cardiac death. Circulation 75:131–138, 1987.

47. Neerincx MA, Griffoen E: Cognitive task analysis: Harmonizing tasks to human capacities. Ergonomics 39:543–561, 1996.
48. Olsen O, Kristensen TS: Impact of work environment on cardiovascular diseases in Denmark. J Epidemiol Community Health 45:4–10, 1991.
49. Orth-Gomer K: International epidemiological evidence for a relationship between social support and CVD. In Shumaker SA, Czajowski SM (eds): Social Support and Cardiovascular Disease. New York, Plenum Press, 1994, pp 97–117.
50. Orth-Gomer K, Eriksson I, Moser V, et al: Lipid lowering through work stress reduction. Int J Behav Med 1:204–214, 1994.
51. Peter R, Hallqvist J, Reuterwall C, et al: Psychosocial work environment and myocardial infarction: Improving risk prediction by combining two alternative job stress models in the SHEEP Study. (Submitted), 1999.
52. Peter RW, McQuillan S, Resnick SK, Gold MR: Increased Monday incidence of life-threatening ventricular arrhythmias: Experience with a third-generation implantable defibrillator. Circulation 94:1346–1349, 1996.
53. Rabkin SW, Mathewson FAL, Tate RB: Chronobiology of cardiac sudden death in men. JAMA 44:1357–1358, 1980.
54. Richardson D, Loomis D: Trends in fatal occupational injuries and industrial restructuring in North Carolina in the 1980s. Am J Public Health 87:1041–1043, 1997.
55. Rosamond WD, Chanbless LE, Folsom AR, et al: Trends in the incidence of myocardial infarction and in mortality due to coronary heart disease, 1987 to 1994 [abstract]. New Engl J Med 339:863, 1998.
56. Rozanski A, Blumenthal JA, Kaplan J: Impact of psychological factors on the pathogenesis of cardiovascular disease and implications for therapy. Circulation 99:2192–2217, 1999.
57. Schnall PL, Landsbergis PA, Baker D: Job strain and cardiovascular disease. Annu Rev Public Health 15:381–411, 1994.
58. Schnall PL, Landsbergis PA, Schwartz J, et al: A longitudinal study of job strain and ambulatory blood pressure: Results from a 3-year follow-up. Psychosom Med 60:697–706, 1998.
59. Schnall PL, Pieper C, Schwartz JE, et al: The relationship between job strain, workplace diastolic blood pressure, and left ventricular mass index. Results of a case-control study [published erratum appears in JAMA 1992 Mar 4;267(9):1209]. JAMA 263:1929–1935, 1990.
60. Siegrist J: Threat to social status and cardiovascular risk. Psychother Psychosom 42:90–96, 1984.
61. Siegrist J, Peter R: Measuring effort-reward imbalance at work: Guidelines. Dusseldorf, University of Dusseldorf, 1996.
62. Stansfeld SA, North FM, White I, Marmot MG: Work characteristics and psychiatric disorder in civil servants in London. J Epidemiol Commun Health 49:48–53, 1995.
63. Stokols D, Pelletier KR, Fielding JE: Integration of medical care and worksite health promotion. JAMA 273:1136–1142, 1995.
64. Sytkowski PA, D'Agostino RB, Belanger A, Kannel WB: Sex and time trends in cardiovascular disease incidence and mortality: The Framingham Heart Study, 1950–1989. Am J Epidemiol 143:338–350, 1996.
65. Theorell T, de Faire U, Johnson J, et al: Job strain and ambulatory blood pressure profiles. Scand J Work Environ Health 17:380–385, 1991.
66. Theorell T, Karasek R: Should heart attack patients return to stressful jobs? Stress Med 11:219–220, 1995.
67. Tofler GH: Triggering and the pathophysiology of acute coronary syndromes. Am Heart J 134:S55–S61, 1997.
68. Tuchsen F: Working hours and ischaemic heart disease in Danish men: A 4-year cohort study of hospitalization. Int J Epidemiol 22:215–221, 1993.
69. Tuchsen F, Endahl LA: Increasing inequality in ischaemic heart disease morbidity among employed men in Denmark 1981–1993: The need for a new preventive policy. Int J Epidemiol 28:640–644, 1999.
70. Uehata T: Long working hours and occupational stress-related cardiovascular attacks among middle-aged workers in Japan. J Human Ergol 20:147–153, 1991.
71. U.S. Departments of Labor and Commerce: Fact Finding Report. Commission on the Future of Worker-Management Relations. Washington, DC, U.S. Departments of Labor and Commerce, 1994.
72. Vahtera J, Kivimaki M, Pentti J: Effect of organizational downsizing on health employees. Lancet 350:1124–1128, 1997.
73. Walters D: Health and safety strategies in a changing Europe. Int J Health Services 28:305–331, 1998.
74. Weinberg D: A brief look at postwar U.S. income inequality. Washington, DC, U.S. Census Bureau, Current Population Reports, 1996.
75. Wilkinson RG: Unhealthy Societies: The Afflictions of Inequality. London, Routledge, 1996.
76. Willich SN, Lewis M, Lowel H, et al: Physical exertion as a trigger of myocardial infarction. Triggers and mechanisms of myocardial infarction study group. N Engl J Med 329:1684–1690, 1993.
77. Willich SN, Lowel H, Lewis M, et al: Weekly variation of acute myocardial infarction: Increased Monday risk in the working population. Circulation 90:87–93, 1994.
78. Wilson PWF, D'Aostino RB, Levy D, et al: Trends in coronary heart disease: A comparison of the original (1956–1968) and offspring Framingham Study cohorts. Anaheim, CA, American Heart Association, 1991.
79. Wing S, Dargent-Molina P, Casper M, et al: Changing association between community structure and ischaemic heart disease mortality in the United States. Lancet 2:1067–1070, 1987.
80. Wolff E: Top heavy: A study of wealth inequality in America. New York, Twentieth Century Fund Press, 1995.

INDEX

Entries in **boldface type** indicate complete chapters.